World leaders adopted Sustainable Development Goals (SDGs) as part of the 2030 Agenda for Sustainable Development. Providing in-depth knowledge, this series fosters comprehensive research on these global targets to end poverty, fight inequality and injustice, and tackle climate change.

The sustainability of our planet is currently a major concern for the global community and has been a central theme for a number of major global initiatives in recent years. Perceiving a dire need for concrete benchmarks toward sustainable development, the United Nations and world leaders formulated the targets that make up the seventeen goals. The SDGs call for action by all countries to promote prosperity while protecting Earth and its life support systems. This series on the Sustainable Development Goals aims to provide a comprehensive platform for scientific, teaching and research communities working on various global issues in the field of geography, earth sciences, environmental science, social sciences, engineering, policy, planning, and human geosciences in order to contribute knowledge towards achieving the current 17 Sustainable Development Goals.

This Series is organized into eighteen subseries: one based around each of the seventeen Sustainable Development Goals, and an eighteenth subseries, "Connecting the Goals," which serves as a home for volumes addressing multiple goals or studying the SDGs as a whole. Each subseries is guided by an expert Subseries Advisor.

Contributions are welcome from scientists, policy makers and researchers working in fields related to any of the SDGs. If you are interested in contributing to the series, please contact the Publisher: Zachary Romano [Zachary.Romano@springer.com].

More information about this series at http://www.springer.com/series/15486

Musa Touray · Aisha Touray

Clinical Work and General Management of a Standard Minimal-Resource Facility

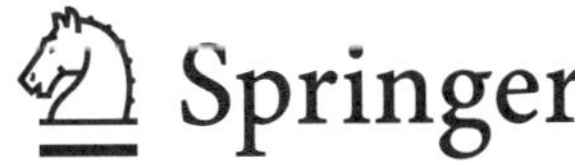

Springer

Musa Touray
Centre Medical Epalinges
Epalinges
Switzerland

Aisha Touray
Faculty of Biology and Medicine
University of Lausanne
Lausanne
Switzerland

ISSN 2523-3084 ISSN 2523-3092 (electronic)
Sustainable Development Goals Series
ISBN 978-3-030-71034-7 ISBN 978-3-030-71032-3 (eBook)
https://doi.org/10.1007/978-3-030-71032-3

This Springer imprint is published by the registered company Springer Nature Switzerland AG
The registered company address is: Gewerbestrasse 11, 6330 Cham, Switzerland

Foreword

The last decade has borne witness to significant improvement in the availability and dissemination of clinical literature. Access is now facilitated in the form of electronic files, regularly updated reference websites, web seminars, and paperbound books. Despite this gigantic step forward in the global availability and management of medical literature, easy and efficient access to clinical literature that can improve the management of patients remains a global challenge in low-income regions where pragmatic clinical literature is most needed. It is an acknowledged fact that economically disfavored areas, in particular Africa south of the Sahara, are disproportionally affected, and the disease burden takes its highest toll.

This book provides straightforward, relevant clinical information to facilitate access to standards of care for healthcare workers in the areas of the world where the clinical approach to disease assessment and management is the norm in regard to healthcare provision. This book presents guidelines to enable provision of quality and standard healthcare for common medical conditions in a minimal-resource facility setting. The presented information is detailed enough not to compromise quality of care. Effective clinical management by judicious use of limited resources is demonstrated. It further enables the clinical practitioner and students of medicine, nursing and other health providing disciplines to rapidly overview this vast subject and stay abreast.

Relevant information as to how to establish, maintain, and further develop health facilities in low-income regions is provided.

This book will certainly be a useful pocket company and reference for healthcare workers including students of medicine, nursing, pharmacy/drug dispensation, laboratory medicine, and public health. Administrators of health facilities may find it useful, as the book contains several practical and readily modifiable healthcare-related administrative documents.

I am confident that the book may gain a significant place in the healthcare terrain of The Gambia and beyond. It may equally be valuable for international students and healthcare workers from Europe, the Americas, and elsewhere who intend to do internships in similar geographic regions.

Banjul, The Gambia   Ousman Nyan

Preface

We write this book to share our experience in establishing, directing, and practicing clinical work in Bijilo Medical Centre (BMC), a prototype minimal-resource facility in a low-income region. The book is intended for all healthcare workers, in the hope that they will be able to use our experiences with BMC to improve healthcare delivery in The Gambia and other low-income regions.

North-South collaborations in the health sector have a significant impact on the evolution of healthcare systems in sub-Saharan Africa. A multitude of factors must be considered for the sustainability of established facilities. Often the sustainability and development of established facilities depend on the fragile North-South cooperation. Here, we underline the importance of local diligence and discipline. The significance of in-house training is outlined. South-South collaboration is mentioned and should be fostered.

This book provides a roadmap to self-reliance and sustainable development for established health facilities in low-income regions. The book contains tools essential to provide quality healthcare in a standard minimal-resource setting. Emphasis is placed on the importance of good communication between the healthcare provider and the patient as well as among the healthcare providers themselves: "doctoring together."

The significance of a good administrative unit in a standard minimal-resource healthcare facility is demonstrated. Tools necessary for the smooth operation of a developing healthcare facility are provided in the form of quality tables as well as many practical charts reproduced within the document.

Epalinges, Switzerland
Lausanne, Switzerland

Musa Touray
Aisha Touray

Acknowledgments

Our sincere gratitude goes to the following people, without whose contribution this book would never have come into being:

- The 35-plus dedicated staff members of the BMC "Dream Team"
- Professor Ousman Nyan, Professor of Medicine and Deputy Vice Chancellor (Academic)/Provost, AF SMAHS, Banjul campus, University of The Gambia
- Mr. Bouba Baldeh, state registered nurse, The Gambia
- Mr. Ousainou Ceesay, senior medical student, American University, The Gambia
- Dr. Yaya Sankareh, medical officer, Edward Francis Small Teaching Hospital, The Gambia
- Dr. Lamin Jaiteh, surgical consultant, Edward Francis Small Teaching Hospital, Banjul, The Gambia
- Dr. Mariama Touray, medical officer, Department of Internal Medicine, University Hospital of Vaud, Lausanne, Switzerland
- Dr. Jarai Touray, medical officer, Department of Pediatrics, Hospital Riviera-Chablais, Rennaz, Switzerland
- Ms. Leoni Limbach for the illustrations
- Ms. Karen McWilliams and Ms. Phyl Good for editorial and layout assistance

About the Book

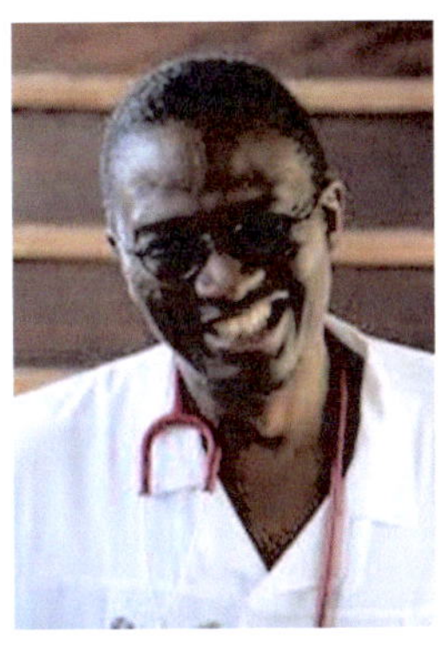

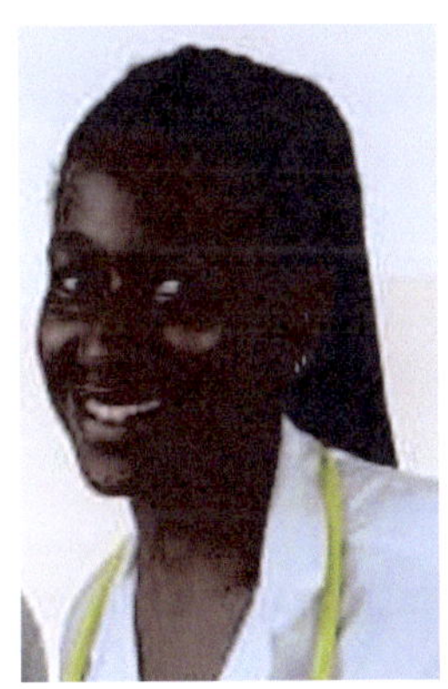

We wrote this book to share our experience in establishing, directing, managing, administrating, and practicing standard clinical work at the Bijilo Medical Centre (BMC), The Gambia, West Africa. Bijilo Medical Center is a prototype standard minimal-resource healthcare facility in a low-income region. The book is intended for all scopes of healthcare workers, in the hope that they will be able to use our experiences with BMC to improve healthcare delivery in The Gambia and other low-income regions globally. As the saying goes, "science has no borders."

The book does not claim to be comprehensive. It cannot replace standard reference textbooks, which should remain the mainstay of initial learning during both undergraduate and postgraduate training. However, the book can be a handy reference guide during clinical work. It may also serve as guiding summary literature for revisiting material already learned in the lecture rooms.

According to the dictum of "doctoring together," this book is intended to be used by a large scope of healthcare workers including:

- Students of medicine
- Medical residents
- Students of nursing (BSc, state registered nursing, enrolled nursing, and community nursing)
- Students of pharmacology and drug dispensing
- Established practicing pharmacists and drug dispensers
- Established public health workers
- Students of public health
- Students of laboratory technology
- Established laboratory technicians
- Students of physiotherapy

- Established practicing physiotherapists
- Health facility administrators

In addition to addressing local needs, we hope that this book may appeal to international healthcare workers who are involved in clinical programs in low-income countries. Too, medical and nursing students from Europe and North America may want to do internships in minimal-resource facilities as described herein.

Guided by the principle "think global, act local," this book is intended to be an evolving dynamic reference material in both national and international contexts. Constructive critical comments are welcome in order that we may update and improve subsequent editions.

Epalinges, Switzerland   Musa Touray
Lausanne, Switzerland   Aisha Touray

Contents

Part I   Introduction and Purpose of This Book

1   Introduction... 3
  1.1   Healthcare Systems in The Gambia, a Prototype
         Low-Income Region 4
  1.2   Pertinent Health Facts About a Typical Low-Income Region:
         The Gambia, West Africa........................... 6
  Bibliography 7

2   A Clinical Approach to Diagnosis and Treatment 9
  2.1   Medical History Taking 9
  2.2   Physical Examination.............................. 11
  2.3   Diagnostic Workup: Laboratory Tests, Radiography,
         Ultrasound, and ECG.............................. 13
  2.4   Final Diagnosis 14
  2.5   Formulation of a Treatment Plan 14
  2.6   Medical Prescription 15
  2.7   Medical Documentation............................ 15
  2.8   Clinical Red Flags 15
  Bibliography 16

**3   The Periodic Medical Checkup: A Clinical Approach
   to Preventive Medical Care** 17
  3.1   Medical History During a Checkup Visit............. 18
  3.2   Physical Examination During a Checkup Visit 19
  3.3   Laboratory/Paramedical Workup During a Checkup....... 20
  3.4   Optional Further Workup During a Checkup............ 20
  3.5   Review of Immunization Status During a Checkup........ 20
  Bibliography 21

Part II   Major Diagnoses and Treatment Regimens

4   Neurology... 25
  4.1   History: Questions to Ask 25
  4.2   Physical Examination............................. 25
      4.2.1   Cardinal Paramedical Neurology Investigations 27
  4.3   Neurology Red Flags 27

5 Ear, Nose, and Throat (ENT) and Stomatology 43
   5.1   History: Questions to Ask 43
   5.2   Physical Examination. 44
   5.3   Cardinal Paramedical Ear, Nose, and Throat Examinations . . 44
   5.4   Ear, Nose, and Throat Red Flags 44

6 Cardiovascular 55
   6.1   History: Questions to Ask 55
   6.2   Physical Examination. 56
   6.3   Cardinal Paramedical Cardiovascular Investigations. 56
   6.4   Cardiovascular Red Flags 57

7 Respiratory Diseases 73
   7.1   History: Questions to Ask 73
   7.2   Physical Examination. 74
   7.3   Cardinal Paramedical Respiratory System Examinations 74
   7.4   Respiratory System Red Flags. 74

8 Gastroenterology 85
   8.1   History: Questions to Ask 87
   8.2   Physical Examination. 87
   8.3   Cardinal Paramedical Gastroenterology Examinations 87
   8.4   Gastroenterology Red Flags. 87

9 Urology and Nephrology 107
   9.1   History: Questions to Ask 108
   9.2   Physical Examination. 108
   9.3   Cardinal Paramedical Urology and Nephrology
         Examinations 109
   9.4   Urology and Nephrology Red Flags 109

10 Obstetrics, Gynecology, and Antenatal Care 123
   10.1 Common Gynecology Diagnostic Procedures. 123
   10.2 Pregnancy Diagnosis 125
   10.3 Antenatal Visits 125
   10.4 Laboratory Tests to Be Done During Routine
         Antenatal Visits 125
   10.5 Guidelines for Referral to Specialized Care 125

11 Musculoskeletal 149
   11.1 History: Questions to Ask 150
   11.2 Physical Examination. 151
   11.3 Clinical Features That Differentiate Inflammatory from
         Mechanical Pain. 151
   11.4 Cardinal Paramedical Musculoskeletal Examinations. 151
   11.5 Musculoskeletal Red Flags 151

12 Dermatology 157
   12.1 History Taking in Dermatology: Questions to Ask 157
   12.2 Physical Examination in Dermatology 158

13 Hematology 171
   13.1 History: Questions to Ask 171

13.2 Physical Examination. 171
13.3 Cardinal Paramedical Hematology Examinations 172
13.4 Hematology Red Flags. 172

14 Endocrinology 179
14.1 History: Questions to Ask 180
14.2 Physical Examination. 180
14.3 Cardinal Paramedical Endocrinology Examinations 180
14.4 Endocrinology Red Flags. 180

15 Ophthalmology 189
15.1 History: Questions to Ask 190
15.2 Physical Examination. 191
15.3 Cardinal Paramedical Ophthalmology Examinations 191
15.4 Ophthalmology Red Flags 191

16 Psychiatry 203
16.1 History: Questions to Ask 204
16.2 Physical Examination. 204
16.3 Cardinal Paramedical Psychiatry Examinations 204
16.4 Psychiatry Red Flags 204
Bibliography 215

17 Pediatric Conditions and Their Treatment. 217
17.1 History Taking 217
17.2 Physical Examination. 219
17.3 Laboratory Investigation 219
17.4 Initial Care After Birth. 219
17.5 Pediatric Developmental Milestones 220
17.5.1 Red Flags Signifying Developmental
Retardation. 220
17.5.2 Correlating Acquired Skills with Age 220
17.6 Management of a Sick Child: Key Elements. 222
17.7 General Pediatric Management Plan 222
Bibliography 234

18 Palliative Care. 235
18.1 Key Elements of Palliative Care 235
18.2 Healthcare for the Terminal Patient 237
18.3 Suggestions for Delivery of Difficult News. 238
Bibliography 238

Part III Organization and Services

19 Organization of Regular Standard Health Care 241
19.1 Outpatient Triage and Patient Flow Within the Facility. 241
19.1.1 Standard Nursing Shifts. 242
19.1.2 Nursing Duties During a Shift
and How the Outgoing Shift Hands
Over to the Incoming Shift 242

19.1.3 The Pharmacy: How to Dispense Prescribed
Drugs to Outpatients 242

19.2 Patient Admission to the Hospital Wards
and Inpatient Care 244

19.2.1 Patient Admission to the Hospital Wards. 244

19.2.2 Administration of Medication to Inpatients. 245

19.2.3 Inpatient Monitoring and Vital Signs
Measurement 246

19.3 Discharging an Inpatient from the Wards
to His/Her Home 246

19.4 Medical Follow-Ups After Initial Ambulatory or Inpatient
Patient Management. 247

19.5 Physiotherapy Services 247

19.5.1 Basic Requirements to Establish
a Physiotherapy Unit 250

19.5.2 Scheduling Physiotherapy Sessions. 251

References. 251

20 **The Surgical Unit: Organization and Management** 253

20.1 Organization of the Surgical Unit 253

20.1.1 Personnel 254

20.1.2 Equipment 255

20.1.3 Consumables 255

20.1.4 Costing of Surgical Procedures 256

20.2 The Surgical Procedure 256

20.2.1 Preoperative Stage 256

20.2.2 Intraoperative Stage 257

20.2.3 Postoperative Stage 258

20.2.4 Blood Transfusion Unit in a Standard
Minimal-Resource Facility 259

21 **Behind the Scenes: Pharmacological Services** 265

21.1 Local Factors that Must Be Considered When Adapting
the WHO Essential Medicine List 265

21.2 The Pharmacy and the Medicine Dispenser. 266

21.2.1 Basic Knowledge Needed for Medicine
Dispensing. 267

21.2.2 Routes of Administration of Medicines. 267

21.2.3 Medicines with Age or Weight Restrictions 267

21.2.4 The Art of Prescribing a Medication
and the BMC-EML 269

Bibliography 269

22 **Adapted Essential Medicines List for a Standard
Minimal-Resource Health Facility** 271

22.1 Essential Medicines for Neurological Conditions
in a Standard Minimal-Resource Facility 272

22.2 Essential Medicines for Ear, Nose, and Throat (ENT)
Conditions in a Standard Minimal-Resource Facility 272

22.3 Essential Medicines for Cardiology Conditions
in a Standard Minimal-Resource Facility 272
22.4 Essential Medicines for Respiratory Conditions
in a Standard Minimal-Resource Facility 272
22.5 Essential Medicines for Gastrointestinal Conditions
in a Standard Minimal-Resource Facility 272
22.6 Essential Medicines Used in Urology and Nephrology
Conditions in a Standard Minimal-Resource Facility 280
22.7 Essential Medicines Used in Gynecology-Obstetrics
Conditions in a Standard Minimal-Resource Facility 280
22.8 Essential Medicines Used in Musculoskeletal Conditions
in a Standard Minimal-Resource Facility 283
22.9 Essential Medicines Used in Dermatology and Allergic
Conditions in a Standard Minimal-Resource Facility 283
22.10 Essential Medicines Used for Hematology Conditions
in a Standard Minimal-Resource Facility 283
22.11 Essential Medicines Used in Infectious Disease
Conditions in a Standard Minimal-Resource Facility 283
22.12 Essential Medicines Used in Endocrinology
Conditions in Standard Minimal-Resource Facility 292
22.13 Essential Medicines Used in Ophthalmology
Conditions in a Standard Minimal-Resource Facility 292
22.14 Essential Medicines Used in Psychiatry Conditions in a
Standard Minimal-Resource Facility 295
22.15 Essential Medicines Used for Palliative Care
in a Standard Minimal-Resource Facility 295
Bibliography 298

23 Immunization and Vaccines 301
Bibliography 310

**24 Basic Clinical Laboratory Services in a Standard
Minimal-Resource Facility** 311
References 319

25 Hospital Administration and Management 321
25.1 Administration of a Standard Minimal-Resource Facility ... 322
25.1.1 Costing Hospital Products and Services 323
25.1.2 Hospital Equipment and Material Inventory 323
25.1.3 Organization of the Reception 323
25.1.4 Accountancy, the Cashier, and Bookkeeping 324
25.1.5 Security of the Facility 324
25.2 Stationery 325
25.3 Hospital Stock Management 325
25.4 Hospital Rules and Regulations 325
25.4.1 Hospital Rules 326
25.4.2 Hospital Staff Regulations 326
25.5 Continuous Training Sessions and Staff Meetings 327

25.6 Job Descriptions, Primary Staff Responsibilities, and
Employment Procedures 327
25.6.1 Medical Staff Job Descriptions in a Standard
Minimal-Resource Facility 327
25.6.2 Paramedical Staff........................... 329
25.6.3 Administrative Staff.......................... 331
25.7 Hospital Maintenance Unit in a Standard
Minimal-Resource Facility 333
25.7.1 Electricity................................ 333
25.7.2 Plumbing 333
25.7.3 Construction.............................. 334
25.7.4 Carpentry 334
25.7.5 Gardening 334
25.7.6 Housekeeping and Laundry.................... 334
25.8 Appendix: Checklists of Hospital Chores and Duties by
Classified Department and Position.................... 334
25.8.1 Routine Hospital Chores 335
25.8.2 Human Resource Management Checklist 336
25.8.3 Facility Management Checklist................. 337
25.8.4 Nursing Team Management Checklist............ 337
25.8.5 Groundsman Management Checklist............. 338
25.8.6 Housekeeping Management Checklist............ 338

26 Essentials of Effective Clinical Communication 339
26.1 Patient Card 341
26.2 Medical Report................................. 342
26.3 Certificate of Good Health......................... 343
26.4 Attestation of Fit to Fly 344
26.5 Attestation of Birth 345
26.6 Referral Form for Outside Treatment 347
26.7 Surgical and Medical Procedure Informed Consent Form. . . 348
26.8 Retroviral (HIV) Test Consent Form 349
26.9 Surgical Operation Report......................... 350
26.10 Request for Maternity Leave 351
26.11 Excused Duty Certificate.......................... 352
26.12 Antenatal Card................................. 353
26.13 Obstetrical Delivery Chart......................... 355
26.14 Child Health Card 357
26.15 Essential Medication List.......................... 361
26.16 Available Vaccines/Infant Immunization Schedule 362
26.17 Laboratory Request Form 363
26.18 X-ray Request Form.............................. 364
26.19 Medical Prescription Form 365
26.20 Self-Discharge Form 366
26.21 Certificate of Death 367
26.22 Job Application Form............................. 368

26.23 Cash Transaction Receipts............................370
26.24 Institutional Affiliations............................373
       Bibliography...374

Appendix 375

Glossary 377

Bibliography 385

Index...387

Abbreviations and Acronyms

3TPR MOB	Mnemonic for priority care in a pediatric emergency situation: Tiny, temperature, trauma; Pallor, poisoning, pain; Respiratory distress, restless; Malnutrition, (O)edema; Burns
5 Fs	Mnemonic for cholecystitis screening: Female, Fat, Fair, Family, Fertile, over Forty
5 Ps	Mnemonic for urogenital treatment: Partners, Prevention of Pregnancy, Protection from STDs, Practices, Past history of STDs
AAA	Abdominal aortic aneurysm
ABCD	Mnemonic for emergency signs: Airway; Breathing; Circulation, coma, convulsing; Dehydration, diarrhea
ABCDE	Mnemonic for addressing problems in a severely unwell patient: Airway, Breathing, Circulation, Disability, Exposure OR
ABCDE	Mnemonic for describing skin lesions: Asymmetrical, Borderless, Color change, Diameter, Evolving
ABO	The major human blood group system
ACE	Angiotensin-converting enzyme
ACIP	Advisory Committee on Immunization Practices (U.S.)
ACS	Acute coronary syndrome
ACT	Artemisinin-based combination therapy
ADH	Antidiuretic hormone
AF	Atrial fibrillation
AFB	Acid fast bacillus
AHA	American Heart Association
AIDS	Acquired immune deficiency syndrome
ALP	Alkaline phosphatase
ALT	Alanine amino transferase
amp	Ampoule
AN	Autonomic neuropathy
AOM	Acute otitis media
AP	Anterior-posterior OR angina pectoris
AR	Aortic regurgitation
ARB	Angiotensin receptor blocker
ARDS	Acute respiratory distress syndrome
ARF	Acute rheumatic fever
ART	Assisted reproductive technology OR antiretroviral therapy
AST	Aspartate amino transferase

ATA/AACE	American Thyroid Association (ATA) and American Association of Clinical Endocrinologists (AACE)
ATLS	Advanced trauma life support
ATS	Australasian triage scale
AVB	Atrioventricular block
AVS	Aortic valve stenosis
BCG	Bacillus Calmette–Guérin
BD	Twice daily
BHCG	Beta human chorionic peptide
BMC	Bijilo Medical Centre
BMI	Body mass index
BP	Blood pressure
BPD	Biparietal distance
BPH	Benign prostatic hypertrophy
BUN	Blood urea nitrogen
CAT	Computed tomography
cc	Cubic centimeter
CCF	Congestive cardiac failure
CCN	Critical care nurse
CDC	Centers for Disease Control and Prevention (U.S.)
CEA	Carcinoembryonic antigen
CFC	Chlorofluorocarbon
CN	Cranial nerve
CNS	Central nervous system
COPD	Chronic obstructive pulmonary disease
CRD	Chronic renal disease
CRP	C-reactive protein
CSF	Cerebrospinal fluid
CT	Computed tomography
CVA	Cerebrovascular accident
D&C	Dilatation and curettage
D, d	Day(s)
DDPRT	Mnemonic for the right Drug, Dose, Patient, Route, and Time
Ddx	Differential diagnosis
DIC	Disseminated intravascular coagulation
DM	Diabetes mellitus
DOB	Day of birth
DOT	Direct observed treatment
DPT	Diphtheria, pertussis, tetanus (vaccine)
DRE	Digital rectal examination
DTaP	Diphtheria, tetanus, and/or pertussis (vaccine)
DVT	Deep venous thrombosis
Dx	Diagnosis
EAC	External auditory conduit
ECG	Electrocardiogram
ED	Excused duty medical certificate
EEG	Electroencephalogram
EFSTH	Edward Francis Small Teaching Hospital (The Gambia)

EMG	Electromyogram
EML	Essential medicines list
ENT	Ear, nose, (and) throat
EPTB	Extrapulmonary tuberculosis
ERASME	Mnemonic for writing medical prescriptions: effective, rational, adjusted, secure, monitored, and economical
ESR	Erythrocyte sedimentation rate
ETEC	Enterotoxigenic *Escherichia coli*
EUP	Extrauterine pregnancy
FBC	Full blood count
FEV1	Forced expiratory volume in the first second
FGM	Female genital mutilation
FP	Facial paralysis
FSH	Follicle-stimulating hormone
FUO	Fever of unknown origin
FVC	Forced vital capacity
g/L	Grams per liter
GALS	Mnemonic for musculoskeletal evaluation: Gait, Arms, Legs, Spine
GBS	Guillain-Barré syndrome
GD	Gestational diabetes
GERD	Gastro-esophageal reflux disease
GFR	Glomerular filtration rate
GI	Gastrointestinal
GOLD	Global Initiative for Chronic Obstructive Lung Disease, used to determine the severity of COPD
GT	Gamma transferase
GTD	Gestational trophoblast disease
GTN	Gestational trophoblastic neoplasm
HART	Highly active retroviral treatment
Hb	Hemoglobin
HbsAg	Hepatitis B surface antigen
HBV	Hepatitis B virus
HCC	Hepatocellular carcinoma
HCG	Human chorionic gonadotropin
HDL	High-density lipid
HEEADSSS	Mnemonic for adolescent medical history taking: Home, Education, Eating, Activities, Drugs, Sexuality, Suicide, Safety
HELLP	Hemolysis, Elevated Liver enzymes, Low Platelet count (syndrome)
Hg	Mercury, used to measure blood pressure
HIV	Human immunodeficiency virus
HP	Hyperglycemia in pregnancy
HPV	Human papilloma virus
h, Hr(s)	Hour(s)
HSV	Herpes simplex virus
HZV	Herpes zoster virus
IBD	Irritable bowel disease

IBS	Irritable bowel syndrome
ICP	Intracranial pressure
ICU	Intensive care unit
IgG	Immunoglobulin G
IgM	Immunoglobulin M
IM	Intramuscular
INR	International normalized range OR ratio
IOP	Intraocular pressure
IPT	Intermittent preventive treatment
IPV	Inactivated polio vaccine
IU	International units
IUFD	Intrauterine fetal death
IUGR	Intrauterine growth restriction/retardation
iv	Intravenous
IVF	In vitro fertilization
JE	Japanese encephalitis
JEV	Japanese encephalitis virus
JVP	Jugular venous pressure
KCl	Potassium chloride
L	Liter
LDL	Low-density lipid
LSHTM	London School of Hygiene and Tropical Medicine
MAO	Monoamine oxidase inhibitor
MCH	Mean corpuscular hemoglobin
MCHC	Mean corpuscular hemoglobin concentration
MCV	Mean corpuscular volume
mEq/L	Milliequivalents per liter
mg	Milligram
MI	Myocardial infarction
MIP	Maternal intermittent prophylaxis
ml	Milliliter
mm	Millimeter
mmol/L	Millimoles per liter (also μmol/L)
MMR	Measles, mumps, and rubella vaccine
MOF	Multiple organ failure
mOsm	Osmolarity, or milliosmoles per liter
MR	Mitral regurgitation
MRC	Medical Research Council at LSHTM
MRI	Magnetic resonance imaging
MS	Multiple sclerosis
MVP	Mitral valve prolapse
NaCl	Sodium chloride
NAS	No added salt
NG	Nasogastric
NRT	Nicotine replacement therapy
NSAID	Nonsteroidal anti-inflammatory drug
NSTEMI	Non-ST-elevation myocardial infarction
OAC	Oral anticoagulant

OPQRST	Mnemonic for a systematic description of a patient's chief complaint: Onset, Palliation/provocation, Quality, Region/radiation, Severity, Time
OPV	Oral polio vaccine
ORS	Oral rehydration solution
PCA	Posterior communicant aneurysm
PCM	Paracetamol
PCOS	Polycystic ovary syndrome
PCP	Pneumocystis carinii pneumonia
PE	Pulmonary embolism
Pen G	Penicillin Grunenthal
PICT	Provider-initiated counseling and testing
PID	Pelvic inflammatory disease
PO, po	Per Os, refers to medication taken orally
POP	Plaster of Paris
PPD	Purified protein derivative
PPI	Proton pump inhibitor
PR	Pulmonic regurgitation
PROM	Premature rupture of membranes
PSA	Prostate-specific antigen
PTB	Pulmonary tuberculosis
RBC	Red blood cell count
RHD	Rheumatic heart disease
RTA	Road traffic accident
RVTH	Royal Victoria Teaching Hospital, now called EFSTH (The Gambia)
SAS	Sleep apnea syndrome
SBP	Systolic blood pressure
SC	Subcutaneous
SDHSW	State Department of Health and Social Welfare (The Gambia)
SEN	State-enrolled nurse
SGOT	Serum glutamate oxalate transferase
SGPT	Serum glutamate pyruvate transferase
SIDS	Sudden infant death syndrome
SLE	Systemic lupus erythematosus
SMAHS	School of Medicine and Allied Health Sciences (The Gambia)
SpA	Spondyloarthritis
SRN	State-registered nurse
SSRI	Selective serotonin reuptake inhibitor
stat	Unique dose OR, urgent or rush, from "statum" (Latin)
STD	Sexually transmitted disease
STEMI	ST-elevation myocardial infarction
STI	Sexually transmitted infection
SZRECC	Shaikh Zayed Regional Eye Care Centre (The Gambia)
TAA	Thoracic aortic aneurysm
tab	Tablet
TB	Tuberculosis bacillus
tinct	Tincture
TM	Tympanic membrane

TMD	Temporomandibular joint disorder
TMP/SMX	Trimethoprim sulphametoxine
TMVL	Transient monocular visual loss
TOF	Tetralogy of Fallot
TORCH	Mnemonic for early pregnancy screening: Toxoplasmosis, Other (Syphilis), Rubella, Cytomegalovirus, Herpes simplex virus
TPHA	Treponema pallidum hemagglutination assay
TSCI	Traumatic spinal cord injury
TSH	Thyroid-stimulating hormone
URTI	Upper respiratory tract infection
UTI	Urinary tract infection
VAPP	Vaccine-associated paralytic poliomyelitis
VDRL	Venereal Disease Research Laboratory
VINDICATE	Mnemonic for a range of differential diagnosis categories: Vascular, Inflammatory, Neoplastic, Degenerative/Deficiency, Idiopathic/Intoxication, Congenital, Autoimmune/Allergic, Traumatic, Endocrine
VZV	Varicella zoster virus
w/w	"Weight per weight," a measure of chemical concentration
WBC	White blood cell count
WHO	World Health Organization
WILD	Mnemonic for substance addiction evaluation: usage interferes with obligations at Work, school or at home; continued usage despite Interpersonal or social consequences; Legal problems related to substance usage; and usage in Dangerous situations

Part I

Introduction and Purpose of This Book

Contents

1.1   **Healthcare Systems in The Gambia, a Prototype Low-Income Region** 4

1.2   **Pertinent Health Facts About a Typical Low-Income Region:**
      The Gambia, West Africa 6

Bibliography 7

This book is intended to aid medical personnel in practicing evidence-based health care in a minimal-resource setting. Furthermore, the book outlines how to establish, direct, and sustain a standard minimal-resource health facility in low income regions. An overview of the fundamental factors that must be addressed to successfully establish and operate such a facility is provided.

Three main sections comprise this book, and each section is organized into chapters that break down specific topics. Part I introduces the reader to the challenges unique to healthcare provision in a minimal-resource setting. Bijilo Medical Centre (BMC), a standard minimal-resource health facility in a low-income African region, serves as a model in this regard throughout the book.

Chapters 2 and 3 describe BMC's clinical approach to the diagnosis and treatment of patients, including the method and concept behind the periodic medical checkup. The primary goal of our clinical approach is to achieve the best possible clinical outcome under the given conditions, judiciously using the limited available resources. To that end, only essential paramedical exams that will have direct impact on the management of the patient are ordered, respecting the World Health Organization (WHO) paradigm, "to test is to treat." Cultural, religious, psychosocial, and national administrative factors that challenge healthcare providers in impoverished regions are addressed (Fig. 1.1a).

Part II delves into diagnoses and recommended treatment regimens for most pathologies that medical personnel are likely to encounter. Diseases and conditions are sorted according to system (neurologic, respiratory, etc.) and a chapter is devoted to each. Every chapter offers guidance on history taking and conducting a thorough physical examination to make an accurate diagnosis. For each system, specific information regarding treatment regimens is also offered in tabular form.

Part III pulls back somewhat from the fundamentals of patient care to offer a workable model

© The Author(s), under exclusive license to Springer Nature Switzerland AG 2021

M. Touray, A. Touray, *Clinical Work and General Management of a Standard Minimal-Resource Facility*, Sustainable Development Goals Series, https://doi.org/10.1007/978-3-030-71032-3_1

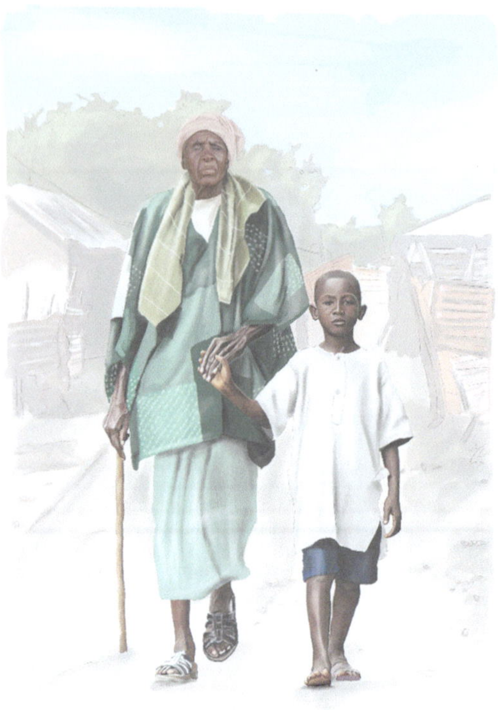

Fig. 1.1a *Health determinants*: Poverty is a significant health determinant (Fig. 1.1a). It is a socioeconomic condition in which an individual, family or community lacks the essential resources to ensure reasonable livelihood. Poverty may manifest as hunger, malnutrition, limited access to healthcare, education, and other basic services. Consequently, poverty perpetuates ill health and other social ailments. A vicious cycle thus establishes. Standard minimal healthcare facilities may be instrumental in breaking this devastating vicious cycle

for managing the important internal organizations and routine hospital services that support patient care. Chap. 19 covers the organization and patient flow from intake, to treatment, to discharge and follow-up care, while the organization and management of the surgical unit is covered in Chap. 20.

Chapters 21, 22, 23, and 24 elaborate aspects of pharmacological services, essential medicines, preventative health measures, and the diagnostic capabilities of laboratory medicine. Chap. 22 offers a comprehensive essential medicines list (EML) based on that of the WHO. BMC's EML was adapted from the original to be a pragmatic tool for low-resource medical facilities.

The use of expensive auxiliary medication that does not conform with evidence-based clinical practice is discouraged, and facilities should adhere to the WHO essential drug list when prescribing drugs. The effects of local epidemiological factors, economic impacts, cultural norms, legal considerations, and national regulations on drug availability are considered. The need to maintain the rigors of evidence-based medical practices for drug usage is not compromised.

Finally, Chap. 25 offers guidance for administrators regarding establishing best practices for hospital administration and management (costing, equipment and material inventory, accountancy, etc.), job descriptions and staff responsibilities, and maintenance of the physical facility (electricity, plumbing, housekeeping, etc.).

Three appendices follow the main text. They consist of a glossary of common terms, samples of many common medical forms, and a list of referral centers used by BMC.

It is hoped that BMC may serve as a prototype health facility and that this book will be a valuable supplement to governmental efforts to improve the health of underprivileged communities.

1.1 Healthcare Systems in The Gambia, a Prototype Low-Income Region

Health is "a state of complete physical, mental and social well-being and not merely the absence of disease or infirmity."
– World Health Organization, July 1946

Nations adopt several systems to meet their healthcare demands; they maintain and improve health through the affordable application of health science and through the adoption of healthy lifestyle choices by both individuals and societies. The key to designing national healthcare delivery systems is to effectively address the main determinants of health. The World Health Organization (WHO) identifies these as the social and economic environment, the physical environment, and the person's individual characteristics and behaviors. Specifically, health determinants include the following:

- Culture and beliefs
- Social support networks
- Education and literacy
- Social environments
- Physical environments
- Personal health practices and coping skills
- Healthy childhood development
- Employment/working conditions
- Income and social status
- Biology and genetics
- Healthcare services
- Gender

Healthcare delivery is organized into institutions and facilities that attend to the health needs of individuals, families, and communities in diverse forms. The healthcare delivery facilities may provide varying health services that require specific human resources, equipment, and infrastructure. Based on the complexity of the medical condition to be cared for, the delivered healthcare services may be considered to be primary, secondary, tertiary, or quaternary healthcare.

Primary healthcare is an approach to health and well-being centered on the needs and circumstances of individuals, families, and communities. It addresses comprehensive and interrelated physical, mental, and social health and well-being.

Primary healthcare aims to provide whole-person care for health needs throughout people's lives. It ensures that they receive comprehensive care, ranging from promotion and prevention to treatment, rehabilitation, and palliative care in a location as close as feasible to their everyday environment. The approach of merely treating a set of specific diseases is grossly inadequate.

A well-structured primary healthcare system aims at honoring the Universal Declaration on Human Rights: "Everyone has the right to a standard of living adequate for the health and well-being of himself and of his family, including food, clothing, housing and medical care and necessary social services." Primary healthcare is typically delivered in ambulatory circumstances or visitations.

Secondary healthcare includes necessary treatment for a short period of time for a brief but serious illness, injury, or other health condition in an acute or subacute setting. This care is often found in a hospital emergency department. Secondary care embraces skilled attendance during childbirth, intensive care, and medical imaging services. The term "secondary care" is often equivalent to "hospital care."

In The Gambia, both large and small health centers provide secondary medical care. There are about seven main health centers, either government-run or private, and 12 smaller centers, each providing inpatient and outpatient treatment.

Tertiary healthcare is specialized consultative healthcare, usually for inpatients and on referral from a primary or secondary health professional. It is provided in a facility that has personnel and facilities for advanced medical investigation and treatment. Examples of tertiary care services include cancer management, neurosurgery, cardiac surgery, plastic surgery, treatment for severe burns, advanced neonatology services, palliative care, and other complex medical and surgical interventions.

For an example, in The Gambia, tertiary care services are delivered by four main referral hospitals, the Medical Research Council (MRC), several private clinics, and nongovernmental organization (NGO)-operated clinics. The main referral hospital countrywide is the Edward Francis Small Teaching Hospital (EFSTH).

Quaternary healthcare is an extension of tertiary care in reference to advanced levels of medicine that are highly specialized and not widely accessed eg Fig. 1.1b. Experimental medicine and some types of uncommon diagnostic or surgical procedures are considered quaternary healthcare. These services are usually offered only sporadically by NGOs that dispatch medical missions from abroad.

Bijilo Medical Center/Hospital (BMC, www.bijilomedical.org) is a nongovernmental health facility with the goal of delivering affordable, quality healthcare. The types of healthcare services provided, based on attendance statistics, are

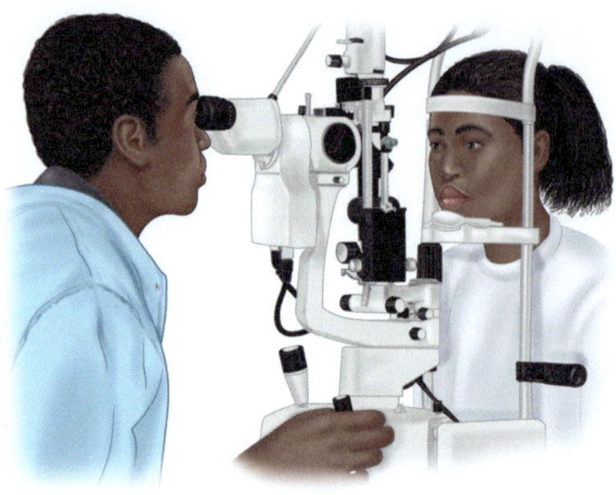

Fig. 1.1b Health facilities may be categorised based on their main attendance, their geographic location, or their establishing principles. It is a common practice to categorise health facilities as primary, secondary, tertiary or quaternary healthcare facilities, with quaternary health care facilities being an extension of tertiary care. At the summit of the referral chain, quaternary care provides advanced levels of medicine that are highly specialized and not widely accessed

about 60% primary, 20% secondary, and 20% tertiary care.

BMC was founded in 2002 through a series of coordinated steps, which can serve as a foundation for establishing other new healthcare facilities. To set up a facility in The Gambia entails the following steps:

1. Determine the legal framework of the facility which may involve seeking advice from a registered legal practitioner.
2. Purchase (or rent) an appropriate piece of land or a building.
3. Register the facility with the State Department of Health and Social Welfare (SDHSW), to which all health care facilities are answerable.
4. Draft and sign a memorandum of understanding with the SDHSW.
5. Purchase and install the needed equipment.
6. Employ the necessary human resources.

Note that the abovementioned steps may not be sequential.

1.2 Pertinent Health Facts About a Typical Low-Income Region: The Gambia, West Africa

Healthcare workers should be guided by basic demographic, epidemiological, socioeconomic, and geographic knowledge. A health survey conducted between 1997 and 2016 revealed the following about The Gambia:

- The total population (2016) is 2,039,000.
- Life expectancy at birth, m/f (years, 2016) is 61/63.
- The probability of dying between 15 and 60 years of age (m/f, per 1000 population, 2016) is 290/235.
- Public spending on health was 3–7% of GDP in 2010–2014.
- There are four doctors and 57 nurses/midwives per 100,000 people.
- There are three pharmaceutical personnel per 100,000 people.
- Fifty-seven percent of births are attended by qualified health staff.
- Ninety-one percent of one-year-olds are immunized with one dose of measles vaccine (2011).
- Eighty-nine percent of the country's population is using an improved drinking water source.
- Sixty-eight percent of the population has access to adequate sanitation facilities.
- There are four government-run referral hospitals, eight health centers, 16 minor health centers, and one research health center.
- Approximately 12 NGOs, private clinics, and mobile clinics operate countrywide.
- The Edward Francis Small Teaching Hospital, located in Banjul, is the main referral hospital and offers specialist consultant services.
- Quite often, a healthcare provider may suggest "overseas treatment" because of the lack of an appropriate management scheme for a given disease condition. Presently, disease conditions requiring overseas treatment are mainly oncological, cardiological, or dysmorphic malformation.

Bibliography

1. https://www.who.int/violence_injury_prevention/road_safety_status/country_profiles/en/.
2. Preclinical and clinical lecture notes of the curriculum of medical studies, Faculty of Medicine, University of Lausanne, Course year 2015–2021.
3. Scientific-Units-Recommendations-Formulas (SURF), guidelines, Médecine Interne General, Philippe Furger en collaboration avec Thierry Fumeaux et le SURF-team. 2020.
4. The Gambia standard drug treatment guidelines, 2nd ed. Department of State for Health and Social Welfare, The Republic of the Gambia; 2001. http://apps.who.int/medicinedocs/documents/s22418en/s22418en.pdf.
5. Cornuz J, Pasche O, Kermode-Noppel T. Compas: Stratégies de prise en charge clinique, Médecine interne générale ambulatoire: Institute of Social and Preventive; 2010.

Contents

2.1 **Medical History Taking** 9

2.2 **Physical Examination** 11

2.3 **Diagnostic Workup: Laboratory Tests, Radiography, Ultrasound, and ECG** 13

2.4 **Final Diagnosis** 14

2.5 **Formulation of a Treatment Plan** 14

2.6 **Medical Prescription** 15

2.7 **Medical Documentation** 15

2.8 **Clinical Red Flags** 15

Bibliography 16

The fundamental task of a medical facility is to care for patients: to assess, diagnose, and treat illness and injury.

The clinical approach (described in detail later in the chapter) is composed of six general components:

1. History taking
2. Physical examination
3. Diagnostic workup
4. Diagnosis
5. Formulation and execution of a treatment plan
6. Follow-up visit

Information gathered in the first three steps should be utilized to derive a diagnosis and to formulate a cost-effective treatment. The execution of the treatment plan can be either on an outpatient or an inpatient basis.

2.1 Medical History Taking

The goal of taking the patient's history is to obtain the maximum amount of clinically relevant information possible in a short period of time, while reassuring the patient that he or she is very important

M. Touray, A. Touray, *Clinical Work and General Management of a Standard Minimal-Resource Facility*, Sustainable Development Goals Series, https://doi.org/10.1007/978-3-030-71032-3_2

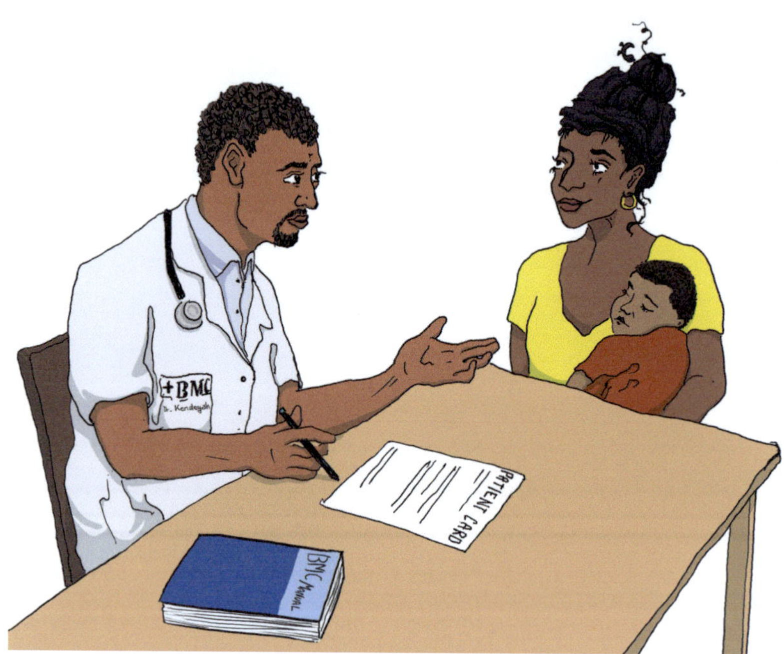

Fig. 2.1 *History taking* is crucial. Adopt the Balint patient-doctor positioning as shown. Politely ask nonessential escorts to leave the consultation room. Reassure the patient that confidentiality is guaranteed. Show empathy. Ask relevant questions whose answers have a pertinent impact on confirming a specific diagnosis that is related to the chief complaint. Be systematic. Remember and make use of the OPQRST mnemonic

and is being listened to fully. The patient's medical history should be taken directly from the patient when possible. To put the patient at ease, the patient and the healthcare provider should be situated diagonally to each other rather than directly face to face (Fig. 2.1). Patients' escorts should be excused from the consultation room during this time in order to allow the patient to speak freely.

The room should be well lit and ventilated, with a ceiling fan and/or open windows so the patient is comfortable and at ease. The consultation should take place in the patient's native language if possible. An interpreter should be brought in only if absolutely necessary. The information received should be treated with confidentiality and written down on the patient's record card carefully and concisely.

Using the head-to-toe method of assessment described in the following section aids in developing an accurate assessment of the patient's condition. The following systematic method has proven useful at BMC:

1. Chief Complaint: "Why Did You Come to the Hospital Today?"
   This question should be explored fully to understand the medical problem of the patient

and to gauge what he or she expects from the healthcare provider. For a systematic description of the chief complaint, the OPQRST mnemonic may be useful to discern reasons for a patient's symptoms and history. The parts of the mnemonic are as follows:

(a) *Onset of the event*
   What the patient was doing when it started (active, inactive, or stressed), whether the patient believes that activity prompted the pain, and whether the onset was sudden, gradual, or part of an ongoing chronic problem.

(b) *Provocation or palliation*
   Does any movement, pressure (such as palpation), or other external factors make the problem better or worse? This can also include whether the symptoms relieve with rest.

(c) *Quality of the pain*
   This is the patient's description of the pain. Questions can be open-ended or leading. Ideally, this will elicit descriptions of the patient's pain: is it sharp, dull, crushing, burning, tearing, or some other feeling? Is there the pattern such as intermittent, constant, or throbbing?

(d) *R*egion and *R*adiation

Where the pain is located on the body, and whether it radiates or moves to any other area.

(e) *Severity*

The pain score (usually on a scale of 0–10). Zero is no pain, and ten is the worst possible pain ever.

(f) *Time* (history)

How long has the condition been going on and how has it changed since onset (better, worse, different symptoms)? Determine whether it has ever happened before, whether and how it may have changed since onset, and when the pain stopped if it is no longer currently being felt.

2. *Systemic history:* The clinician should ask if the patient has experienced or is experiencing problems in any of the following areas:

   (a) *Neurological:* headache, dizziness, and vision anomalies

   (b) *Ear, nose, throat (ENT):* dysphagia, odynophagia, dysphonia, dry throat, discharge (otorrhea, rhinorrhea), tinnitus, hear loss, and vertigo

   (c) *Cardiovascular:* chest pain, pedal edema, and dyspnea

   (d) *Respiratory/pulmonary:* cough and hemoptysis

   (e) *Digestive:* abdominal pain, diarrhea, nausea, vomiting, loss of appetite, and recent weight loss

   (f) *Urogenital:* dysuria, hematuria, urethral discharge, and dyspareunia

   (g) *Osteoarticular:* joint pain and muscle pain

   (h) *Dermatological:* ulcers, macules, papules, and squamous lesions

   (i) *Psychosocial history:* marital status, how many siblings, description of present living conditions, and number of children

   (j) *Medical history:* list of current medications, history of chronic diseases (hypertension, diabetes, sickle-cell disease, asthma, etc.), prior hospital admissions, surgeries, and current significant hard drug use

2.2 Physical Examination

After the chief complaint has been stated and the patient's systemic history has been taken, the clinician should begin the physical examination by looking at the patient from head to toe in order to assess his or her general condition (Fig. 2.2). The patient's overall clinical condition, nutritional status, and facial expression should be assessed. The patient's weight, temperature, blood pressure, pulse, and respiratory rate should be taken, and the results should be noted on the patient's record card.

Next, the clinician should perform a complete physical exam, paying special attention to the system corresponding to the chief complaint (Fig. 2.3). Again, the head-to-toe approach will aid in conducting a thorough assessment:

- *Neurological:* determine level of consciousness, orientation (time, space, and personal information), pupillary reaction, movement of limbs, and gait.

- *Otorhinolaryngology/ear, nose, and throat:* examine nose for signs of rhinorrhea, polyps; check pharynx with tongue depressor. Palpate to determine cervical and peritragal adenopathy.

- *Cardiovascular:* Inspect, auscultate, then palpate; check for lower limb edema and perform auscultation of the heart.

- *Respiratory/pulmonary:* Inspect, auscultate, then palpate the thoracic cage, checking for deformations of the thorax and upper abdomen, pain on palpation; examine hands (cyanosis, clubbing), lips, and mouth; auscultate the lungs.

- *Gastroenterology/digestive:* Inspect, auscultate, then palpate; examine contour of abdomen; check for presence of mass, scars, tenderness on palpation.

- *Urology and nephrology:* check for any lesion on the external genitalia.

- *Gynecology:* check for any lesion on the external genitalia and perform colposcopy.

- *Osteoarticular/musculoskeletal:* identify any limping indicating pain in muscles and/or joints; check for swollen or warm joints, any functional deficits.

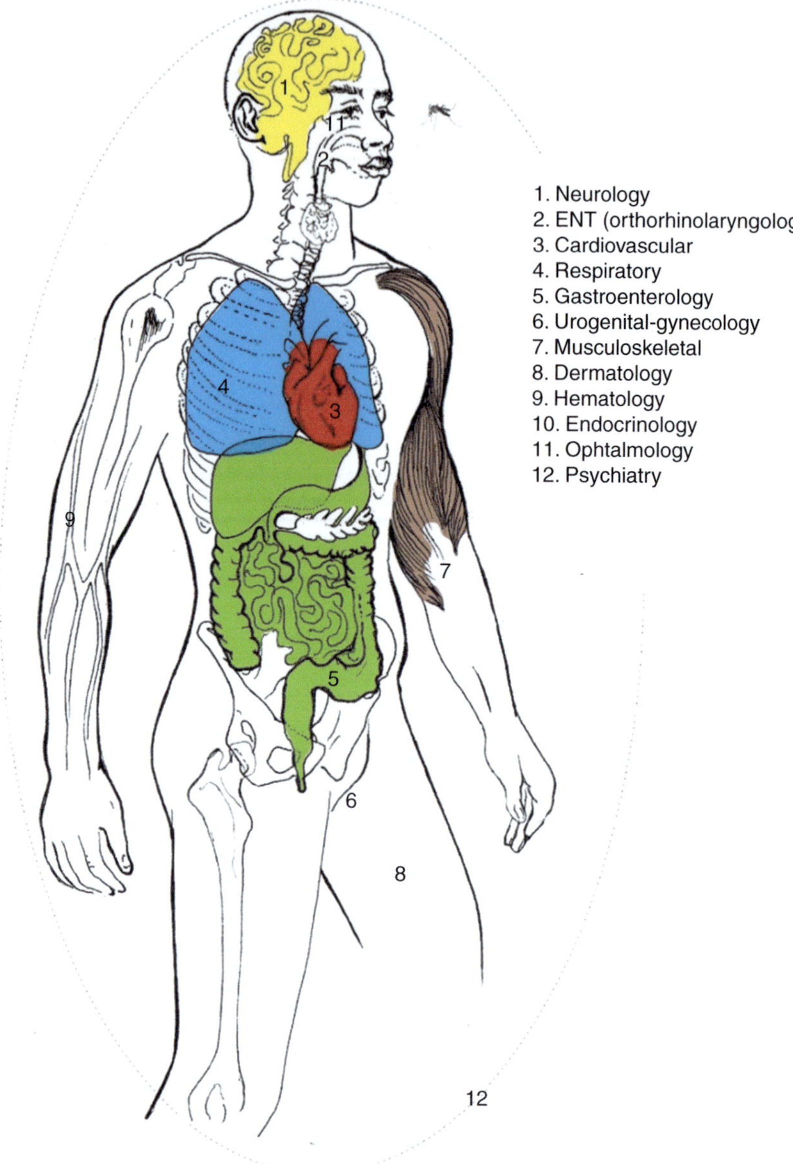

Fig. 2.2 The "head-to-toe" systemic presentation of clinical topics, starting from the head of the patient to his/her toes. The systems are sequentially evaluated

- *Dermatology/skin*: determine general condition; check for macules, pustules, squamous lesions, scratch marks, ulcerations, or other lesions.
- *Hematology*: check for parasitic infection (e.g., malaria) or anemia, conjunctival pallor, presence of petechia, presence of conjunctival pallor.
- *Endocrinology*: check for occult signs; diabetes, for example, minor peripheral neurologic dysfunctions, afflictions of the thyroid or pituitary axis, and pathologies of the suprarenal gland.
- *Ophthalmology*: check for structural anomalies; test ocular motor skills, visual field, and visual acuity. Palpate the ocular globe.
- *Psychiatry*: appreciate the general appearance of the patient including dress code, personal hygiene, facial expression, and language; assess patient for mental health issues such as depression, suicidal risk, anxiety, or substance abuse.

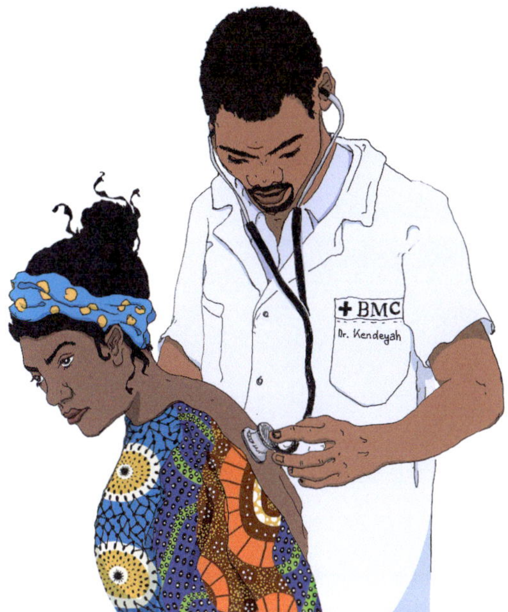

Fig. 2.3 The *physical* examination is the second pillar of a routine clinical workup. Examine the patient from head to toe by sequentially inspecting, palpating, and auscultating. Pay special attention to systems related to the chief complaint. Ensure the patient's safety and security, and always respect the patient's sense of modesty. The patient may be examined while he or she is lying down, sitting, or standing

2.3 Diagnostic Workup: Laboratory Tests, Radiography, Ultrasound, and ECG

One must always remember that the economic status of most patients is low. It is important that all diagnostic procedures and treatment be cost-effective (Fig. 2.4). The dictum "to test is to treat" should be a guiding principle when determining which tests to order to confirm or discard a differential diagnosis (Ddx). The chief complaint of the patient must be thoroughly considered when reaching a diagnosis. With that in mind, we use the VINDICATE mnemonic to provide a reasonable range of chief-complaint-related differential diagnosis categories:

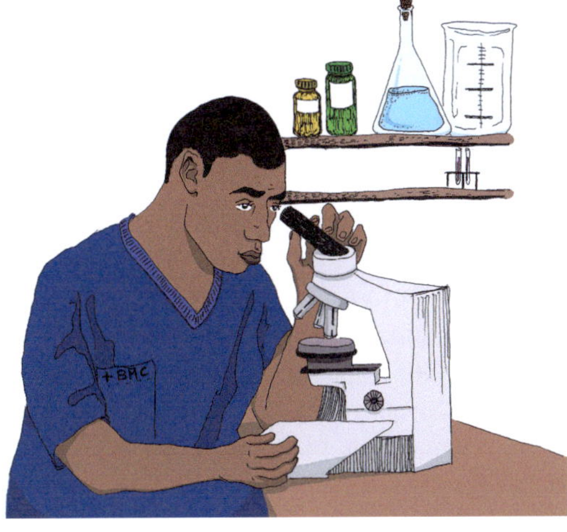

Fig. 2.4 *Paramedical* examinations are carefully selected to confirm or discard differential diagnoses. Only investigations that will have a direct impact on the management of the patient should be performed. Remember, "to test is to treat." Avoid unnecessary, expensive paramedical examinations

- *V*ascular
- *I*nflammatory
- *N*eoplastic
- *D*egenerative/*D*eficiency
- *I*diopathic/*I*ntoxication
- *C*ongenital
- *A*utoimmune/*A*llergic
- *T*raumatic
- *E*ndocrine

The diagnostic workup should rely primarily on historical and physical findings rather than on costly paramedical procedures; only pertinent paramedical procedures should be performed to confirm or discard a differential diagnosis (Fig. 2.4).

Based on the patient's history, the physical examination, and results obtained from paramedical examination, the clinician should reflect on the case history and establish a list of problems. Under each item on the list of problems, the differential diagnosis should be noted. Results of any significant paramedical examinations performed should also be included.

Case Example A 13-year-old schoolgirl presented with 3 days' history of headache, fever, delayed menses, nausea, and vomiting. Temperature was 38.2 °C and chest was clear.

List of problems and Ddx:

1. Headache/fever
   (a) Malaria:
       Att: perform Hb, WBC, BF
   (b) Meningitis:
       Att: thorough history, seek nuchal rigor at physical examination, directed neurological physical. PL not available
2. Amenorrhea
   (a) Unwanted teenage pregnancy
       Att: more history taking, do urinary B-HCG
   (b) Urinary tract infection
       Att: urine stix
       TTT: Treat underlining diagnosis accordingly

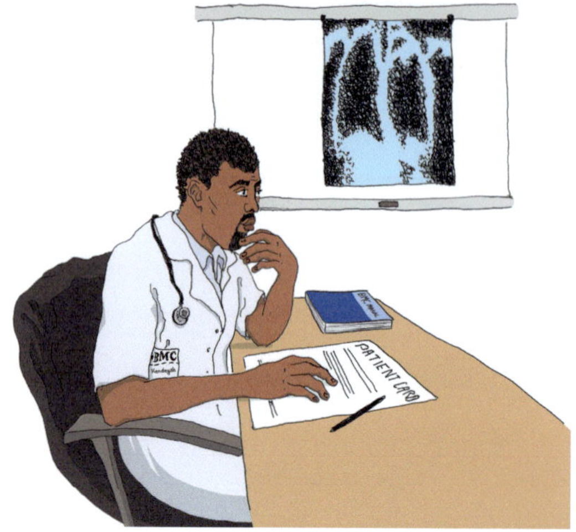

Fig. 2.5 To propose a *diagnosis*, the physician needs to take a quiet moment to think, reflect, and make the best use of his/her medical knowledge. All relevant historical, physical, and paramedical examination findings should be considered when proposing a diagnosis. Based on the forgoing findings, the most probable diagnosis is retained

2.4   Final Diagnosis

On the basis of patient history, physical examination, and paramedical examinations, a diagnosis may be made. For this, the physician should take a quiet intellectual moment (Fig. 2.5) during which time he/she reflects and combines all acquired data to make a diagnosis. The final diagnosis should be disclosed and explained to the patient, and it should be clearly noted on the patient's record card.

2.5   Formulation of a Treatment Plan

A clear therapeutic management plan should be designed and explained to the patient. If hospitalization is recommended, this should be explained to the patient. The arguments for inpatient treatment should be explained in simple and understandable language.

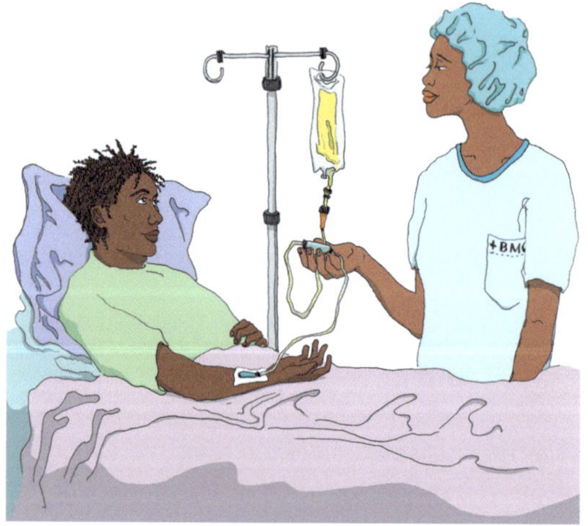

Fig. 2.6 Once the diagnosis is retained, the physician formulates an evidence-based *management* plan to provide the most optimal therapy for the patient. Execution of this plan requires clear and ongoing communication with the nursing and dispensing team: "doctoring together." A concerted team effort must be maintained between various healthcare workers to ensure proper implementation of the management plan

Evidence-based medical treatment should be prescribed and dispensed (Fig. 2.6).

2.6 Medical Prescription

After formulating an evidenced-based medical diagnosis, the attending physician may write a medical prescription. The prescription should include the identity of the patient, date of prescription, the precise dosage, and mode and duration of administration.

Efforts should be made by the prescribing physician to limit the treatment regimen to medications found in Chap. 22, which is adapted from the WHO Essential Drug List. Costly auxiliary medications that have no evidence-based, proven benefit to the patient should be avoided.

2.7 Medical Documentation

Written communication is a regular and significant part of routine clinical practice. The generated reports may be intended for other healthcare workers, for employers, for the various legal systems, or for personal records (Table 2.1). All written documentation has legal value and consequences, so the signatory of the document must assure him/herself of the accuracy of the entire document. BMC is keen on generating high-quality medical documents, having learned that these documents may have a significant impact on patient outcome.

Table 2.1 delineates the pertinent information that should be included in each type of document.

2.8 Clinical Red Flags

Clinical red flags are signs and symptoms discovered while taking a patient's medical history, or performing a physical examination or paramedical investigation that may indicate a possible serious pathology.

Quality healthcare provision requires particular attention when taking medical history, when performing physical examination, and when evaluating laboratory results. Clinical features

Table 2.1 Medical documents: clinical management often requires writing documents for the patient or for other healthcare providers

Medical document	Pertinent information and format
Attestation of birth	Identity of baby, gender, date and time of birth, birth weight and height, identity of mother
Certificate of death	Identity of patient, date of birth (DOB) (or age if not known), cause of death. State whether death is natural or violent (if unsure, you may omit the word "natural"), providing date, time, and place of death
Certificate of good health	Patient identity, DOB, summary of state of mental and somatic well-being. Confirm absence of evidence of contagious diseases
Comprehensive medical report	Patient identity, DOB, current diagnosis, comorbidities, current anamnesis, treatment plan and evolution, laboratory results, proposition, and discussion
Fit to fly certificate	Verify the capacity to fly without foreseeable medical complication, giving the date, and, if possible, the duration of flight that can be undertaken
Medical and surgical procedure consent form	This document provides evidence that the surgical procedure has been explained to the patient by a qualified healthcare giver in simple, plain language. The patient's signature on the document is legal evidence that he or she both accepts that the procedure will be done and has been informed of possible consequences that could result from the procedure
Medical referral report	Name and DOB of patient, diagnosis or suspected diagnosis, synopsis of the case, and its management. Outline clearly the reason for the referral. Attach lab and imaging results, if any
Request for maternity leave	Patient identity, DOB, expected due date, first and last day of maternity leave. Specify date to return to work
Surgical operation report	The surgeon documents his or her procedure meticulously by describing the procedure performed. This report contains all technical surgical details, instruments used, support staff present, and the condition of the patient at the end of the procedure. It also contains instructions regarding care to be provided in the postsurgical period

Key elements that must be included are shown

and symptoms characterized by high mortality and morbidity incidences should be rigorously searched for and promptly attended to. This may be achieved either by intensifying the care with appropriately trained personal and equipment or by referring speedily to an appropriate care center.

Clinical red flags are outlined systematically in the chapters dealing with diagnosis and treatment.

Bibliography

1. Papadakis MA, McPhee SJ, Rabow MW. Current medical diagnosis and treatment. New York, NY: McGraw-Hill Education; 2019. https://accessmedicine.mhmedical.com/book.aspx?bookID=2449.
2. Preclinical and clinical lecture notes of the curriculum of medical studies, Faculty of Medicine, University of Lausanne, Course year 2015–2021.
3. Scientific-Units-Recommendations-Formulas (SURF), guidelines, Médecine Interne General, Philippe Furger en collaboration avec Thierry Fumeaux et le SURF-team. 2020.
4. Pocket Book of Hospital Care for Children. Guidelines for the management of, common, childhood illnesses, 2nd ed, World Health Organization; 2013.
5. Essential med notes, 2020 Comprehensive medical references and review for the United States Medical Licensing Exam (USMLE) step II and the Medical Council of Canada Qualifying Exam (MCCQE) Part 1, 36th ed., Sara Mirali and Ayesh Seneviratne.
6. WHO model list of essential medicines, 20th list. World Health Organization; March 2017, Amended August 2017. https://apps.who.int/iris/bitstream/handle/10665/273826/EML-20-eng.pdf?ua=1.
7. The Gambia standard drug treatment guidelines, 2nd ed. Department of State for Health and Social Welfare, The Republic of the Gambia; 2001. http://apps.who.int/medicinedocs/documents/s22418en/s22418en.pdf.
8. Cornuz J, Pasche O, Kermode-Noppel T. Compas: Stratégies de prise en charge clinique, Médecine interne générale ambulatoire. Lausanne: Institute of Social and Preventive Medicine; 2010.

The Periodic Medical Checkup: A Clinical Approach to Preventive Medical Care

Contents

3.1   **Medical History During a Checkup Visit** 18

3.2   **Physical Examination During a Checkup Visit** 19

3.3   **Laboratory/Paramedical Workup During a Checkup** 20

3.4   **Optional Further Workup During a Checkup** 20

3.5   **Review of Immunization Status During a Checkup** 20

Bibliography 21

Medical checkups, defined as general examinations of a person's overall health condition, comprise a significant number of visits to BMC. Checkup visits offer good opportunities to provide appropriate preventive care to community members.

Other synonyms of the medical checkup are periodic health check, periodic health review, or preventive health check.

A medical checkup is typically a request from an individual or institution to a physician to use his or her knowledge, skills, and available paramedical investigations to determine an individual's current state of health. The procedure is similar to the diagnostic clinical approach described in Sect. 3.2, but the purpose of the checkup is to assess a patient's overall health rather than to diagnose and treat a specific problem.

Medical checkups consist of taking a patient's medical personal and family history, conducting a thorough physical examination, and perhaps ordering carefully selected paramedical investigations. On putting these findings together, a firm conclusion may be made regarding the individual's current state of health, and in some cases, a prognosis may be made vconcerning his or her future health status. The medical checkup is a mainstay of preventive medical services, and these services constitute a significant component of general primary care.

The medical checkup visit should be coordinated and systematic, so as not to miss any significant pathology. For the checkup to be effective, it is important to provide a convivial and secure history-taking and examination environment. The patient must be given the opportunity to express his or her reason for coming on that visit at that given time.

The medical checkup is called differently depending on regions, institutions, culture, and

M. Touray, A. Touray, *Clinical Work and General Management of a Standard Minimal-Resource Facility*, Sustainable Development Goals Series, https://doi.org/10.1007/978-3-030-71032-3_3

other factors. The basic practice is the same despite the varying terms. Commonly used terms include:

- Periodic health evaluation
- Annual physical
- Comprehensive medical examination
- General health check
- Preventive health examination

3.1   Medical History During a Checkup Visit

The first step in a checkup is to determine why the patient has chosen to come in at that specific point in his or her life. Depending on the patient's situation, appropriate questions must be asked to define the person's motivation in order to tailor the visit to meet the needs of the patient. Typical motivations include the following:

- Death in the family or neighborhood.
- Diagnosis of STD in a partner.
- Feeling of aging on turning 30, 40, or 50.
- Requirement for beginning a fitness program.
- Requirement imposed by an employer.

Once the patient's motive is clear, then direct, systematic questions should be asked in order to discover the patient's medical and family history and to uncover past issues regarding all systems. Proceeding from head to toe, the clinician should inquire and document all historical elements.

Personal medical history:

- Childhood disease, past hospitalizations, trauma, involvement in accidents, etc.
- Past and current substance use (alcohol, tobacco, cannabis, heroin, etc.)
- Hobbies, sports (frequency, regularity, and intensity)
- Interrogate presence of allergies (determine severity: whether limited to skin or if it affects breathing)

- Travel history
- Sexual behavior to determine exposure risks
- Professional background and exposure
- Gauge level of formal education

Family history: limit your interrogation to first-degree relatives and note presence of:

- Metabolic diseases (diabetes, hyper- or hypothyroidism, lipid disorder, asthma).
- Cardiovascular conditions (sudden death syndrome, hypertension, stroke, coronary artery disease, myocardial infarction, peripheral arteriopathy, etc.).
- Oncologic (breast, prostate, colon cancer) disease, etc. Make an effort to determine age of onset of the disease conditions.
- Musculoskeletal disorder (rheumatoid arthritis, congenital muscle diseases, or myopathies).
- Skin diseases (e.g., vitiligo, tinea versicolor).

Neurologic history: interrogate

- Headache
- Dizziness
- Visual acuity and visual field
- Hearing issues

Ear, nose, and throat history: interrogate

- Pain on swallowing, voice tone, and voice quality issues
- Presence of mass in the neck region
- Sense of smell

Cardiovascular history: interrogate as precisely as possible

- Chest pain, shortness of breath, palpitation
- Pedal edema, occurrence of paroxysmal nocturnal dyspnea
- Cold hands and feet
- Changes in exercise intolerances, etc.

Respiratory history: interrogate any occurrence of

- Difficult of breathing at rest or during physical exercise
- Any wheezing, cough
- Contact history for tuberculosis

Digestive history:

- Abdominal pain, signs of reflux disease, food intolerance
- Transit (diarrhea-constipation), aspect of the feces (consistency, color, presence of blood, etc.)
- Weight loss, weight gain, whether voluntary or involuntary, kinetics of the loss or gain

Urogenital history:

- Dysuria, presence of urethral discharge, odor, dyspareunia, etc.
- Past history of urinary tract infection, circumcision, female genital mutilation, sexual orientation, and habits
- Regularity, duration and intensity of menses, and date of last menstruation

3.2 Physical Examination During a Checkup Visit

Physical examination should be systematic and structured.

Vital physical signs: take the patient's

- Blood pressure (BP) and pulse
- Temperature
- Weight
- Height

A routine physical examination should then be performed that encompasses all clinical systems in the spirit of "head-to-toe":

Neurology physical examination: qualify

- Gait
- Check visual acuity by confrontation test and hearing loss by whispering
- Occulomotricity

Gross motor or sensitivity losses: paresis and dysesthesia.

Ear, nose, and throat physical examination: inspect, auscultate, and palpate:

- Inspect general morphology of neck, nose, and ears, appreciate scars and adenopathy.

Cardiovascular physical examination: inspect, auscultate, and palpate:

- Inspect neck veins.
- Auscultate the heart and note regularity of heart beat and pulse.
- Feel peripheral pulses.

Respiratory physical examination: inspect, auscultate, and palpate:

- Inspect morphology of the thoracic cage.
- Inspect general respiratory rate and pattern.
- Appreciate AP distance of the thorax.
- Auscultate and appreciate quality of air entry and exit in all pulmonary fields. Note presence of hypoventilation, wheezing, and crepitations.
- Percuss all lung fields and note presence of tympanism or dullness.

Digestive physical examination: inspect, auscultate, and palpate:

- Note appearance of the abdomen (protuberant, flat, protrusions, herniations).
- Note scars, masses, and tenderness.
- Qualify bowel movements/noises: frequency, tonality distribution.

Urogenital physical examination: note

- General form of external genital organs, scars, signs of mutilation, malformations, etc.
- Rectal examination should be considered based on history, gender, and age. Rectal examination should be systematically proposed to men over 50 years of age.

Musculoskeletal physical examination: inspect and test

- Gait, general muscle tone.
- Appearance of main joints (shoulder, hip, knee, ankle, elbow, and wrist). Appreciate the hands/feet and interphalangeal joints.

Dermatological physical examination: inspect and palpate

- General appearance of skin and personal hygiene, texture and state of skin hydration, scars, scratches or other lesions.

More detailed information regarding the head-to-toe examination procedure may be found in Chap. 2.

3.3 Laboratory/Paramedical Workup During a Checkup

Based on the medical history and physical examination, and conforming to the wishes of the patient, some or all of the following paramedical tests may be ordered:

- FBC
- Fasting blood sugar
- Aspartate aminotransferase (AST)
- Alanine aminotransferase (ALAT)
- Bilirubin
- Creatinine
- Urinalysis
- Electrocardiogram (ECG)
- Chest X-ray

3.4 Optional Further Workup During a Checkup

Based on the history, age, physical examination, and basic laboratory findings as well as the general clinical impression, the checkup may be further tailored to address the individual's clinical requirements. Further evaluations that may be required include the following:

- Extending serological tests to cover STDs (hepatitis B, HIV, syphilis, gonorrhea, and chlamydia).
- TSH to probe thyroid dysfunction.
- PSA, alpha-fetoprotein for cancer.
- Hormone panels for infertility or erectile dysfunction: testosterone, estrogen, progesterone, luteinizing hormone, and prolactin.
- Exercise ECG, MRI, CT or CAT scan, and ultrasound evaluations.

3.5 Review of Immunization Status During a Checkup

Immunization is the process of preventing an organism to contract a disease or pathogenic agent. On perfroming this act, the organism is said to be *immune* to that pathogen. Vaccination is the administration of an immune-producing substance (vaccine) to an individual.

Immunization is one of the most effective preventive health measures, and routine immunization schedules constitute a central pillar in all national health systems. The vaccination schedules vary from country to country depending on the local epidemiological, demographic, and microbiological realities. Other factors affecting national vaccination schemes are availability of trained staff, availability and maintenance of cold-chain resources, logistical challenges, and religious and cultural issues.

Scientific data and statistics demonstrate dramatic declines in rates of vaccine-preventable diseases when compared with the prevaccine era.

Table 3.1 Vaccines: During a checkup, the vaccination status of the patient should be reviewed

Vaccine	Disease	Recommended schedule
BCG	Tuberculosis	At birth or soon after
DPT	Diphtheria Pertussis Tetanus	At the age of 2 months, 3 months, 4 months, and 1 year
Haemophilus influenzae	Haemophilus influenzae	At the age of 2 months, 3 months, and 4 months
Hepatitis B vaccine	Hepatitis B infection	At birth, age of 2 months, 3 months, and 4 months
OPV	Poliomyelitis	At birth, age of 2 months, 3 months, 4 months, 9 months, and 18 months
Pneumococcal vaccine	Pneumonia	At the age of 2 months, 3 months, and 4 months
Tetanus toxoid	Both neonatal and adult tetanus	At the age of 2 months, 3 months, 4 months, and 1 year
Yellow fever vaccine	Yellow fever	At the age of 9 months

Compliance to the standard recommended schedule should be encouraged

Typical diseases that are effectively prevented by well-designed vaccination schemes are listed:

- Diphtheria
- Invasive *H. influenzae* in children below 5 years of age
- Hepatitis A
- Hepatitis B (acute)
- Measles
- Meningococcal disease, all serotypes
- Mumps
- Pertussis
- Pneumococcal disease, invasive below 5 years of age
- Polio (paralytic)
- Rotavirus
- Rubella
- Congenital rubella syndrome
- Smallpox
- Tetanus
- Varicella

During a checkup visit, the person's vaccination history can also be reviewed, and subsequently booster doses can be advised and/or administered (Table 3.1).

Standard minimal-resource health facilities adhere to the national immunization scheme (e.g., BMC in The Gambia). A sustainable cold chain is maintained, and the vaccines are stored strictly adhering to cold-chain requirements. All freeze-dried vaccines are reconstituted with the indicated diluents. A special day is selected to dispense and record the vaccination (immunization clinic). The vaccines are administered to the patients by a trained public health officer. Most minimal-resource centers may obtain the vaccines in the national scheme from the national health officer at a minimal cost.

Bibliography

1. Papadakis MA, McPhee SJ, Rabow MW. Current medical diagnosis and treatment. New York, NY: McGraw-Hill Education; 2019. https://accessmedicine.mhmedical.com/book.aspx?bookID=2449.
2. Preclinical and clinical lecture notes of the curriculum of medical studies, Faculty of Medicine, University of Lausanne, Course year 2015–2021.
3. Scientific-Units-Recommendations-Formulas (SURF) guidelines, Médecine Interne General, Philippe Furger en collaboration avec Thierry Fumeaux et le SURF-team. 2020.
4. Pocket Book of Hospital Care for Children. Guidelines for the management of, common, childhood illnesses, 2nd ed. World Health Organisation; 2013.
5. Essential med notes, 2020 Comprehensive medical references and review for the United States Medical Licensing Exam (USMLE) step II and the Medical Council of Canada Qualifying Exam (MCCQE) Part 1, 36th ed., Sara Mirali and Ayesh Seneviratne.

6. WHO model list of essential medicines, 20th list. World Health Organization; March 2017, Amended August 2017. https://apps.who.int/iris/bitstream/handle/10665/273826/EML-20-eng.pdf?ua=1.
7. The Gambia standard drug treatment guidelines, 2nd ed. Department of State for Health and Social Welfare, The Republic of the Gambia; 2001. http://apps.who.int/medicinedocs/documents/s22418en/s22418en.pdf.
8. Cornuz J, Pasche O, Kermode-Noppel T. Compas: Stratégies de prise en charge clinique, Médecine interne générale ambulatoire. Lausanne: Institute of Social and Preventive Medicine; 2010.
9. Diseases and conditions: comprehensive guides on hundreds of conditions. Mayo Clinic. https://www.mayoclinic.org/diseases-conditions.
10. https://www.uptodate.com.
11. https://www.cdc.gov/ncbddd/actearly/milestones.
12. https://www.who.int/biologicals.

Part II

Major Diagnoses and Treatment Regimens

Different approaches to teaching, presenting, and practicing clinical medicine have been elaborated in previous sections. Each medical teaching facility tends to choose a system that corresponds to the experience of medical instructors active in that facility.

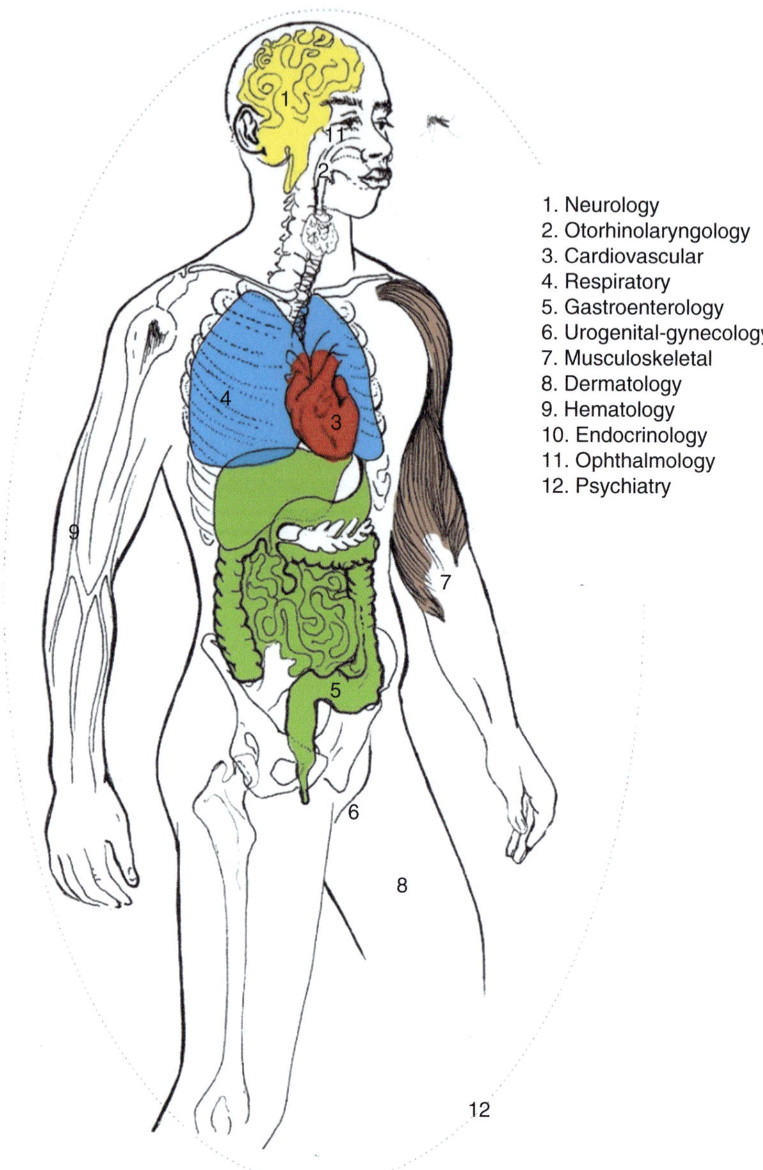

The "head-to-toe" systemic presentation of clinical topics, starting from the head of the patient to his/her toes. The systems are sequentially evaluated

Part II is organized according to the "head-to-toe" systemic method of elaborating medical data (see the reproduction of Fig. 2.2 above). As the name suggests, the head-to-toe method presents medical topics systemically, starting from the head of the patient to the neck, chest, abdomen, the urogenital system, the musculoskeletal system, and the skin. This systemic, sequential method enables the clinician to be thorough and not miss any system. When properly adopted, the head-to-toe method has a powerful inherent mnemotechnical character.

Contents

4.1   **History: Questions to Ask** 25

4.2   **Physical Examination** 25
4.2.1 Cardinal Paramedical Neurology Investigations 27

4.3   **Neurology Red Flags** 27

Neurological disorders are diseases of the brain, spine, and the nerves that connect them. Structural, biochemical, or electrical abnormalities in the brain, spinal cord, or other nerves can produce a range of *symptoms*. There are more than 600 diseases of the nervous system, notably brain tumors, epilepsy, spinal cord disorders, and peripheral nerve disorders, just to mention a few (Fig. 4.1). In this section, we address neurological disorders that are encountered in minimal-resource facilities (Table 4.1).

To treat the myriad of neurologic cases presenting at a typical standard minimal-resource facility, it is important to differentiate generalized neuropathies from focal conditions. Presenting conditions may be secondary to underlying systemic diseases such as malaria, diabetes, dysthyroid, substance abuse, intracranial lesions, HIV-AIDS, neurosyphilis, toxic encephalopathies, posttraumatic lesions, and congenital conditions. It is important to ask the right questions and to perform a directed neurologic examination. Remember to appreciate the general condition of the patient, for example,

whether he or she is oriented in the three modes (time, person, and space), with the Glasgow score. Evaluate any motor and sensory deficits.

Detecting meningeal signs in time can be lifesaving.

Abusive use of marijuana, alcohol, tobacco, and traditional medication may also be contributing etiologic factors.

4.1 History: Questions to Ask

- Does your head hurt?
- Are you dizzy? Is your vision blurred?
- Any muscle weakness? Any numbness?
- Any episode of unconsciousness?
- Has any family member had a seizure disorder?

4.2 Physical Examination

- Gauge the level of consciousness (in person, space, and time).
- Watch the gait.

© The Author(s), under exclusive license to Springer Nature Switzerland AG 2021
M. Touray, A. Touray, *Clinical Work and General Management of a Standard Minimal-Resource Facility*, Sustainable Development Goals Series, https://doi.org/10.1007/978-3-030-71032-3_4

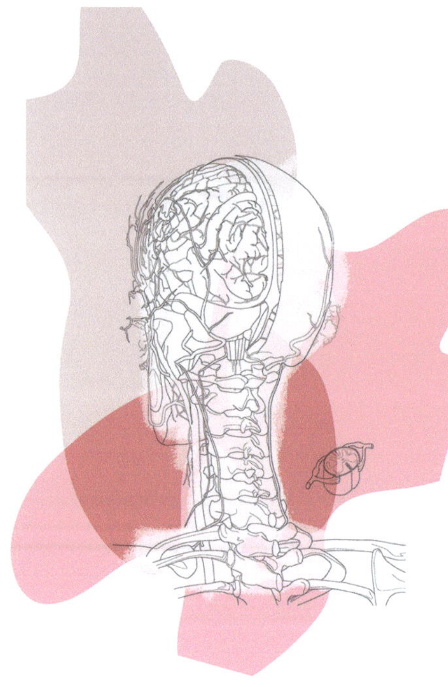

Neurology

List of neurology disorders that are described in the text.
For easy reference, the corresponding page on which the
disease condition is described is in brackets.

Acute confusional state (p207 and p209)
Brain tumors (p27)
Cerebrovascular accident (p28)
Chronic pain syndrome (p28)
Congenital neurological defects (p29)
Cranio Facial pain (p31)
Dementia (p29)
Dysautonomia (p29)
Epilepsy/seizure (p30)
Essential tremor (p30)
Facial paralysis (p31)
Falls in older persons (p32)
Fibromyalgia (p32)
Gait disorders (p33)
Guillain Barré syndrome (p33)
Headache (p34)
Hiccup (p35)
Intracranial abscess (p35)
Intracranial aneurysm (p35)
Meningitis (bacterial) (p36)
Multiple sclerosis (p36)
Neurocutaneous diseases (Neurofibromatosis) (p37)
Neurologic manifestations of systemic diseases (p37)
Parkinsonism: (p37)
Peripheral neurologic deficit (p38)
Polyneuropathy (p39)
Stupor and coma (p39)
Transient ischemic attack (p39)
Tremor (p37)

Fig. 4.1 Neurology: A mnemonic illustration representing main Neurological anatomic structures and their corresponding pathologies

- Perform tests of orientation.
- Test motor skills and sensitivity.
- Exclude meningism.
- Use the *Glasgow coma scale*:
  - *Eye opening*:
    spontaneous (4)
    to speech (3)
    to pain (2)
    nil (1)
  - *Verbal response*:
    oriented (5)
    confused conversation (4)
    inappropriate words (3)
    incomprehensible sounds (2)
    nil (1)
  - *Motor response*:
    obeys (6)
    localized (5)
    withdraws (4)
    abnormal flexion (3)
    extensor response (2)
    nil (1)

- Obtain the *Blantyre coma score*: Apply a standardized stimulus, for example, pinching, then sum up the response
  - Verbal response
  - Visual response
  - Physical response

4.2.1 Cardinal Paramedical Neurology Investigations

- Full blood count (FBC)
- Erythrocyte sedimentation rate
- Lumbar puncture
- Computed tomography (CT) scan of brain
- Magnetic resonance imaging (MRI)
- Electroencephalogram (EEC)
- Electromyogram (EMG)

4.3 Neurology Red Flags

- Sudden onset of severe headache, peaking in less than 1 minute; explosive sensation in the head
- Recent unhabitual neurologic symptoms
- Headache with associated fever in the absence of infectious focus
- Hypertension >180/120, malignant hypertension
- Recent head or cervical injury, recent cervical manipulation
- Cutaneous rash and/or meningism
- Suspicion of glaucoma
- Anticoagulation: patient on oral anticoagulant and history of fall

Table 4.1 Neurological conditions and their treatment

Diagnosis and classification	Treatment and relevant clinical features: neurological conditions
Brain tumors Heterogeneous group of neoplasms originating from different cells within the central nervous system (CNS) or from systemic cancers that have metastasized to the CNS *Primary brain tumors* Includes various cell types with significantly different tumor growth rates • High-grade glioma • Low-grade glioma • Primary CNS lymphoma • Meningioma • Brain metastasis *Intracranial mass lesions* • Meningioma • Glioblastoma • Astrocytoma • Ependymoma • Medulloblastoma	*Treatment* • Control pain • Educate patient and family • Dexamethasone, tab, 4 mg, 1–2 tab/d, 3 d, to reduce cerebral edema • Refer for tertiary care *Diagnostic evaluation* • History • Physical examination • Laboratories (comprehensive metabolic panel) • Imaging (MRI) *Note*: Neurologic symptoms and signs may result from local brain invasion, compression of adjacent structures, and increased intracranial pressure. Clinical manifestations are determined by the function of the involved areas of the brain and the histology of the tumor *Clinical manifestations* • Headache • Seizures • Focal deficits • Sensory loss • Aphasia • Visual spatial dysfunction • Cognitive dysfunction • Increased intracranial pressure (nausea and projectile emesis) *Systemic cancers with predilection to metastasize to the CNS include* • Lung cancer • Melanoma • Breast cancer

(continued)

Table 4.1 (continued)

Diagnosis and classification	Treatment and relevant clinical features: neurological conditions
Cerebrovascular accident (CVA), stroke Occurs when the blood supply to part of the brain is interrupted or severely reduced *Classification* • 90% ischemic: Cardiogenic emboli: occlusion of small vessels • 10% hemorrhagic *Risk factors* • High blood pressure • Atherosclerosis • Hypercholesteremia • Atrial fibrillation • Prior heart attack • Sickle cell anemia • Clotting disorders • Congenital heart defects • Diabetes • Smoking • Obesity • Heavy alcohol misuse • Drugs, such as cocaine or methamphetamine	*Acute treatment* *Ischemic stroke (represents 90% of stroke)* • Thrombolysis in the first 6 h after onset of symptoms tissue plasminogen activation tPA, Actilyse Cathflo, dry substance 2 mg, slow iv after excluding counter indications • Secondary preventive treatment • Antiplatelet: Aspirin 100–300 mg daily *Thrombotic CVA* • Aspirin 300 mg 14 d • Simvastatin, 20 mg daily *Hemorrhagic CVA* Reduce blood pressure gradually over several days *Note: No iv glucose solution, as it worsens cerebral edema* *Etiology* • Atherosclerosis of large vessels • Cerebral infarction from thrombosis of a cerebral vessel • Embolism from a distant site (e.g., atrial fibrillation, infections) • Intracerebral hemorrhages • Subarachnoid hemorrhage *Diagnostic features* • Sudden onset of neurologic deficit due to cerebrovascular dysfunction • Patient often has hypertension, diabetes mellitus, tobacco use, atrial fibrillation, or atherosclerosis
Chronic pain syndrome More than 3 months of pain as follows: back pain, leg/foot pain, arm/hand pain, headache, chronic regional pain, widespread pain	*Treatment* • Pharmacologic medicine: Paracetamol *and* • Ibuprofen, tab, 400 mg, 2 × 1 tab/d, • Physiotherapy • Psychological support: empathic listening, motivation • Behavioral therapy • Neuromodulation • Interventional approaches: moderately spaced psychology consultation • Gabapentin tabs, 100 mg, 2 × 1 tab/d • Amitriptyline, 25 mg tabs, 1 tab/d to be taken in the evening, for 1–6 months • TENS: Transcutaneous Electrical Stimulation where available • Refer to tertiary pain unit when no significant pain relief is attained *Classification* • *Neuropathic pain*: peripheral, including postherpetic neuralgia, diabetic neuropathy; or central, including post-stroke pain or multiple sclerosis • *Musculoskeletal pain*: back pain, myofascial pain syndrome, ankle pain • *Inflammatory pain*: For example, inflammatory arthropathies, infection • *Mechanical/compressive pain*: For example, renal calculi, visceral pain from expanding tumor masses *Patient assessment* • History: characterize pain, remember OPQRST mnemonic • Physical examination • Diagnostic testing: FBC, erythrocyte sedimentation rate (ESR), imaging, EMG where needed

Table 4.1 (continued)

Diagnosis and classification	Treatment and relevant clinical features: neurological conditions
Congenital neurological defects Neural tube defects are congenital anomalies of neural development with a spectrum of clinical manifestations; they can affect the cranium or spine *Hydrocephalus* Abnormal increase in the amount of cerebrospinal fluid within the ventricles of the brain, usually resulting in an increase in size of the head of an infant *Meningocele/meningomyelocele* Defect in the spinal cord involving only the meninges (Meningocele) or both the meninges and neural tissue *Spina bifida* Defect in the formation of the spinal column *Sacrococcygeal teratoma* Malformation with a mass protruding from the sacral end of the neonate	*Treatment* • Patient education • May involve surgery to remove the tumor or derivation of the excess cerebrospinal fluid by way of implanted stents • Refer for neurosurgical consultation *Treatment* • Educate patient and parent • Provide pain relief • Psychological support • Physical therapy where needed *Prevention* Because it may be challenging to obtain the recommended amount of folic acid (400 µg/d) through natural folate-rich foods, acid folic supplements are recommended to all women planning to have a baby for as long as 12 weeks after conception *Clinical symptoms* • Morning headache • Paralysis of cranial nerve VI • Setting sun phenomenon • Bulging fontanelle • Nausea • Ataxia • Fecal-urinary incontinence
Dementia Progressive intellectual decline Age is the main risk factor, followed by family history and vascular disease risk factors *Classifications* • Alzheimer's disease • Vascular dementia • Dementia with Lewy bodies • Frontotemporal dementia	*Treatment* • Provide psychosocial support • Strengthen the family and community support by educating them about the disease condition • Ensure personal hygiene of the patient • Avoid stigmatization • "Brain jogging": engage in conversations, puzzles, simple arithmetic exercises *Clinical features* • Age-related neurodegenerative disease • Short-term memory impairment • Visuospatial, language, and executive function deficits • Neuropsychological assessment, neuropsychiatric evaluation by a trained neuropsychologist
Dysautonomia (autonomic neuropathy, AN) Caused by pathological process in the central or peripheral nervous system. The disease condition results to symptoms related to abnormalities of blood pressure regulation, thermoregulatory sweating, gastrointestinal function, sphincter control, and sexual function *Classification* • Cardiovascular AN • Gastrointestinal AN • Diabetic AN • Hereditary AN • Urologic AN	*Treatment* • Identify and treat the underlying disease process • Adapted physiotherapy • Refer to tertiary center for specialized consultations *Diagnostic features* • Postural hypertension or abnormal heart rate regulation • Abnormalities of sweating, intestinal motility, sexual function, or sphincter control • Syncope may occur • Symptoms may occur in isolation or in any combination

(continued)

Table 4.1 (continued)

Diagnosis and classification	Treatment and relevant clinical features: neurological conditions
Epilepsy/seizure Disorder of the central nervous system characterized by spontaneous recurrent motor and/or sensory neuronal discharge	*Treatment* *Acute seizure*: • Diazepam, tab, 5 mg, 1 tab/d, (in general 0.2 mg/kg) • Diazepam ampoule 5 mg, 1 amp iv (or im) bolus • Maintenance with maximum 3 amps in 24 h.
Classification • Generalized • Partial • Absence (petit mal)	*Prophylaxis and oral maintenance treatment* • Phenytoin, tab, 100 mg, 1 tab/d, increase progressively, maximum 3 tab/d • Valproate acid, tab, 200 mg, 1/d, increase gradually as needed to maximum 4 × 1 tab/d • Carbamazepine, tab, 200 mg, 1 tab/d, increase progressively, maximum dose 2 × 2 tab/d • Phenobarbital, tab, 15 mg, 2 × 1 tab/d • Place the patient on the left lateral side *Tips for clinical management* • History should be completed by witnesses of the seizure where possible • Patient education is important • Stigmatization should be discussed • Carpenters should be warned when working at heights • Professional drivers should be warned and monitored for compliance of drug treatment • Rule out eclampsia if pregnant
Essential tremor Involuntary repetitive movement brought about by arm movement and sustained antigravity postures, affecting common daily activities such as writing, drinking from a glass, and handling eating utensils	*Treatment* • Patient education • Propranolol, tab, 40 mg, 1 × 1 tab/d *Diagnostic features* • Postural tremor of hands, head, or voice • Positive family history • May improve temporarily with alcohol consumption • No abnormal findings other than the tremor • Beginning at any age
Differential diagnosis • Enhanced physiologic tremor • Parkinson's disease • Dystonic head tremor • Spasmodic dystonia	*Signs and symptoms* • Tremor is enhanced on emotional stress • Lower limbs are usually spared • Tremor is not present at rest but emerges from action

Table 4.1 (continued)

Diagnosis and classification	Treatment and relevant clinical features: neurological conditions
Craniofacial pain Painful sensation of the head and neck regions often mediated by sensory fibers carried by corresponding nerves: *Classification/Nomenclature* • Trigeminal neuralgia • Painful trigeminal neuropathy • Postherpetic neuralgia • Painful post-traumatic trigeminal neuropathy • Trigeminal trophic syndrome • Cluster-tic syndrome • Glossopharyngeal neuralgia • Occipital neuralgia	*Treatment* • Address any underlying cause • Paracetamol, tab, 500 mg, 3 × 2 tabs/d • Ibuprofen 400 mg 2 × 1 tab/d *Or* • Gabapentin (or Pregabalin), tab, 100 mg, 2 × 1 tab/d can be gradually increased up to 3 × 2 tabs/d • TENS: Transcutaneous Electrical Stimulation where available *Etiology* • Nerve injury may induce peripheral and central changes that contribute to persistent pain and dysesthesia • Pathologic mechanisms: inflammation, nociceptor activation, tissue injury, primary afferent fibers and sensitized central structures *Secondary causes* • Cancer pain • Dental pain • Temporomandibular joint syndrome • Giant cell arteritis • Post-traumatic and postoperative pain *Main implicated nerves* • Trigeminal • Nervus intermedius • Glossopharyngeal • Vagus • Upper cervical spinal cord roots via the occipital nerves and great auricular nerve *Clinical features* • May be paroxysmal quality, which is typically maximal at onset and is • Often described as lancinating, electrical shock-like, or jabbing. A single sharp pain or repetitive pains in succession • Pain may be of variable duration: a fraction of a second or endure for several seconds • Some neuralgic conditions have trigger zones (areas that when stimulated provoke an attack) or other triggers
Facial paralysis (FP) *Central* • Stroke • Brain tumor • Multiple sclerosis *Peripheral* • 80% idiopathic • Viral (herpes HIV) • Syphilis • Lyme disease • Posttraumatic, etc.	*Treatment* *Idiopathic facial paresis* • Prednisolone, 5 mg tabs, 10 tabs/morning, 5 d • Omeprazole 10 mg tab, 1 tab/d 7 d *Lyme disease-induced facial paresis* • Doxycycline, 100 mg tabs, 2 × 1 tab/d, 14 d • If Herpes simplex virus (HSV) suspected • Valaciclovir, tab, 500 mg, 2 × 1 tab/d, 5 d *or* • Acyclovir, tab, 200 mg, 4 × 1 tab/d, 7 d *Clinical tips* • Otoscopy is always indicated (might show vesicles in Ramsay Hunt's zone, indicating a herpetic infection) • Protective eyeglasses and eye care are recommended if patient is unable to close eyes • Differentiate central FP from peripheral FP

(continued)

Table 4.1 (continued)

Diagnosis and classification	Treatment and relevant clinical features: neurological conditions
Falls in elderly person A person coming to rest on the ground or another lower level	*Treatment* • Address suspected etiologies • Adapted and tailored physical therapy: muscle strengthening, and proprioception training • Review of medication: omit suspected medication • Assure proper vital signs especially blood pressure, for example, iatrogenic orthostatic hypotension *Etiology* Usually caused by a complex interaction among the following: • Intrinsic factors: age-related decline in function, disorders, and adverse drug effects • Extrinsic factors: environmental hazards, cumbersome furniture, extending carpets, situation in bathrooms • Situational factors: related to the activity being done, for example, rushing to catch a bus or to the rest room *Risk factors* • Muscle weakness, arthritis, balance, and gait problems • Visual impairments • Medication inducing hypotension • Medication-induced sleepiness/dizziness • Environmental hazards • Chronic conditions: Heart disease, brain disease, diabetes, inner ear problems, alcoholism
Fibromyalgia Chronic widespread musculoskeletal pain accompanied by fatigue, psychiatric symptoms (depression, anxiety, cognitive dysfunction, and sleep disturbance) as well as multiple somatic symptoms, including tender points found on physical examination The most common areas of reported pain in patients with this condition are the low back, neck, shoulders, and hips	*Treatment* • Empathic psychological support • Thorough patient education on the notion of pain • Paracetamol, tab, 500 mg, 3 × 2 tab/d as needed • Amitriptyline, tab, 25 mg, 1 tab/in the evening, 1–3 months • TENS: Transcutaneous Electrical Stimulation where available *Clinical manifestations* • Widespread musculoskeletal pain • Fatigue • Cognitive disturbances • Depression and anxiety and sleep disorder • Headache • Paresthesia *FIBROW (useful mnemonic)* • *F*atigue, fog (cognitive disturbance) • *I*nsomnia • *B*lues (depression) • *R*igidity • *O*w! Widespread pain

Table 4.1 (continued)

Diagnosis and classification	Treatment and relevant clinical features: neurological conditions
Gait disorder Abnormal pattern of walking *Common underlying causes* • Vascular disorder: Cerebral ischemia, cerebella hemorrhage • Medications and toxins: Antiepileptic drugs, chemotherapy	*Treatment* • Address underlying cause • Physiotherapy and/or ergotherapy: muscle strengthening, coordination exercises and proprioception training • Supplementation in case of vitamin deficiencies *Etiology* Locomotion/walking involves balance and coordination of muscles so that the body is propelled forward in a rhythm (stride). Common causes of gait imbalance: • A degenerative disease (such as arthritis) • An inner ear disorder • Stroke • Foot conditions • A neurologic condition • Poorly fitting shoes *Classification* • *Propulsive gait*: a stooping, rigid posture, and the head and neck are bent forward. Steps tend to become faster and shorter. For example, Parkinsonism • *Scissors gait*: the knees and thighs hit or cross in a scissors-like pattern when walking. For example, spastic cerebral palsy. • *Spastic gait*: one leg is stiff and drags in a semicircular motion on the side most affected by long-term muscle contraction • *Steppage gait*: a "high stepping" type of gait in which the leg is lifted high, the foot drops (appearing floppy), and the toes points downward, scraping the ground, when walking. Peroneal muscle atrophy or peroneal nerve injury, as with a spinal problem (such as spinal stenosis or herniated disc), can cause this type of gait • *Waddling gait*: movement of the trunk is exaggerated to produce a waddling, duck-like walk. Progressive muscular dystrophy or hip dislocation present from birth can produce a waddling gait
Guillain-Barré syndrome Acute immune-mediated polyneuropathies is a heterogeneous condition with several variant forms, mostly presenting as an acute, monophasic paralyzing illness provoked by a preceding infection	*Treatment* • Address underlying cause • Provide respiratory support: Oxygen • Hydrocortisone ampoule, 100 mg, 3 amps, 1 x/d, iv, for 5 d, to be given in the morning • Omeprazole tab, 20 mg, 1 tab/d, 10 d *Etiology* An immune response to a preceding infection that cross-reacts myelin or the axon of peripheral nerve components as a result of molecular mimicry, resulting in demyelinating and axonal forms Common preceding infections: *campylobacter jejuni*, influenza, HIV

(continued)

Table 4.1 (continued)

Diagnosis and classification	Treatment and relevant clinical features: neurological conditions
Headache Pain in any region of the head, and may occur on one or both sides of the head, be isolated to a certain location, radiate across the head from one point, or have a constricting quality A headache may appear as a sharp pain, a throbbing sensation, or a dull ache. Headaches can develop gradually or suddenly and may last from less than an hour to several days *Classification* Based on history and physical examination, the headache can be classified into one of two groups: primary (~95%) and secondary (~5%) headaches *Primary headache* • Tension headache • Migraine headache • Trigeminal neuralgia • Cluster headache • Other primary headaches *Secondary headache* • Head/neck trauma • Vascular affection • Withdrawal syndrome • Drugs/medication • Infection, for example, meningitis • Homeostasis anomalies • Cranium, neck, ENT, or other facial structural anomalies, for example, temporomandibular joint disorder (TMD), cervical spondylosis, dental diseases, sinusitis • Psychiatric affection • Headache induced by intracranial tension • Hypertension	*Treatment* • Paracetamol, tab, 500 mg, 3 × 2 tab/d, 5 d • Naproxen, tab, 500 mg, 2 × 1 tab/d • Ibuprofen, 400 × mg, 2 × 1 tab/d, 5 d • Diclofenac, tab, 25 mg, 2 × 1 tab/d • Physiotherapy: relaxation methods *Migraine headache* In addition to the above regimen, add: • Domperidone, tab, 10 mg, 3 × 1 tab/d, 5 d • Propranolol, tab, 40 mg, 1 tab/d *or* • Sumatriptan, tab, 50 mg, 1 tab/d (during crises) • TENS: Transcutaneous Electrical Stimulation where available *Etiology* • Dehydration • Emotional and physical exhaustion, hypertension • Trauma • Intracranial lesions • Malaria *Note:* Be on the alert for red flags: SNOOPS (useful mnemonic) • *S*ystemic symptoms • *N*eurologic signs/symptoms • *O*nset: abrupt or explosive • *O*ld age • *P*rior history of *S*econdary illness *Cranial neuropathies and facial pain* • Bell's palsy: Seventh cranial nerve is affected • Microvascular cranial nerve palsy: Go to the eye; common in diabetes and hypertension • Third nerve palsy: Oculo-motricity and regulation of pupilar size • Fourth nerve palsy: Superior oblique palsy • Sixth nerve palsy: VI or abducens palsy *Migraine headache* Diagnostic features • Usually pulsatile, lasting 4–72 h • Pain is typically but not always unilateral • Nausea, vomiting, photophobia, and phonophobia are common accompaniments • Pain is aggravated with routine physical activity • An aura of transient neurologic symptoms, commonly visual, may precede the head pain • Head pain may occur with no aura • Depression *Clinical tips* • Good history taking and physical examination is indicated to ensure an etiologic approach to treatment • Always assess neurological status

Table 4.1 (continued)

Diagnosis and classification	Treatment and relevant clinical features: neurological conditions
Hiccup Involuntary contractions of the diaphragm followed by a sudden closure of vocal cords, which produces the characteristic "hic" sound	*Treatment* • Treat underlying cause • Patient education • Diazepam, tabs, 5 mg, max 2× d *Etiology* • Large meal • Alcoholic • Carbonated beverages • Sudden excitement • Sign of an underlying medical condition, such as irritation of the vagus nerves or phrenic nerves, which serve the diaphragm muscle; for example, eardrum inflammation, tumor, cyst, or goiter in the neck, gastroesophageal reflux, sore throat, or laryngitis • Central nervous pathologies: encephalitis, meningitis, multiple sclerosis, stroke, traumatic brain injury, tumors *Clinical tips* • Differentiate neurological hiccups from nonneurological hiccups: associated with other neurological signs vs. isolated
Intracranial abscess Focal collection within the brain parenchyma, which can arise as a complication of a variety of infections, trauma, or surgery	*Treatment* • Combination of antibiotics and surgical drainage for both diagnostic and therapeutic purposes • Penicillin G, ampoule, 1 MU, 3 × 2 amp iv/d *or* • Ceftriaxone, ampoule, 2 g, 2 × 1 amp iv/d, 5 d *and* • Metronidazole iv bags for infusion, 500 mg, 3 × 1 bag iv daily *and* • Dexamethasone ampoule, 2 mg, 2 amp/d, iv *Poor prognostic factors* for recovery from a brain abscess include: • Rapid progression of the infection before hospitalization • Severe mental status changes on admission • Stupor or coma (60–100% mortality) • Rupture into the ventricle (80–100% mortality)
Intracranial aneurysm Localized dilation of any of the cerebral arteries *Good to know* • Most subarachnoid hemorrhages are caused by ruptured intracranial saccular aneurysms • Twenty percent of strokes are hemorrhagic	*Treatment* • Intracranial aneurysms are mostly incidental finding on brain imaging • Reassure patient • Ensure normal blood pressure • Regular brain imaging (1×/year) to monitor size • Address to tertiary center for appropriate care *Clinical presentation* • Asymptomatic • Sudden severe headache • Loss of consciousness • Nausea and vomiting • Meningism • Photophobia

(continued)

Table 4.1 (continued)

Diagnosis and classification	Treatment and relevant clinical features: neurological conditions
Meningitis (bacterial) Infection of the meningeal structures lining the cranium and spinal cord *Differential diagnosis* • Cerebral malaria • Extrapyramidal syndrome (drug-induced, e.g., metoclopramide) • Encephalitis • Septicemia • Febrile convulsions • Intracranial hemorrhage in neonates	*Treatment* • Ceftriaxone, ampoule, 2.0 g, 1 amp/d, 3 d *or* • Penicillin G ampoule, 1.0 M, 1 amp 4×/d • Followed by oral treatment • Pen G, tab, 500 mg, 3 × 1 tab/d, 7 d *or* • Cephalexin, tab, 500 mg, 3 × 1 tab/d 7 d • Adequate fluid and calorie maintenance • Optimal care of unconscious patient • Appropriate posture to avoid aspiration pneumonia • Nasogastric (NG) tube feeding • Frequent turning to avoid bedsores *Clinical tips* • Oral intake is contraindicated in unconscious patients • Isolation: meningococcal meningitis is highly contagious • Concomitant empirical treatment of severe malaria is recommended • Prevention: vaccination of people exposed • Corticoid before or at the same time as the antibiotic • Immunoglobulin G (IgG) ampoules not readily available in most minimal-resource facilities
Multiple sclerosis (MS) Immune-mediated inflammatory demyelinating disease of the central nervous system *Classification* • Relapsing-remitting MS • Relapsing and progressive MS • Secondary progressive MS • Primary progressive MS	*Treatment* • Adapted physiotherapy • Psychological support • Refer to appropriate facility for tertiary care • During a typical relapse: Hydrocortisone ampoule, 100 mg, 3 amps 1×/d (to be diluted in 500 ml 9% NaCl) 3 d *Diagnostic features* • Episodic neurologic symptoms • Patients usually under 50 years of age at onset • Single pathologic lesion cannot explain clinical findings • Multiple pathologic foci best visualized by MRI of the brain *Signs and symptoms* • Abnormal neurologic signs without disability • Ataxia: truncal or limb ataxia • Loss of coordination • Moderate nystagmus or other mild disability nystagmus, marked extraocular weakness • Marked dysarthria • Inability to swallow • Loss of bowel and bladder function, incontinence • Loss of visual acuity, optic neuritis *Clinical findings* • Weakness • Numbness, tingling, or unsteadiness in the limb • Spastic paraparesis • Retrobulbar optic neuritis • Diplopia • Disequilibrium • Sphincter disturbance; for example, urinary urgency, or hesitancy *Good to know*: There has been a long history of controversy pertaining to vaccinations causing MS. It is now an established scientific fact that vaccines do not cause MS. In fact, certain vaccines (e.g., Hepatitis B) may have protective effective on the onset of MS

Table 4.1 (continued)

Diagnosis and classification	Treatment and relevant clinical features: neurological conditions
Neurocutaneous diseases A multiorgan disorder inherited as an autosomal dominant trait. It is characterized by dyspigmented brown spots on the skin, and deformities of subcutaneous tissue and bone *Neurofibromatosis* • Type 1 is Recklinghausen disease; multiple hyperpigmented macules, Lisch nodules, neurofibroma • Type 2; bilateral VIII cranial nerve tumor often accompanied by other intracranial or intraspinal tumors	*Treatment* • Patient education about nature and prognosis of condition • Control pain • Surgical excision of nodules only when causing significant compression effects *Pathogenesis* The nervous system develops from the epithelial layer of the embryo, as a result of this common origin, a number of congenital diseases include both neurologic and cutaneous manifestations *Signs and symptoms* • Documented nodules • Mobile nodules over cutaneous nerves • May overgrow subcutaneous tissue
Neurologic manifestations of systemic diseases Involvement of the nervous system is frequently observed in patients across a vast number of systemic diseases *Classification* • Encephalopathies • Cranial nerve palsy • Retinopathy • Inflammatory myopathy • Oculopathy	*Treatment* • Identify and treat the etiology *Etiology* • Hypertension • Diabetes • Vasculitis • Disseminated lupus erythematosus • Assess and evaluate condition individually
Parkinsonism: Parkinson's disease Movement disorder resulting from degeneration and malfunction of the central nervous system common in old age	*Treatment* • Madopar 120 mg, tab, 3 × 1 tab/d *Diagnostic features* • Any combination of tremor, rigidity, bradykinesia, and progressive postural instability (Parkinsonism) • Cognitive impairment is sometimes prominent

(continued)

Table 4.1 (continued)

Diagnosis and classification	Treatment and relevant clinical features: neurological conditions
Peripheral neurologic disorder peripheral nervous system refers to parts of the nervous system outside the brain and spinal cord. It includes the cranial nerves and spinal nerves from their origin to their end *Classification* • Mononeuropathy: one nerve • Multiple mononeuropathy, or mononeuritis multiplex: several discrete nerves • Polyneuropathy: multiple nerves diffusely • Plexopathy: a plexus, for example, brachial plexus • Radiculopathy: nerve root	*Treatment* • Treat underlying cause • Supportive: physiotherapy, ergotherapy • Pain control *Etiology* A result of damage to the nerves outside of the brain and spinal cord (peripheral nerves) causing weakness, numbness and pain, usually in hands and feet or other areas • Medical conditions: tumors, diabetes, bone marrow disorders, nephropathies, hepatopathies • Traumatic injuries • Infections • Metabolic problems, for example, diabetes • Inherited causes • Exposure to toxins • Medication • Vitamin deficiencies (B vitamins) • Substance abuse: For example, alcohol *Characteristics of pain* • Stabbing • Burning • Tingling *Classification of peripheral nerves* • Sensory nerves: temperature, pain, vibration or touch, from the skin • Motor nerves: control muscle movement • Autonomic nerves: control functions such as blood pressure, heart rate, digestion, and bladder *Clinical signs and symptoms* • Gradual onset of numbness, prickling or tingling in feet or hands, which can spread upward into legs and arms (hands and feet paresthesia) • Sharp, jabbing, throbbing, or burning pain • Extreme sensitivity to touch • Pain during activities that should not cause pain • Lack of coordination and falling • Muscle weakness • Feeling as if wearing gloves or socks • Paralysis if motor nerves are affected • Autonomic nerves are affected: heat intolerance excessive sweating or not being able to sweat, bowel, bladder or digestive problems, fluctuations in in blood pressure causing dizziness or light-headedness

Table 4.1 (continued)

Diagnosis and classification	Treatment and relevant clinical features: neurological conditions
Polyneuropathy A specific term that refers to a generalized, homogeneous process affecting peripheral nerves, with the distal nerves usually affected most prominently	*Treatment of the underlying process* • Reducing exposure to endogenous or exogenous toxins • Gabapentin (Neurontin) 300 mg tabs, 2 × 1 tab/d • Tramadol tab, 100 mg, 2 × 1 tab/d as needed • Duloxetine (Cymbalta) tab, 30 mg, 2 × 1 tabs/d • Carbamazepine (Tegretol), tabs, 100 mg, 2 × 1 tab/d • Phenytoin tabs, 100 mg, 2 × 1 tab/d
Classification *Peripheral neuropathy* refers to any disorder of the peripheral nervous system, including radiculopathies and mononeuropathies *Neuropathy* refers even more generally to disorders of the central and peripheral nervous system *Pathophysiologic classification* Axonal versus demyelinating	*Clinical presentation* Symmetric distal sensory loss, burning sensations, or weakness, for example, Guillain Barré syndrome or GBS (demyelinating) *Etiology and pathogenesis* • Diabetic • Longstanding human immunodeficiency virus (HIV) infection • Vasculitic neuropathy • Critical illness • Amyloidosis • Hypothyroidism • Vitamin deficiencies • Lyme disease • Autoimmune • Toxic • Hereditary • Environmental • Idiopathic
Stupor and coma Clinical states in which patients have impaired responsiveness (or are unresponsive) to external stimulation and are either difficult to arouse or are unarousable *Coma* is *defined* as "unarousable unresponsiveness"	*Treatment* • Apply life support principles: ABCDE (Airway, Breathing, Circulation, Dolor-pain, Environment) • Identify and treat underlying cause • Maintain lateral decubitus position to avoid broncho-aspiration • Provide information to patient and family *Diagnostic features* • Level of consciousness is depressed • Stuporous patients respond only to vigorous stimuli • Comatose patients are unarousable and unresponsive
Transient ischemic attack A transient episode of neurologic dysfunction caused by focal brain, spinal cord, or retinal ischemia, without acute infarction *Differential diagnosis* • Seizures • Migraine with aura • Syncope • Transient global amnesia • Hypoglycemia • Multiple sclerosis • Brain tumors • Subdural hematomas • Hepatic, renal, and pulmonary encephalopathies • Peripheral vestibulopathies • Hysteria	*Treatment* • Comprehensive assessment • Address underlying etiology • Address to appropriate facility for tertiary care • Advice on appropriate lifestyle modification: regular physical exercise, for example, walk 1 h/d, low-fat diet, body weight reduction and/or stabilization *Diagnostic features* • Focal neurologic deficit of acute onset • Clinical deficit resolves completely within 24 h • Risk factors for vascular disease are often present • Pathophysiology • Decreased blood flow to a local portion of the brain, due to blockage of blood flow to a brain region from an in situ occlusion of a supply artery, or from embolism to that artery The neurologic signs and symptoms are *focal* and *transient*

(continued)

Table 4.1 (continued)

Diagnosis and classification	Treatment and relevant clinical features: neurological conditions
Traumatic spinal cord injury Spinal cord injuries may result from damage to the vertebrae, ligaments or disks of the spinal column or to the spinal cord itself. A traumatic spinal cord injury may stem from a sudden, traumatic blow to the spine that fractures, dislocates, crushes or compresses one or more of the structures named *Diagnostic features* • History of preceding trauma • Development of acute neurologic deficits	*Treatment* • Provide essential first aid by applying life support principles: ABCDE (Airway, Breathing, Circulation, Dolor-pain, Environment) • Safeguard posture using appropriate immobilization techniques • Refer promptly to tertiary center *Advanced trauma life support (ATLS) management (ABCDE mnemonic):* • *A*irway management: rigid collar to immobilize neck, en bloc mobilization • *B*reathing and ventilation: malperfusion can lead to multiple organ failure; fluid resuscitation (nor)epinephrine, atropine • *C*irculation and hemorrhage control, neurogenic shock • *D*isability, neurologic deficit: motor and sensory functions • *E*xposure and environmental control *Etiology* • Motor vehicle accidents • Falls at workplace and home and from trees • Violence, fights, and use of weapons • Sports accidents *Clinical presentation* • Complete cord injury • Incomplete injury • Central cord syndrome • Anterior cord syndrome • Transient paralysis and spinal shock *Pathophysiology* • Fracture of one or more of the bony elements • Dislocation at one or more joints • Tearing of ligament(s) • Disruption and/or herniation of the intervertebral disc *Complications* • Varying impaired sensory and motor functions • Sphincter dysfunction (urine and feces) • Priapism • Decubitus ulcers • Thromboembolism • Reactional mood disorder impact

Table 4.1 (continued)

Diagnosis and classification	Treatment and relevant clinical features: neurological conditions
Vestibular dysfunction (vertigo) Symptom of illusory movement. Vertigo is a symptom, not a diagnosis *Benign paroxysmal positional vertigo (BPPV)* A common form of vertigo, accounting for nearly one half of patients with peripheral vestibular dysfunction. It is most commonly attributed to calcium debris within the posterior semi-circular canal, known as canalithiasis	*Treatment* • Dix-Hallpike maneuver • Head impulse test • Vestibular rehabilitation • Betahistine, tab, 24 mg, 2 × 1, tab, daily, 5 d *Pathophysiology* It arises because of asymmetry in the vestibular system due to damage to or dysfunction of the labyrinth, vestibular nerve, or central vestibular structures in the brainstem *Clinical features* • Vertigo • Nausea and vomiting • Postural and gait instability • Tilt illusion • Drop attacks • Spatial disorientation *Evaluation* • History (time course aggravating and provoking factors) • Metabolic panel • Brain imaging when clinically indicated (red flags) • Otoscopy • Cranial nerve (CN) examination *Red flags* • Age • Consciousness alteration • Focal neurological signs • Headache • Medical history • Multidirectional or vertical nystagmus

Contents

5.1   History: Questions to Ask 43

5.2   Physical Examination 44

5.3   Cardinal Paramedical Ear, Nose, and Throat Examinations 44

5.4   Ear, Nose, and Throat Red Flags 44

ENT, also known as oto-rhino-laryngology, is a medical specialty that deals principally with diseases affecting the ear, nose, and throat (Fig. 5.1 and Table 5.1).

Within the structures of the ear, nose, and throat (ENT) are complex and interrelated mechanisms that allow a person to produce sound, hear, maintain balance, smell, breathe, and swallow.

When diagnosing and treating ear, nose, and throat disorders, it is important to differentiate genetic disorders from those due to environmental influences. This is challenging because similar clinical features may be produced by different environmental factors or by different genetic influences.

Specific ENT conditions comprise pathologies of the upper respiration system, the oropharyngeal cavity, the lobe of the ear, the auditive canal, and the middle and inner ear. These afflictions are mostly infectious. Infectious conditions may be predilected by underlying congenital defects, poor personal hygiene, and dietary deficiency conditions. Iron, folic acid, and vitamin D deficiencies are endemic. Good history taking and a thorough physical examination are mandatory and revealing.

5.1   History: Questions to Ask

- Do you have pain when swallowing fluid or liquid?
- Have you or your relatives noticed a change in your voice?
- Does your nose run? Do your nose/eyes itch? Do you sneeze? Do you experience nasal obstruction?
- Have you noticed a change in your sense of smell? Hyposmia? Anosmia? Cacosmia?
- Do you have headaches or facial pain?
- Do you cough? Dry? Productive? Bloody?
- Does your ear hurt? Does it ring?
- Do you experience vertigo?

43
M. Touray, A. Touray, *Clinical Work and General Management of a Standard Minimal-Resource Facility*, Sustainable Development Goals Series, https://doi.org/10.1007/978-3-030-71032-3_5

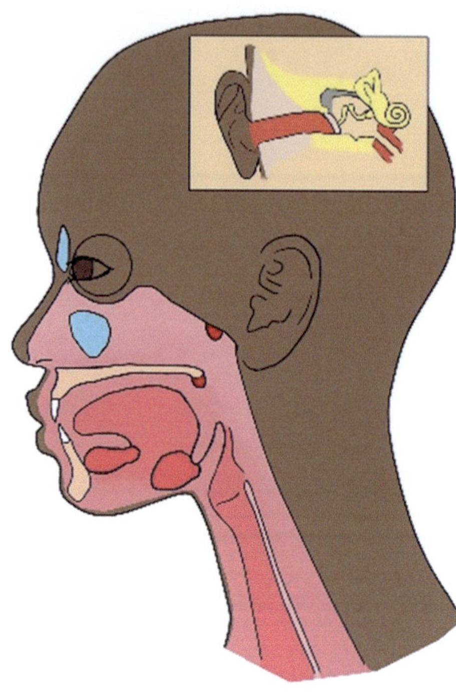

Ear Nose Throat

List of ENT disorders that are described in the text.
For easy reference, the corresponding page on which the
disease condition is described is in brackets.

Acute dental abscess (p45)
Acute rhinitis/sinusitis (p46)
Acute sinusitis (p46)
Acute tonsillitis (p47)
Adenopathy (p47)
Allergic rhinitis (p47)
Chronic sinusitis (p48)
Dental caries (p49)
Dysphonia (p49)
Epistaxis (p49)
External otitis (p49)
Gingivitis (p50)
Hearing loss (p45)
Malocclusion (p50)
Otitis media (p50)
Periodontal abscess (p51)
Pharyngitis/tonsillitis (p51)
Poor oral hygiene (p51)
Pulpitis (p51)
Retropharyngeal abscess (p53)
Stridor (p53)
Temporomandibular joint disorders (p48)
Traumatic spinal cord injury (p40)
Vertigo (p54)
Vestibular dysfunction (p41, p54)

Fig. 5.1 ENT: A mnemonic illustration representing main ENT anatomic structures and their corresponding pathologies

- Do you have secretions from your ear, for example, on your pillow?
- Do you hear properly?

5.2   Physical Examination

- Appreciate quality of voice.
- Palpate neck for adenopathy.
- Look at the tongue and throat.
- Test swallowing and cough.
- Test hearing by whispering words in the ear and asking them to repeat them, at the left and then right ear, one at a time.
- Look in the ear with the naked eye or with an otoscope.
- Palpate the periauricular region and the sinuses.

5.3   Cardinal Paramedical Ear, Nose, and Throat Examinations

- Full blood count
- Chest X-ray

5.4   Ear, Nose, and Throat Red Flags

- Voluminous tumefied and erythematous tonsil
- Progressive odynodysphagia
- Dysphonia: accompanied by other symptoms, fluctuating, high - or low-pitched, hoarse, socially inconvenient
- Chronic cervical adenopathy
- Disfiguring maxillofacial trauma, malocclusion

Table 5.1 Ear, nose, and throat (ENT) and stomatology conditions and their treatment

Diagnosis and classification	Treatment and relevant clinical features: ear, nose, and throat (ENT) conditions
Acute dental abscess Mixed bacterial infection of periapical teeth region mainly by *Staphylococcus* spp.	*Treatment* • In the absence of systemic signs and symptoms, antimicrobial therapy is usually not indicated • Drainage and relief of the tooth out of occlusion • Consider extraction of infected tooth • Endodontic therapy (root canal treatment) of affected tooth If associated systemic signs and symptoms are present, consider adjunct antibiotherapy • Amoxicillin, tab, 500 mg, 3 × 1 tab/d, 3 d, *and* • Metronidazole, tab, 500 mg, 3 × 1 tab/d, 3 d *Prevention* • Prevention and early management of dental caries • Dietary advice: Advise patient to avoid sugary foods and soft drinks and have adequate fresh fruit and vegetables in their diet • Oral hygiene instructions • Patient should regularly brush their teeth after meals *Signs and symptoms* • Severe pain that disturbs sleep • Facial swelling may be localized or extending to adjacent tissues • Abscesses of the mandibular incisors or molars may discharge extra orally • Affected tooth is mobile and tender to percussion • Fever and headache may be present
Hearing loss Commonly experienced by everyone from time to time *Classification* • Sensorineural: inner ear, cochlea, or the auditory nerve • Conductive: limits the amount of external sound from gaining access to the inner ear, for example, cerumen impaction, middle ear fluid, or ossicular chain fixation • Mixed loss: combination of conductive and sensorineural hearing loss *Acute hearing loss* is an acute sensorineural hearing loss, mostly unilateral, occurring within a 72-hour period often idiopathic. The prognosis for hearing recovery depends largely upon the severity of the hearing loss	*Treatment* • Identify underlying cause • Ear rinsing if cerumen impaction and inspect the external auditory canal by otoscopy • Refer to appropriate tertiary center if needed for audiometry and further work-up for hearing aid *Clinical features* • Gradual or immediate or rapid hearing loss, • Sensation of a blocked ear or aural *Etiology* • Congenital: microtia, atresia of external auditory canal, • Infection: AOM (Acute Otitis Media) meningitis • Trauma: tympanic membrane perforation, barotrauma • Tumor: Squamous cell carcinoma, exostosis, osteomas, eighth nerve Neuroma, polyps, cholestomas, osteosclerosis • Cerumen • Eustachian tube dysfunction • Presbycusis • Meniere disease • Noise exposure • Endocrine, systemic, or metabolic diseases • Autoimmune • Iatrogenic • Ototoxic substances: heavy metals, antibiotics (gentamycin and neomycin), antimalarial (quinine) *Clinical evaluation* • Whispering: Office hearing evaluation • Weber and Rinne tests • Formal audiologic assessment: speech and impedance audiometry

(continued)

Table 5.1 (continued)

Diagnosis and classification	Treatment and relevant clinical features: ear, nose, and throat (ENT) conditions
Acute rhinitis/sinusitis Rhinitis and rhinosinusitis refer to inflammation in the nasal cavity and paranasal sinuses. Acute rhinosinusitis lasts less than 4 weeks *Classification* • Allergic • Infectious (viral and/or bacterial) • Irritative	*Treatment* • Nasal rinsing with 0.9% NaCl solution • Oral antihistamine: Chlorphenamine (Piriton), tabs, 25 mg 2 × 1 tab/d, 5 d, *or* Cetirizine tab, 10 mg 1 × 1 tab/d, 5 d • Paracetamol, tab, 500 mg, 3 × 2 tab/d 5 d *and* • Ibuprofen, tab, 400 mg, 2 × 1 tab/d 5 d for the pain and fever When bacterial infection is suspected:Amoxicillin, tab, 500 mg, 3 × 1 tab/d, 5 d *Complications* • Pre-septal cellulitis • Orbital cellulitis • Subperiosteal abscess • Intracranial abscess • Meningitis • Septic cavernous sinus thrombosis • Osteomyelitis *Clinical tips* • Avoid allergen where possible • Maintain good nasal hygiene *Signs and symptoms* • Nasal congestion and obstruction • Purulent nasal discharge • Maxillary tooth discomfort • Facial pain or pressure that is worse or localized to the sinuses when bending forward • Fever, fatigue, cough • Hyposmia or anosmia • Ear pressure or fullness, headache • Halitosis • Eustachian tube dysfunction (e.g., ear pain, fullness, or pressure, hearing loss, or tinnitus)
Acute sinusitis Infection of the air spaces in the bones of the head which are connected to the nose, so that infections in the nose, for example, colds, catarrh, can spread to these spaces *Etiology* • Acute infective rhinitis (common cold) • Dental infection or dental extraction • Fractures involving the sinuses	*Treatment* • Nasal rinsing with 0.9% NaCl solution • Paracetamol, tab, 500 mg, 3 × 2 tab/d, 5 d • Oral antihistamine: Hydro chlorphenamine (Piriton), tab, 25 mg, 1 tab/d, 5 d *or* Cetirizine, tab, 10 mg, 1 tab/d, 5 d Where antibiotherapy is indicated: • Amoxicillin, tab, 500 mg, 3 × 1 tab/d, 5 d *Indication for oral antibiotic* • Persisting sinusitis (>10 d) • Signs of bacterial infection (purulence, bloody rhinorrhea, green expectorations) • Biphasic evolution (symptom aggravation after 5–6 d) • Fever and other symptoms >3 d • Dental or jaw pain *Management tips* • Teach patient how to make saline water at home: 1 tsp full of cooking salt in a mug full of clean water. This is normally about 200 ml • Teach how to rinse nose regularly (4× daily) during the acute phase

Table 5.1 (continued)

Diagnosis and classification	Treatment and relevant clinical features: ear, nose, and throat (ENT) conditions
Acute tonsillitis Symptomatic infection of the tonsils and peritonsillar tissues. Infection is mostly viral, but suppuration may be by Group A *streptococcus* *Nomenclature* • Tonsillopharyngitis caused by Group A *Streptococcus*, or *Streptococcus pyogenes* • Suppurative tonsillitis • Tonsillar abscess • Peritonsillar cellulitis	*Treatment* • Penicillin, tab, 1.2 million units, 3 × 1 tab/d, 7 d *or* • Amoxicillin, tab, 500 mg, 3 × 1 tab/d, 5 d *or* • Cephalexin, tab, 500 mg, 3 × 1 tab/d, 5 d *or* • Erythromycin, tab, 500 mg, 4 × 1 tab/d, 5 d When judged necessary: • Paracetamol, tab, 500 mg, 3 × 2 tab/d, 5 d *and/or* • Ibuprofen, tab, 400 mg, 3 × 1 tab/d, 5 d *Clinical tips* • Mononucleosis: caution against physical activity such as boxing, due to risk of spleen rupture • When strepto-test is positive, institute antibiotherapy promptly to avoid rheumatic fever • Strepto-test if available
Adenopathy Any disease or inflammation that involves glandular tissue or lymph nodes. The term is usually used to refer to lymphadenopathy or swollen lymph nodes. Adenopathy: lymph node >1.5–2 cm *Nomenclature of lymph nodes of the head and neck* • Posterior auricular • Occipital • Superficial cervical • Deep cervical • Posterior cervical • Supraclavicular • Preauricular • Parotid • Tonsillar • Submental • Submandibular	*Management tips* • Differentiate benign from malignant • Reassure the patient • Follow-up at one month to see evolution when no etiology found • Ultrasonographic characterization and biopsy when needed *Etiology* • Inflammatory-infectious: TB, animal bites, infected ulcers • Neoplastic: lymphomas, breast cancer, metastasis • For generalized adenopathy, think of systemic disease such as HIV *Clinical signs* • Tenderness or pain when touched • Redness and warmth on the skin over and around them • Visible lumps under the skin *Features suggestive of infectious etiology (benign):* • Fever • Chills • Fatigue • Runny nose • Sore throat • Earache • Headache *Red flags* • Rapidly growing nodes • Nodes that remain swollen for more than 2 weeks • Unexplained weight loss • Long-lasting fevers or night sweats • Easy bleeding or bruising • Stiff nodes that do not move when pushed
Allergic rhinitis Intermittent sneezing, rhinorrhea, and nasal obstruction, itching of the eyes, nose, and palate	*Treatment* • Eviction of the allergen • Cetirizine, tab, 10 mg, 1 tab/d during crises *or* • Loratadine, tab, 10 mg, 1 tab/d, during crises *Associated conditions* • Allergic conjunctivitis • Sinusitis • Asthma • Atopic dermatitis (eczema) • Oral allergy syndrome • Eustachian tube dysfunction • Anosmia

(continued)

Table 5.1 (continued)

Diagnosis and classification	Treatment and relevant clinical features: ear, nose, and throat (ENT) conditions
	Risk factors • Family history of atopy (i.e., the genetic predisposition to develop allergic diseases) • Male sex • Birth during the pollen season • Firstborn status • Early use of antibiotics • Maternal smoking exposure in the first year of life • Exposure to indoor allergens, such as dust mite allergen • Serum immunoglobulin E (IgE) >100 U/ml • Presence of allergen-specific IgE *Clinical features* • Clear rhinorrhea, sneezing, tearing, and itching • Postnasal drip • Cough, bronchospasm, eczematous dermatitis • Irritability • Fatigue • History of environmental allergen exposure
Temporomandibular joint disorders Abnormal structural, biologic, behavioral, environmental, and cognitive factors leading to symptoms related to temporomandibular joint	*Treatment* • Paracetamol, tab, 500 mg, 3 × 2 tab/d, 5 d *and/or* • Naproxen, tab, 500 mg, 3 × 1 tab/d, 5 d • Advice to eat soft food *Etiology* • Joint trauma • Behavioral factors • Head and cervical posture *Clinical manifestation* • Pain • Ear discomfort or dysfunction • Headache • Temporomandibular joint discomfort or dysfunction
Chronic sinusitis A complex inflammatory-infectious condition involving the paranasal sinuses and linings of the nasal passages that lasts 12 weeks or longer, despite attempts at medical management	*Treatment* • If >3 weeks • Same as acute sinusitis • Nasal rinsing • Mometasone, spray, 4× daily • Co-amoxicillin, tab, 1 g, 2 × 1 tab/d, 5 d *Etiology* • Exposure to allergens and irritants • Defects in muco-ciliary function • Immunodeficiency • Infections with bacteria, viruses, and fungus *Clinical tips* Efforts should be made to identify any underlying causes: • Allergy • Polyps • Asthma • Pneumonia • Malformations • Immunologic deficiency • Poor ENT hygiene

Table 5.1 (continued)

Diagnosis and classification	Treatment and relevant clinical features: ear, nose, and throat (ENT) conditions
Dental caries A sugar-dependent infectious disease resulting in cavities or holes in the teeth	*Treatment* • Paracetamol, tab, 500 mg, 3 × 2, tab, as needed *Dietary advice* • Advise patient to avoid sugary foods and soft drinks and include adequate fresh fruit and vegetables in their diet • Reduction in the availability of a microbial substrate by regular brushing, preferably after every meal • Tooth strengthening and protection of teeth through use of fluoride. Rinse and apply sealants to susceptible sites *Signs and symptoms* • Localized toothache • Cavitation in the teeth • Tooth sensitivity to hot and cold stimuli • Susceptible sites are those areas where plaque accumulation can occur unhindered, for example, pits and fissures of the posterior teeth, interproximal surfaces, and teeth in malocclusion *Pathogenesis* Poor oral hygiene results in accumulation of bacteria in a plaque on the tooth surface. Acid is produced as a by-product of the metabolism of dietary carbohydrate by the plaque bacteria, causing demineralization of the tooth surface. The weakened tooth structure disintegrates, resulting in a cavity in the tooth
Dysphonia Vocal disorder perceived by patients or their relatives	*Treatment* • Treat underlying cause • Logopedics where needed *Laryngeal symptoms* • Functional (~70%) • Neurologic (neurodegenerative diseases, paralysis, stroke, trauma) • Organic
Epistaxis Bleeding from a unilateral anterior nasal cavity Posterior cavity or bilateral. Large-volume epistaxis needs specialized care	*Treatment* • Treat underlying cause • Compression of the nasal alae together to apply pressure to the Kiesselbach plexus • Nasal packing with clean cotton wool *Predisposing factors* • Nose picking • Foreign bodies • Forceful nose blowing • Rhinitis • Nasal mucosal drying form, from low humidity or supplemental nasal oxygen • Deviation of nasal septum • Hereditary hemorrhagic telangiectasia (Osler-Weber-Rendu Syndrome) • Poorly controlled hypertension
External otitis Inflammation of the external auditory canal. Infectious, allergic, and dermatologic disease may all lead to external otitis	*Treatment* • Treat/remove precipitating factor: diabetes, dermatitis, trauma • Ciproxin, tab, 500 mg, 2 × 1 tab/d, 5 d • Paracetamol, tab, 500 mg, 3 × 2, tab, daily *and/or* • Ibuprofen, tab, 400 mg 3 × 1 tab/d, 5 d *Risk factors* • Swimming or other water exposure • Any trauma, for example, from excessive cleaning or aggressive scratching of the ear canal • Devices that occlude the ear canal such as hearing aids, earphones • Allergic contact dermatitis • Psoriasis, atopic dermatitis *Management tips* • Educate about ear hygiene • Stop poking sticks and cotton wool in the ear • Discourage the use of loud music and especially earphones on high volume

Table 5.1 (continued)

Diagnosis and classification	Treatment and relevant clinical features: ear, nose, and throat (ENT) conditions
Gingivitis Inflammatory process characterized by gingival redness, swelling, and bleeding provoked by a periodontal probe, brushing, or flossing *Classification* • Acute necrotizing • Ulcerative gingivitis • Chronic gingivitis	*Treatment* • Proper oral hygiene • Exclude deficiencies (iron) • Paracetamol, tab, 500 mg, 3 × 2 tab/d, as required • Refer to specialized dental care • Teach good oral hygiene • Exclude iron deficiency *Management tips* • Advice on good oral hygiene • Well-balanced diet: 5 fruits per day, adequate carbohydrate and protein intake • Smoking is a precipitating factor (periodontitis)
Malocclusion Failure of proper closure of the mouth resulting in irregular contact of opposing teeth in the upper and lower jaws	*Treatment* • Attempt gentle manual reduction 30 min after administration of Diazepam, tab, 10 mg • Refer for specialized dental care *Clinical features* • Could be acute or chronic • May result from luxation or subluxation of the temporomandibular joint
Otitis media Infection of the middle ear, which communicates with the throat. Bacterial infection of the mucosal lined air-containing spaces of the temporal bone *Chronic otitis media* Chronic infection of the middle ear with perforation of the tympanic membrane (TM) and pus discharging from the ear for more than 2 weeks • Chronic otorrhea with or without otalgia • Tympanic membrane perforation with conductive hearing loss • Surgical attention is often needed	*Treatment* • Amoxicillin, tab, 500 mg, 3 × 1 tab/d, 5 d • Paracetamol, tab, 500 mg, 3 × 2 tab/d, 5 d *and/or* • Ibuprofen, tab, 400 mg, 2 × 1 tab/d, 5 d *Indications for systemic antibiotics* • Acute otitis media (AOM) lasting 4 d • Signs of systemic involvement • Risk of cardiac and other end-organ complications • Immunosuppression • Bilateral AOM • Presence of otorrhea • Topical antibiotics not effective *Complications* • Mastoiditis • Meningitis • Labyrinthitis • Thrombosis of cavernous sinus • Facial paralysis, etc. • Choleostoma *Management tips* Self-limiting and thus a decreased threshold for antibiotic prescription *Signs and symptoms* • Fever • Sudden and persistent earache • Purulent discharge from the ear • Vomiting • Crying and agitation • Impaired hearing • Red eardrum • Pain on touching the ear • Associated inflamed throat • Perforated eardrum • Otalgia • Often upper respiratory tract infection • Erythema and reduced mobility of the tympanic membranes

Table 5.1 (continued)

Diagnosis and classification	Treatment and relevant clinical features: ear, nose, and throat (ENT) conditions
Periodontal abscess Collection of pus within a periodontal pocket	*Treatment* • *Adult:* Amoxicillin tab, 500 mg, 3 × 1 tab/d, 5 d • *Child:* 10–20 mg/kg per dose, 3×/d for 5 d • Teach good oral hygiene: brush at least 3×/d with fluoride-containing tooth paste, rinse mouth with clean water after each meal
Pharyngitis/tonsillitis Infection of the throat and tonsils by virus, bacteria, or fungus	*Treatment* • Amoxicillin, tab, 500 mg, 3 × 1 tab/d, 5 d • If patient is allergic to penicillin, use • Erythromycin, 500 mg tabs, 4 × 1 tab/d, 5 d *and* • Paracetamol, tab, 500 mg, 3 × 2 tab/d, 5 d, *and/or* • Ibuprofen, tab, 400 mg, 2 × 1 tab/d, 5 d *or* • Naproxen, tab, 500 mg, 2 × 1 tab/d, 5 d • Encourage high fluid intake *Signs suggestive of streptococcal pharyngitis:* • Painful enlarged tonsillar lymph glands • Absence of signs suggesting viral nasopharyngitis (running nose, cough, red eyes) • Whitish exudate at the back of the throat as well as whitish tonsillar exudate • Sustained high-grade fever • Occasionally, the rash of scarlet fever • Menthol-containing bonbons may comfort the pharyngeal pain *Signs and symptoms* • Fever • Dysphagia • Rhinorrhea • Posterior dripping • Reddened throat • Enlarged and reddened tonsils • Palpable tonsillar lymph glands (at the angle of the mandible)
Poor oral hygiene Improper oral condition due to lack of regular and proper cleaning of the oral cavity and the teeth	*Treatment* • Brush teeth ideally 3× daily in a circular motion, preferably after food intake, with toothpaste containing fluoride • Check-up at the dentist's 1× every 2 years *Clinical presentation* • Bad malodorous breath • Gingival bleeding • Caries • Discolored teeth *Management tips* Remind patients that it makes more sense to brush teeth after eating and not only before eating: interesting cultural issue
Pulpitis Inflammation of the pulp of a tooth	*Treatment* • Paracetamol, tab, 500 mg, 3 × 2 tab/d as required • Teach appropriate teeth brushing technics • Assure that there is no iron deficiency *Dietary advice* Advise patient to avoid sugary foods and soft drinks and have adequate fresh fruit and vegetables in their diet Refer to dentist for pulpotomy, endodontic (root canal) treatment, or extraction *Management tips* Prevention and early management of dental caries *Oral hygiene instructions* The patient should regularly brush their teeth after meals

(continued)

Table 5.1 (continued)

Diagnosis and classification	Treatment and relevant clinical features: ear, nose, and throat (ENT) conditions
Deep neck infections Polymicrobial infection of cervical compartments and interfacial spaces Infection often originate from the normal resident flora of the oral cavity. The cervical facia is the structure that envelops muscles, vessels, and visceral structures of the neck. There is a superficial and a deep component. Ideal spaces for pus collection, abscess formation *Red flags* • Trismus: the inability to open the jaw) • Induration and swelling below the angle of the mandible • Medial bulging of the pharyngeal wall • Fever and rigors	*Treatment* • Initiate antibiotherapy: Co-amoxicillin, tab, 1 g, 2 × 1 tab/d and • Metronidazole, tab, 500 mg, 3 × 1 tab/d, 7 d, and • Rehydration, for example, Normal saline bag for infusion, 500 cc, 2×/d to assure adequate urine output *Or* • Ceftriaxone ampoule for injection, 1 g, 1 amp 2×/d and Metronidazole bag for infusion 500 3 × 1 bag/d • Prompt referral to tertiary center *Signs and symptoms* • High fever • Sore throat • Difficulty in swallowing • Hyperextension of neck • Labored and noisy breathing • Stridor • Bulge in posterior pharyngeal wall • Reddened throat, large and inflamed tonsils • *Anatomic consideration of deck fascial spaces* Complex anatomic structures delimiting various spaces. The three spaces of the deep cervical fascia that are of major clinical importance, the submandibular, parapharyngeal, and retropharyngeal spaces • *Submandibular space* lies within the submental and submandibular triangles between the mucosa of the floor of the mouth and the superficial layer of the deep cervical fascia • *Parapharyngeal space* located in the lateral aspect of the neck. Synonyms are lateral pharyngeal or pharyngomaxillary space • *Retropharyngeal space* Bounded by buccopharyngeal fascia, the deep cervical fascia at T1 or T2, the hypopharynx, and the esophagus, posterior aspect of the pretracheal fascia • *Danger space* between alar fascia, prevertebral fascia, base of the skull, posterior mediastinum to the level of the diaphragm • *Prevertebral space* adjacent to the prevertebral fascia • *Peritonsillar space* lies between the capsule of the palatine tonsil, the superior constrictor, and the tonsillar pillars • *Parotid space* around and within the superficial and a deep capsule of the parotid gland

Table 5.1 (continued)

Diagnosis and classification	Treatment and relevant clinical features: ear, nose, and throat (ENT) conditions
Stridor High-pitched grunting noise in the inspiratory phase of breathing caused by the oscillation of a narrowed airway, and its presence suggests significant obstruction of the large airways *Anatomy of the airways:* consisting of two main compartments: • *Extra thoracic:* airways above the thoracic inlet • *Supraglottic area;* consisting of nasopharynx, epiglottis, larynx, aryepiglottic folds, and false vocal cords • *Glottic and subglottic area:* extends from the vocal cords to the extra thoracic segment of the trachea, just before it enters the thoracic cavity • *Intrathoracic:* trachea that lies within the thoracic cavity and the mainstem bronchi	*Treatment* • Cephalexin, ampoule for injection, 500 mg, 3 × 1 amp/d • Change to oral after acute phase, *plus* • Metronidazole, bag for infusion, 500 mg 3 × 1 bag iv/d, if anaerobes suspected *Diagnostic entities of stridor* • *Subglottitis* (viral croup) or laryngotracheobronchitis • *Acute epiglottitis*-threatening infection in which the epiglottis and surrounding tissue become acutely inflamed and edematous, causing severe obstruction of the upper airways *Classification and clinical correlates* • *Inspiratory stridor:* originating from obstruction in the *extra thoracic* region is more pronounced during inspiration, when the pressure inside the airway falls below atmospheric pressure, causing airway collapse • *Expiratory stridor:* originating from obstruction in the *intrathoracic* region is more pronounced on exhalation since intrathoracic pressure rises on expiration and causes airway collapse • *Biphasic stridor: inspiratory and expiratory, fixed central* airway obstruction produces noise on both inspiration and expiration • *Stertor or snoring* airway obstruction occurring from the nasal, nasopharyngeal, or oropharyngeal areas (i.e., adenoid hypertrophy, micrognathia, macroglossia, and tonsil hypertrophy), the noise generated is *low pitched*. It is called *snoring* if it occurs when the patient is sleeping and *stertor* if it is present when the patient is awake *Etiology* • Inflammatory obstruction • Infections: viral or bacterial laryngotracheitis croup) tracheitis, epiglottitis, retropharyngeal abscess, peritonsillar abscess • Burns: inhalation of hot fumes (as in fire outbreaks), thermal epiglottitis and upper airways burns, caustic burns • Anaphylaxis: angioneurotic edema • Inhalation of a foreign body • Congenital malformation of the larynx, for example, laryngomalacia

(continued)

Table 5.1 (continued)

Diagnosis and classification	Treatment and relevant clinical features: ear, nose, and throat (ENT) conditions
Vertigo A sensation of motion where there is no motion or exaggerated sense of motion in response to movement *Classification* • Peripheral vertigo • Ventral vertigo *Peripheral vertigo* • Meniere's syndrome • Labyrinthitis • Benign paroxysmal positional vertigo (BPPV) • Vestibular neuronitis • Traumatic vertigo • Peri-lymphatic fistula • Cervical vertigo • Migraine vertigo *Central vertigo* • Vertigo syndrome due to central lesions • Vestibular schwannoma (acoustic neuroma) • Vascular compromise • Multiple sclerosis	*Treatment* • Vestibular rehabilitation • Betahistine, tab, 24 mg, 2 × 1 tab/d, 5 d *Diagnostic testing* • Audiometry • Neuro imaging • Electronystagmography *Differential diagnosis* • Postural hypotension • Chronic unilateral vestibular hypoperfusion • Vestibular migraine • Vestibular paroxysmal

Cardiovascular 6

Contents

6.1 **History: Questions to Ask** 55

6.2 **Physical Examination** 56

6.3 **Cardinal Paramedical Cardiovascular Investigations** 56

6.4 **Cardiovascular Red Flags** 57

Cardiovascular pathologies are disease conditions pertaining to the heart, as well as the blood vessels of the systemic and the pulmonary blood circulatory systems (Fig. 6.1 and Table 6.1). These disease conditions are common causes for presentation at primary healthcare centers. Cardiovascular diseases may be acquired or congenital. A good history and physical examination will help differentiate between these two types.

Acquired cardiovascular pathologies are common among adults and the elderly and include cardiac failure secondary to hypertension, arrhythmias, and valvopathies.

Hypertension constitutes a huge public health burden. Both short-term and long-term complications are encountered. Short-term complications include recurrent headache, dizziness, blurred vision, lethargy, and irritability. Long-term multisystemic effects of poorly managed hypertension include heart failure, cerebrovascular accidents, renal failure, hypertensive retinopathy, and peripheral neurologic defects.

Congenital cardiovascular pathologies are encountered in pediatric patients and among young adults. Congenital cardiopathies may be suspected from the patients' history: frail, crying babies, labored breast feeding delayed development. Cardinal physical signs may include cardiac murmur and edema.

Rheumatic heart disease and its impact on the cardiac function is commonly encountered.

6.1 History: Questions to Ask

- Do you have chest pain?
- Do you have labored breathing during light effort, for example, walking on a flat surface at a slow pace?
- Do you wake up in the night air-hungry?
- Do you frequently wake up at night to urinate?
- Do you notice that your feet or legs swell?
- Do you have palpitations?
- Do you lose consciousness?

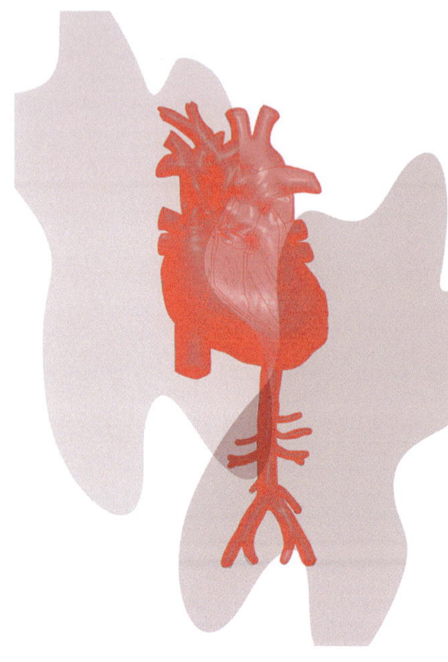

Cardiovascular

List of cardiovascular disorders that are described in the text. For easy reference, the corresponding page on which the disease condition is described is in brackets.

Acute coronary syndrome (p57)
Adult congenital heart disease (p58)
Aortic aneurysm (p58)
Arterial hypertension (p59)
Atrial fibrillation (p60)
Cardiac arrythmias (p61)
Cardiac failure (p61)
Cardiomyopathy (p61)
Cardiovascular arrest (p62)
Chest pain (p63)
Chronic hypotension and orthostatism (p63)
Coronary heart disease (p64)
Deep venous thrombosis (p64)
Endocarditis (p64)
Hypertensive crisis (p65)
Hypertensive emergency (p65)
Lymphedema (p66)
Musculoskeletal chest pain (p66)
Myocardial infarction (p57, p63)
Myocarditis (p66)
Pericardial effusion on tamponade (p67)
Pericarditis (p67)
Peripheral vascular disease Peripheral arterial disease (p67)
Pulmonary embolism (p68)
Refractory arterial hypertension (p69)
Shock (p69)
Syncope (p69)
Valvular heart diseases (p70)

Fig. 6.1 Cardiology: A mnemonic illustration representing main cardiovascular anatomic structures and their corresponding pathologies

6.2   Physical Examination

- Observe the mode of breathing
- Observe skin and mucous tissues: peripheral or central cyanosis
- Look for jugular vein distention
- Palpate the chest to appreciate the heartbeat
- Auscultate the heart and lungs
- Look at the lower limbs (edema) and hands (clubbing)
- Palpate the lower limbs, especially the calf muscles

6.3   Cardinal Paramedical Cardiovascular Investigations

- Full blood count
- Creatinine, microalbuminuria
- Chest X-ray
- ECG
- Echocardiography

6.4   Cardiovascular Red Flags

- Retrosternal chest pain at rest or with minimal effort, suggestive of myocardial event
- Hemodynamic instability
- Symptomatic hypotension without orthostatism
- High clinical index for myocarditis or endocarditis
- Ventricular arrhythmia
- Poorly tolerated supraventricular
- Severe infection (high fever, high white blood cell count [WBC])

Table 6.1 Cardiovascular conditions and their treatment

Diagnosis and classification	Treatment and relevant clinical features: cardiovascular conditions
Acute coronary syndrome (ACS) Acute myocardial ischemia or infarction *Terminology* The terms *STEMI, NSTEMI*, and unstable angina are used in patients who present with clinical characteristics compatible with myocardial ischemia that is, chest pain, diaphoresis, exercise intolerance, associated with typical cardiovascular risk factors *Chronic stable angina pectoris* Precordial chest pain, usually precipitated by stress or exertion, and can be relieved by rest or nitrates *Diagnostic tools* ECG and troponin to differentiate: • Unstable angina pectoris (AP) • ST-elevation myocardial infarction (STEMI) and • Non-STEMI (NSTEMI)	*Acute treatment* • Antiplatelet: Aspirin, tab, 300 mg loading dose, then 100 mg/d • Anticoagulation: heparin 60/70 UI/kg iv bolus maximum 5000 UI iv • Nitrate: Isosorbide mononitrate (if systolic blood pressure >90 mmHg) • Oxygenotherapy, start 2 L/min with target saturation 94% • Analgics: Morphine, 1 mg/ml ampoule, 5–10 mg iv stat dose *or* Tramadol ampoule, 100 mg, 1 amp iv stat • Acute invasive revascularization *or* iv thrombolytic in STEMI *Secondary preventive treatment:* • Antiplatelet: Aspirin, tab, 100 mg, 1 tab/d *Angiotensin-converting enzyme (ACE) inhibitors* • Enalapril, tab, 5 mg, 2 × 1 tab/d, increase progressively, maximum daily dose 40 mg *or* • Lisinopril, tab, 5 mg, 1 tab/d, increase progressively, maximum daily dose 80 mg or • Captopril, tab, 25 mg, 3 × 1 tab/d *Beta blockers* • Atenolol, tab, 50 mg, 1 tab/d, maximal daily dose 100 mg *Aldosterone antagonist* • Spironolactone (Aldactone), tab, 25 mg, 1×/d, maximum daily dose 100 mg *CoA reductase inhibitors (cholesterol reduction)* • Atorvastatin, tab, 10 mg, 1× daily (target LDL-cholesterol 1.8 mmol/L) *Management tips* • Patient education to adopt good hygienic lifestyle • Address cardiovascular risk factors • Stop smoking • Regular physical exercise, for example, walk 30 min daily • Body weight reduction • Compliance for hypertension treatment • With renal failure, heparin is the best anticoagulant *Complications of myocardial infarction* • Post infarction ischemia • Ventricular septal defect • Myocardial dysfunction • Right ventricular infarction • Mechanical defects • Myocardial rupture • Left ventricular aneurysm • Pericarditis • Mural thrombosis

(continued)

Table 6.1 (continued)

Diagnosis and classification	Treatment and relevant clinical features: cardiovascular conditions
Adult congenital heart disease • Detect the condition • Provide adequate information • Recognize and treat associated clinical condition • Write a clear referral medical report	*Treatment* • These conditions need primary clinical assessment and then referral to appropriate tertiary center • All clinicians need to provide essential basic care: diuretic for fluid overload: Bendrofluorothiazide tab, 2.5 mg, 1 tab/d (to be taken in the morning) *Cyanotic congenital heart diseases* Group of disorders associated with hypoxemia caused by right-to-left (intracardiac or extracardiac) shunting of blood *Tetralogy of Fallot* Combination of four different defects: • A hole between the right and left ventricles of the heart • A narrow pulmonary valve • A thickening of the right ventricle muscles • A misplaced aortic valve *Transposition of the great arteries* The pulmonary and aortic valves have switched positions with their arteries, resulting in low-oxygen blood getting pumped out to the rest of the body through the aorta instead of going to the lungs through the pulmonary artery *Tricuspid atresia* The tricuspid heart valve structure is abnormal or is missing entirely, causing disruption to the normal flow of blood. Low-oxygen blood is pumped out to the body as a result *Total anomalous pulmonary venous connection* Occurs when pulmonary veins that bring high-oxygen blood from the lungs to the heart are connected to the right atrium or a systemic vein. The pulmonary veins should be connected to the left atrium. This defect may also be accompanied by a blockage in these veins between the lungs and the heart *Non-cyanotic* • *Atrial septal defect and patent foramen ovale:* Communications in the atrial septum have several distinctive anatomic locations • *Ventricular septal defect:* Communications in the ventricular septum have several distinctive anatomic locations • *Pulmonary valve stenosis:* stenosis or narrowing of the pulmonary valve at any of the three locations: valvular, sub valvular, or supravalvular level • *Coarctation of the aorta:* discrete narrowing of the thoracic aorta just distal to the left subclavian artery
Aortic aneurysm • Thoracic aortic aneurysm TAA: ascending aorta >3.5 cm • Abdominal aorta aneurysm AAA: with a maximal diameter >3.0 cm	*Indication to operate* When diameter >5 cm or rapid progression is seen on the echocardiography because of risk of dissection *Observation* versus *endovascular repair:* Indication of elective repair of asymptomatic abdominal aortic aneurysm relies on risk factors for rupture: • Aneurysm diameter >5.5 cm • Female sex • Patient age • Rapid expansion • Very large aneurysm • Aneurysm morphology

Table 6.1 (continued)

Diagnosis and classification	Treatment and relevant clinical features: cardiovascular conditions
	Management of asymptomatic thoracic aortic aneurysm • Measures to reduce cardiovascular risk • Aggressive blood pressure control • Patient education regarding the symptoms and signs that may indicate the development of complications • Counseling for those suspected of having genetically mediated disease • Screening for associated aneurysmal disease *Clinical facts* • Aneurysm of the aorta: diameter <3 cm • Echocardiographic control indicated • Quit smoking • The natural history of TAA is one of progressive expansion • The rate of expansion depends upon the location and diameter of the aneurysm and its underlying etiology • Most TAAs produce no symptoms • Patients with asymptomatic TAA should be followed for the development of signs and symptoms that may be associated with the TAA • Syphilis is a common underlying cause
Arterial hypertension Definition Arterial blood pressure 140/90 mmHg (*Note*: white coat hypertension!) *Arterial pressure target* <140/90 mmHg, in diabetic patients <130/80 mmHg *Hypertension* • *Normal BP* Systolic <120 mmHg and diastolic <80 mmHg • *Elevated BP* Systolic 120–129 mmHg and diastolic <80 mmHg *Hypertension:* • *Stage 1* Systolic 130–139 mmHg or diastolic 80–89 mmHg • *Stage 2:* Systolic at least 140 mmHg or diastolic at least 90 mmHg *White coat* hypertension: BP that is consistently elevated by office readings but does not meet diagnostic criteria for hypertension based upon out-of-office readings *Masked hypertension* BP that is consistently elevated by out-of-office measurements but does not meet the criteria for hypertension based upon office readings	*Treatment* • Determine patient profile and choose among the following *Calcium channel blockers:* • Nifedipine, tab, 20 mg, 2 x 1 tab/d, maximum daily dose 80 mg *or* • Amlodipine, tab, 5 mg, 1×/d, maximal daily dose 40 mg *Diuretics* • Hydrochlorothiazide, tab, 25 mg, 1 tab/morning, maximum daily dose 100 mg *or* • Torsemide, tab, 2.5 mg, 1 × 1 tab/d *or* • Spironolactone, tab, 25 mg, 1 × 1 tab/d *ACE/angiotensin receptor blocker (ARB) inhibitor* • Enalapril, tab, 5 mg, 2 × 1 tab/d, maximum daily dose 40 mg *or* • Lisinopril, tab, 5 mg, 1 tab/d, maximum daily dose 80 mg *or* • Captopril, tab, 25 mg, 3 × 1 tab/d, maximum daily dose 100 mg *Beta blocker* • Atenolol, tab, 50, 1 tab/d, maximum daily dose 100 mg • Bisoprolol, tab, 5 mg, 1 × 1 tab/d • Propranolol, tab, 10 mg, 1 × 1 tab/d *Combinations* When monotherapy fail, combination therapy (bi-, tri- and quadritherapy possible when target not obtained. The only combination not possible is ACE inhibitor and ARB inhibitor *Risk factors for primary (essential) hypertension* • Age • Obesity • Family history • Race • Reduced nephron number • High-sodium diet • Excessive alcohol consumption • Physical inactivity

(continued)

Table 6.1 (continued)

Diagnosis and classification	Treatment and relevant clinical features: cardiovascular conditions
Clinical evaluation • History • Physical examination • Serum creatinine • Fasting glucose • Urinalysis • FBC • Thyroid-stimulating hormone (TSH) • Lipid profile • Electrocardiogram	*Secondary causes of hypertension* • Oral contraceptives, particularly those containing higher doses of estrogen • Chronic use of NSAID • Antidepressants: Tricyclic, SSRI, and MOI • Corticosteroids • Illicit drug use • Primary renal disease; both acute and chronic kidney disease can lead to hypertension • Primary aldosteronism • Renovascular hypertension often due to fibromuscular dysplasia in younger patients and to atherosclerosis in older patients • Obstructive sleep apnea • Cushing syndrome • Endocrine disorders: hypothyroidism, hyperthyroidism, and hyperparathyroidism may also induce hypertension *Complications of hypertension* • Left ventricular hypertrophy (LVH) • Heart failure, both reduced ejection fraction (systolic) and preserved ejection fraction (diastolic) • Ischemic stroke • Ischemic heart disease, including myocardial infarction and coronary interventions • Chronic kidney disease and end-stage renal disease • Retinopathy • Neuropathy with cognitive decline *Management tips* • Patient education to improve adherence to therapy • Teach the patient: what hypertension is • Short-term and long-term complications • End-organ damages: cardiac, respiratory, eye, brain, kidney, vascular, etc. • Explain about the medication chosen and its mode of action • Lifestyle changes: diet with salt restriction, physical exercises, quit smoking • Encourage sustainable dietary modifications or adjustments: no added salt (NAS)
Atrial fibrillation (AF) Cardiac arrhythmia with the following electrocardiographic characteristics • The R-R intervals follow no repetitive pattern. They have been labeled as "irregularly irregular" • While electrical activity suggestive of P waves is seen in some leads, there are no distinct P waves *Evaluation* • Exclude underlying cause • Evaluate the risk of complications	*Treatment* • Treat underlying cause of atrial fibrillation • Rivaroxaban (Xarelto), tab, 20 mg, 1 tab/d • Marcoumar or Sintrom to target INR 2–3 • If the risk of bleeding is important, start with antiplatelet drug instead of oral anticoagulation: • Aspirin, tab, 100 mg, 1 tab/d • Depending on patient profile, start with frequency control • Atenolol, tab, 25 mg, 1 tab/d, maximal daily dose 100 mg • Cardio selective beta blocker *Note:* AF patients are at increased risk for thromboembolism *Etiology* • Hyperthyroid • Hypertensive heart disease • Chronic obstructive pulmonary disease • Acute coronary syndrome *Complications* • Stroke • Heart failure • Recurrent hospitalization, thromboembolic events • Premature death

Table 6.1 (continued)

Diagnosis and classification	Treatment and relevant clinical features: cardiovascular conditions
	Risk stratification by CHA$_2$DS$_2$VASc score: the score is used to decide whether to administer anticoagulating medication to a patient with AF or not. In patients with score higher than 2, start oral anticoagulation • Congestive heart failure • Hypertension (age > 75) • Diabetes • History of stroke • Vascular disease story (age 65–75) • Sex category (female sex)
Cardiac arrythmias Any rhythm that is not normal sinus rhythm with normal atrioventricular conduction *Normal sinus:* heart rate at rest has been considered to be between 60 and 100 beats/min *Nomenclature* • *Ventricular fibrillation* • *Sudden death* is defined as expected nontraumatic death in the clinically well or stable patient who dies within one hour after onset of symptoms • *Cardiac arrest*	*Treatment* • Identify underlying causes • Characterize precisely the type of arrythmia • Beta blockers are the mainstay of arrythmias encountered in most minimal-resource settings: • Propranolol 40 mg, tab, 1×/d or Atenolol, 25 mg tabs, 1 tab/d *Classification* • Sinus arrythmias, bradycardia, and tachycardia • Atrioventricular block (AVB) • Conduction disturbance between the atria and ventricle that can be physiological (e.g., enhance vagal tonus) pathological • Paroxysmal supraventricular tachycardia: rapid, regular heartbeat commonly seen in young adults, characterized by spontaneous remission
Cardiac failure Structural or functional abnormality that impairs the ability of the heart to pump blood to meet the metabolic needs of the body or Ventricular ejection fraction of less than 40% *Classification (I to IV) ACC/AHA* • *Class 1:* no limitation of physical activity. Ordinary physical activity does not cause undue fatigue, palpitation, dyspnea • *Class II:* slight limitation of physical activity. Comfortable at rest. Ordinary physical activity results in fatigue, palpitation, dyspnea • *Class III:* marked limitation of physical activity. Comfortable at rest. Less than ordinary activity causes fatigue, palpitation, or dyspnea • *Class IV:* unable to carry on any physical activity without discomfort. Symptoms of heart failure at rest. If any physical activity is undertaken, discomfort increases	*Treatment* • Patient education • Dietary salt restriction • Treat underlying causes accordingly *Acute treatment* • Furosemide, tab, 40 mg, 1–2 tab/morning, with weight and BP control *and* • Enalapril, tab, 5 mg, 2 × 1 tab/d • Oxygen, 2 L/min, target saturation 94% *Long-term treatment* Diuretic if signs of hypervolemia: • Torsemide, tab, 5 mg, 1×/morning *or* • Hydrochlorothiazide, tab, 25 mg, 1×/morning *and* • Enalapril, tab, 5 mg, 2 × 1 tab/d *and* • Atenolol, tab, 25 mg, 1×/d, as needed *and* • Spironolacton (Aldactone), tab, 25 mg, 1 tab/d • Classifying heart failure as left-sided, right-sided or global heart failure may affect management strategies *Management tips* • Discontinue calcium-channel blockers (Nifedipine, NSAIDS, etc.) in all heart failure patients • Monitor fluid intake and output • Monitor weight daily to gauge effect of diuretics *Etiology* • Hypertension • Cardiac valve disease • Cardiomyopathy • Severe anemia • Myocardial ischemia/infarction • Thyrotoxicosis • Congenital heart disease • Cardiac arrhythmia • Thyrotoxicosis

(continued)

Table 6.1 (continued)

Diagnosis and classification	Treatment and relevant clinical features: cardiovascular conditions
Cardiomyopathy Heart muscle diseases of unknown cause. Cardiomyopathy is distinct from cardiac dysfunction due to known cardiovascular entities such as hypertension, ischemic heart disease, or valvular disease *Classification* • Dilated • Restrictive • Hypertrophic	*Dilated cardiomyopathy* Heart failure with reduced left ventricular ejection fraction (LVEF), where the left ventricular ejection fraction is defined as less than or equal to 40% *Diagnostic features* • Symptoms and signs of heart failure • Echocardiogram: left ventricular dilation, thinning, and global dysfunction • Severity of right ventricular dysfunction critical to long-term prognosis *Hypertrophic cardiomyopathy* *Clinical features* • May present with dyspnea, chest pain, sudden death • Echocardiogram is diagnostic • Left ventricular wall thickness greater than 1.5 cm defines the disease • Increase the risk of sudden death *Restrictive cardiomyopathy* • Heart failure due to impaired diastolic filling, with reasonably preserved contractile function *Diagnostic features* • Right heart failure tends to dominate over the left heart failure • Pulmonary hypertension is present • Amyloidosis is the most common cause • Echocardiography is key to diagnosis
Cardiovascular arrest Sudden cessation of cardiac activity, so that the victim becomes unresponsive, with no normal breathing and no signs of circulation	*Treatment* Typical clinical scenarios: Patient unconscious and no pulse: • Cardiovascular reanimation with 30 chest compressions and 2 ventilations • Defibrillation if pulseless ventricular tachycardia or ventricular fibrillation • Adenosine 1 mg iv, amiodarone 300 mg iv flush in ml G5% according to ECG *Patient stable with palpable pulse* • Find the underlying cause (6H and 6T, see below) • Anti-arrhythmic treatment if needed *Patient unstable with palpable pulse* • Find the underlying cause (6H and 6T, see below) • Electro cardioversion *Etiology of cardiovascular arrest:* Multiple causes of cardiovascular arrest need to be kept in mind when evaluating a patient with cardiovascular arrest *6H (useful mnemonics):* • Hypoxia • Hypovolemia • Hypo/hyperkaliemia • Hypoglycemia • Hypothermia • Hydrogen (acidosis) *6T: (useful mnemonic)* • Toxins • Tamponade (cardiac) • Tension pneumothorax • Thrombosis coronary (ACS) • Thrombosis pulmonary • Trauma

Table 6.1 (continued)

Diagnosis and classification	Treatment and relevant clinical features: cardiovascular conditions
Chest pain Pain or discomfort in the chest, typically the front of the chest and may be described as sharp, dull, pressure, heaviness or squeezing *Evaluation* • Physical examination • ECG • Chest X-ray • Upper abdominal echography	*Treatment* Determine and treat underlying cause *Epidemiology of chest pain:* • Musculoskeletal chest pain: 30–50% • Gastrointestinal causes 10–20% • Stable angina: 10% • Respiratory conditions: 5% • Myocardial ischemia (including myocardial infarction): 2–4% *Differential diagnosis (life threatening)* • Acute coronary syndrome • Aortic dissection • Pulmonary embolism • Tension pneumothorax • Esophageal rupture, perforation • Cardiac tamponade • Sarcoidosis-related arrythmias *Further differential diagnosis* • *Cardiac*: heart failure, pericarditis, myopericarditis, myocarditis, cardiomyopathy, aortic valve disease, mitral valve disease • *Pulmonary*: pneumothorax, pneumonia, malignancy, pleuritis, sarcoidosis, acute chest pain syndrome (e.g., part of sickle cell crisis), pulmonary hypertension • *Gastrointestinal:* gastrointestinal reflux disease, peptic ulcer disease, esophageal pain, esophagitis, hiatus hernia, acute cholecystitis, biliary colic • *Musculoskeletal:* isolated musculoskeletal chest pain syndrome, rheumatic disease, rib pain trauma, trauma • *Psychiatric:* panic attack-disorder, depression, somatization, fictitious disorder • *Referred pain* • *Herpes zoster* • *Domestic violence*
Chronic hypotension and orthostatic hypotension Impaired autonomic reflexes or depleted intravascular volume, leading to a significant reduction in blood pressure upon standing *Nomenclature* • Postural hypotension	*Treatment* Identify and treat underlying cause Advice on adequate fluid intake, for example, 3 L/24 h, assure clear urine In severe cases, Dobutamine ampoule 250 mg, dilute in 500 ml 0.9% NaCl, infuse iv slowly (2 h) *Etiology* • *Neurogenic*: autonomic failure (vaso-vagal), neurodegenerative disease, neuropathies, autoimmune autonomic impairment, paraneoplastic autonomic neuropathy, familial dysautonomia • *Volume depletion* • *Medication* • *Aging* • *Cardiac pump failure: aortic stenosis, arrythmias* *Clinical presentation* • Dizziness • Syncope • Angina • Stroke

(continued)

Table 6.1 (continued)

Diagnosis and classification	Treatment and relevant clinical features: cardiovascular conditions
Coronary heart disease Narrowing or blockage of the *coronary* arteries usually caused by atherosclerosis (a buildup of fatty material and plaque inside the coronary arteries)	*Primary and secondary prevention coronary heart disease* • Adoption of healthy lifestyle • Regular physical exercise • Body weight control *Risk factors for coronary heart disease* • Positive family history • Gender • Blood lipid abnormalities • Diabetes mellitus • Hypertension physical inactivity • Abdominal obesity • Cigarette smoking • Psychosocial factors • Too few fruits and vegetables • Too much alcohol
Deep venous thrombosis (DVT) Blood clot forms in a deep vein, usually in the lower limbs, which progresses to pulmonary embolism *Clinical assessment* • High-risk embolization during the first week if no treatment • D-dimer • Ultrasound	*Treatment* • Rivaroxaban (Xarelto), tab, 20 mg, 15 mg, 2 × 1 tab/d, 3 weeks, to be followed by Rivaroxaban, tab, 20 mg, 1 tab/d, 3 months • Elastic band-stocking to avoid post-thrombotic syndrome *Risk factors* • Long uninterrupted travel by air (>6 h) • Family history of coagulopathy • Oral contraceptive use • Neoplasm • Pregnancy • Cigarette smoking *Etiology* • Increased tendency of blood in the deep veins to clot, due to: • Stagnation of blood in the vein • Increased viscosity of blood • Inflammation of the blood vessel *Note:* Reason and act as clinically as possible in the approach: History, clinical signs: Homan's
Endocarditis Infection of the endocardial surface of the heart; usually refers to infection of one or more heart valves or infection of an intracardiac device *Diagnosis evaluation* *Duke criteria* • Echocardiography • Electrocardiography (ECG) • Chest radiography • Computed tomography • Blood culture	*Treatment* for 4–6 weeks • Empirical administration of: • Penicillin G amps 2.0 Million U, iv/4× in 24 h, *then* • Amoxicillin, tab, 500 mg, 3 × 1 tab/d 7 d *or* • Cefalexin, tab, 500 mg, 3 × 1 tab/d, 7 d *Signs and symptoms* • Fever, chills • Anorexia, weight loss • Malaise • Headache • Myalgias, arthralgias • Night sweats • Abdominal pain • Dyspnea • Cough • Pleuritic pain • Cardiac murmurs • Splenomegaly as petechiae or splinter hemorrhages *Note: Patients with valvular heart disease need continuous antibiotic prophylaxis*

Table 6.1 (continued)

Diagnosis and classification	Treatment and relevant clinical features: cardiovascular conditions
	Have low threshold for treating coexisting malaria *Complications* • Cardiac: valvular insufficiency, heart failure • Neurologic: embolic stroke, intracerebral hemorrhage, brain abscess, blindness, etc. • Septic emboli: infarction of kidneys, spleen, and other organs. In right-sided endocarditis, septic pulmonary emboli may be seen • Metastatic infection, for example, vertebral osteomyelitis, septic arthritis, psoas abscess • Systemic immune reaction (e.g., glomerulonephritis)
Hypertensive crisis Severely elevated blood pressure BP ≥200/120 mmHg	*Treatment* • Nifedipine, tab, 20 mg, 1, tab, unique dose • To be repeated every 2 h., maximum dose 80 mg in 24 h *Red flags* • Severe chest pain • Severe headache, accompanied by confusion and blurred vision • Nausea and vomiting • Severe anxiety • Shortness of breath • Seizures • Unresponsiveness *Management tips* • Monitor patient with regular BP measurement • When impaired consciousness is suspected, anticipate referral to tertiary center
Hypertensive emergency BP >180/120 mmHg, may be associated with acute neurological, cardiovascular, renal complication. High mortality rate	*Treatment* • Nifedipine, tab, 20 mg, 1-tab sublingual with hourly monitoring of blood pressure *If inadequately managed, may lead to:* • Hypertensive encephalopathy • Left ventricular failure associated with severe hypertension • Hypertension and dissection of aorta • Hypertension with myocardial infarction • Acute glomerulonephritis with severe hypertension • Eclampsia (in pregnant women) *Note: Closely monitor blood pressure, and attend promptly to very rare unpredictable drop in BP* *Complications of untreated hypertension* • Hypertensive cardiovascular disease • Hypertensive cerebrovascular disease • Vascular dementia • Hypertensive kidney disease • Hypertensive retinal disease • Aortic dissection • Atherosclerotic complications

(continued)

Table 6.1 (continued)

Diagnosis and classification	Treatment and relevant clinical features: cardiovascular conditions
Lymphedema Abnormal accumulation of interstitial fluid and fibro-adipose tissues resulting from injury, infection, or congenital abnormalities of the lymphatic system *Classification* • *Primary lymphedema:* congenital developmental abnormalities consisting of hyperplastic or hypoplastic involvement of proximal or distal lymphatic drainage system • *Secondary lymphedema:* involves inflammatory or mechanical obstruction drainage of lymphatic fluid as a result of compressive mass	*Treatment* • Identify and treat the cause • Physiotherapy: lymphatic drainage *Etiology* • Trauma • Regional lymph node resection • Radiotherapy • Extensive involvement of regional nodes by malignant disease • Filariasis • Inflammatory disorder • Obesity • Hereditary syndrome *Diagnostic features* • Painless tumefaction of one or both lower limbs, primarily in women • Pitting edema without ulceration, varicosities, or stasis pigmentation • There may be episodes of lymphangitis on cellulitis
Musculoskeletal chest pain Pain or discomfort felt around the thoracic cage that can be reproduced by palpation and that is typically position-dependent	*Treatment* • Reassure the patient • Paracetamol, tab, 500 mg, 3 × 1 tab/d as needed • Ibuprofen, tab, 400 mg, 3 × 1 tab/d as needed *Nomenclature* • Tietze syndrome: benign, painful, nonsuppurative localized swelling of the costo-sternal, sternoclavicular, or costochondral joints, most often involving the area of the second and third ribs • Xiphoidalgia • Sternoclavicular • Subluxation *Synonym* • Noncardiac thoracic pain *Note:* Avoid over-investigation
Myocarditis Inflammation of the myocardial tissue caused by an acute viral infection or post-viral immune response. Secondary myocarditis is inflammation caused by viral pathogens, medication, chemicals, physical agents, or inflammatory diseases such as Systemic lupus erythematosus	*Treatment* • Bed rest *and* • Aspirin, tab, 500 mg, 3 × 1 tab/d, 7 d *and* • Omeprazole, tab, 20 mg, 2 × 1 tab/d *Clinical findings* • Onset may be several days or weeks after viral infection • Gradual onset of heart failure • Tachycardia on ECG • Evidence of pulmonary edema *Diagnostic features* • Often follows an upper respiratory infection • May present with pleuritic or nonspecific chest pain and signs of heart failure • Echocardiogram documents cardiomegaly and contractile dysfunction

Table 6.1 (continued)

Diagnosis and classification	Treatment and relevant clinical features: cardiovascular conditions
Pericardial effusion on tamponade Accumulation of fluid within the pericardial sac exceeds the small amount that is normally present	*Treatment* Determine and treat underlying cause *Etiology* • Acute pericarditis (the cause is usually viral, bacterial, tuberculous, or idiopathic) • Autoimmune disease • Post myocardial infarction or cardiac surgery • Sharp or blunt chest trauma, including a cardiac diagnostic or interventional procedure • Malignancy, particularly metastatic spread of noncardiac primary tumors • Mediastinal radiation • Renal failure with uremia • Myxedema • Aortic dissection extending into the pericardium • Selected drugs *Clinical presentation* • Clinical impact is determined by the speed of accommodation • May or may not cause pain • Hemodynamic instability • Tamponade • Tachycardia with elevated jugular venous pressure (JVP) and either hypotension or paradoxical pulse
Pericarditis Acute inflammation of the pericardium due to infection or systemic disease, neoplasm, radiation, drug toxicity, prior cardiac surgery, or continuous inflammation process in the myocardium or lung	*Treatment* • Reassure the patient • Aspirin, tab, 500 mg, 3 × 1 tab/d, 10 d • Omeprazole, tab, 20 mg, 2 × 1 tab/d, 10 d *Diagnostic features* • Anterior pleuritic chest pain that is worse supine than upright • Pericardial rub • Fever is common • ESR or CRP usually elevated • ECG reveals a diffuse ST-segment elevation with associated PR depression
Peripheral arterial (vascular) disease Noncoronary arterial syndromes caused by the altered structure and function of the aorta and peripheral arteries due to various pathophysiological processes Peripheral artery disease denotes arterial disease affecting the peripheral (noncoronary) vasculature due to atherosclerosis Complication of reduced or absent blood supply to the distal part of the limbs	*Treatment* • Prompt referral to tertiary center. Usually in cases of total occlusion, it takes 6 h for irreversible complications to occur, for example, permanent loss of affected limb function *Pathophysiology* Narrowing or occlusion of arteries either from atherosclerosis or minor thrombi *Clinical signs and symptoms* • Lower limb extremity pain: intermittent claudication, that is, pain on the calf muscle while walking a distance. Pain is relieved by rest: pelvic and gluteal, thigh, calf and foot claudication may be characterized • May progress to pain at rest to skin darkening and later gangrene • Nonhealing wound-ulcer • Skin discoloration/gangrene: dermite ocre • Reduced pulse: brachial, radial, femoral, popliteal, dorsalis pedis, posterior tibial • Abnormal ancle-brachial index

(continued)

Table 6.1 (continued)

Diagnosis and classification	Treatment and relevant clinical features: cardiovascular conditions
Terminology • Peripheral extremity arteriopathy • Arteriosclerotic disease • Peripheral artery occlusive disease	*Differential diagnosis pf peripheral arterial disease* • Arterial aneurysm • Arterial dissection • Embolism • Popliteal entrapment syndrome • Cystic disease • Thromboangiitis • Radiation arteritis, post traumatic vasculitis, medication (ergot use for migraines)
Pulmonary embolism (PE) Obstruction of the pulmonary artery and its branches by material (e.g., thrombus, tumor, air, or fat) that originated elsewhere in the body *Classification* *Hemodynamically stable PE* or *hemodynamically unstable PE*, causes hypotension *Hypotension*: a systolic blood pressure <90 mmHg or a drop in systolic blood pressure of ≥40 mmHg from the baseline for a period >15 min and which is not explained by other causes, such as sepsis, arrhythmia, left ventricular dysfunction from acute myocardial ischemia or infarction, or hypovolemia *Nomenclature* *Acute PE:* develops symptoms and signs immediately after obstruction of pulmonary vessels *Subacute PE:* develops symptoms within days or weeks following the initial event *Chronic PE:* slowly develops symptoms of pulmonary hypertension over many years (i.e., chronic thromboembolic pulmonary hypertension)	*Treatment* • Heparin (75 units/kg) if DVT clinically suspected • Warfarin, 10 mg, tab, daily at 6 pm, 2d (starting on the same day as Heparin), then 5 mg daily with regular dose adjustment and monitoring of prothrombin time and INR until target of 2.0–3.0 is attained • Xarelto 15 mg tabs, 2 × 1 tab/d, for 3 weeks, then Xarelto y tabs, 1 tab/d, for 3 months • If signs of hemodynamic instability (TAS<90 mmHg) consider thrombolysis if no contraindications *Pathophysiology of pulmonary embolism* Virchow's triad consists of • Venous stasis • Endothelial injury • A hypercoagulable state: alterations in the constituents of the blood (i.e., inherited or acquired hypercoagulable state) *Categories of risk factors* • Genetic: factor V Leiden and the prothrombin gene mutation • Acquired: recent surgery, trauma, immobilization, initiation of hormone therapy, active cancer, obesity, heavy cigarette smoking, oral contraceptives, pregnancy *Risk factors for PE* • Prolonged immobility, for example, hospitalization • Previous PE or DVT • Major surgery, for example, orthopedic, abdominal, or pelvic surgery • Trauma, especially involving the pelvis and lower limbs • In late pregnancy, after Caesarean section and the puerperium • Contraceptive pill or hormone replacement therapy (HRT) use • Certain medical conditions, for example, congestive cardiac failure (CCF), myocardial infarction (MI), stroke, malignancy, etc. • Inherited disorders causing hypercoagulability *Evaluation* • ECG • Chest X-ray • D-dimer • Hypotension sign of severity *Wells score criteria* • Symptoms of deep venous thrombosis • Other diagnosis unlikely • Heartbeat >100/min • Immobilization or surgery if <4 weeks ago • History of DVT • Hemoptysis, neoplasia

Table 6.1 (continued)

Diagnosis and classification	Treatment and relevant clinical features: cardiovascular conditions
Refractory arterial hypertension Hypertension: 140/90 mmHg despite tri-therapy with appropriate dosage for 4 weeks	*Treatment* • Ensure treatment compliance • Prompt referral to appropriate tertiary center • Exclude secondary causes, for example, renal artery stenosis, pheochromatosis, etc. • Most common cause is poor medication compliance *Management tips* • Search for secondary causes of hypertension • Sleep apnea syndrome • Renal parenchymal damage • Renal artery stenosis • Hyperdorism • Primary hyperaldosteronism, pheochromocytoma, dysthyroid
Shock A state of cellular and tissue hypoxia due to reduced oxygen delivery and/or increased oxygen consumption or inadequate oxygen utilization. Commonly caused by circulatory failure with resulting hypotension	*Treatment/clinical management* • Adopt life support approach: airways, breathing, circulation, dolor-pain, safe environment • Recognizing and reversing life-threatening signs and symptoms promptly • Preventing or limiting ongoing blood loss • Restoring intravascular volume where necessary • Maintaining adequate oxygen delivery to vital organs *Clinical classification of shock* • *Hypovolemic:* due to reduced intravascular volume, for example, hemorrhagic • *Cardiogenic:* due to intracardiac causes of cardiac pump failure that result in reduced cardiac output • *Obstructive:* due to extracardiac causes of cardiac pump failure and often associated with poor right ventricle output • *Distributive:* characterized by severe peripheral vasodilatation; septic, neurogenic, endocrine, anaphylactic, shock belong to this category • *Combined:* maximize oxygenation *Diagnostic features* • Hypertension • Tachycardia • Altered mental status • Hypoperfusion and impaired oxygen delivery
Syncope Transient loss of consciousness and postural tone from vasopressor cardiogenic causes with prompt recovery with or without resuscitative measures. High-risk features include abnormal ECG and age older than 60 years *Clinical assessment* • ECG • Shelong's test • Electrophysiologic studies depending on arrythmia detected	*Treatment* • Adopt life support approach: airways, breathing, circulation, dolor-pain, safe environment • Identify and treat underlying cause • Make sure: good fluid intake, no cardiologic or neurologic or psychologic anomalies in the history and physical examination • Address to appropriate tertiary center as needed *Etiology* • Reflex syncope • Orthostatic syncope • Cardiac arrhythmias • Structural cardiopulmonary disease • Pulmonary embolism • Hypersensitivity of carotid sinus • Seizures • Sleep disturbances • Accidental falls • Some psychiatric conditions

(continued)

Table 6.1 (continued)

Diagnosis and classification	Treatment and relevant clinical features: cardiovascular conditions
	Prodrome • Lightheadedness • A feeling of being warm or cold • Sweating • Palpitations • Nausea or nonspecific abdominal discomfort • Visual "blurring" • Diminution of hearing and/or occurrence of unusual sounds • Pallor *Associated clinical symptoms* • Nausea • Vomiting • Feeling cold or clammy • Visual auras or blurry vision • Shortness of breath • Chest pain

Valvular heart diseases
A cardiovascular disease process involving one or more of the four valves of the heart (the aortic, mitral, the pulmonic, and tricuspid valves)
 	
Classification
• Mitral valve stenosis
• Mitral regurgitation
• Mitral valve prolapse syndrome
• Aortic stenosis
• Aortic regurgitation
• Tricuspid valve stenosis
• Pulmonary valve regurgitation
• Damage to cardiac valves may be chronic and progressive, resulting in cardiac decompensation
 	
Clinical manifestations
• Hemoptysis
• Hemoptysis
• Atrial fibrillation
• Thromboembolism
• Chest pain
• Right-sided heart failure
• Hoarseness-dysphonia
• Infective endocarditis
	Treatment
	• Surgical repair or replacement
	• Judicious use of diuretics: Hydrochlorothiazide, tab, 25 mg, 1 tab/d of Bendroflumethiazide tab, 2.5 mg, 1 tab/d
	
	Etiology
	• Rheumatic heart disease
	• Degenerative mitral valve diseases
	• Infective endocarditis
	• Trauma
	• Use of certain drugs, such as ergotamine, bromocriptine
	• Congenital malformations including valve cleft
	• Pathologic calcifications of valve components
	
	Descriptions
	• *Mitral stenosis (MS)* is narrowing of the mitral valve, causing an obstruction to blood flow from the left atrium to left ventricle. This leads to an increase in pressure within the left atrium, pulmonary vasculature, and right side of the heart
	
	Pathomorphology: mitral commissural adhesion; thickened, immobile mitral valve leaflets; and fibrosis, thickening, shortening, fusion, and calcification of the chordae tendineae
	• *Mitral regurgitation* may arise from abnormalities of parts of the mitral valve apparatus, including the valve leaflets, annulus, chordae tendineae, and papillary. The left atrium and ventricle are affected
	
	Pathomorphology: components of the valve apparatus leaflet, chordae tendineae, papillary muscles, and/or annulus may be structurally and functionally altered
	• *Mitral valve prolapse syndrome* (MVP) is the association of a variety of clinical features, including potentially serious arrhythmic and nonrhythmic complications, such as sudden death and infective endocarditis. Nonspecific complaints associated with MVP are:
	  – Atypical chest pain
	  – Palpitations
	  – Dyspnea
	  – Anxiety
	  – Exercise intolerance
	  – Dizziness or syncope
	  – Panic and anxiety disorders
	  – Numbness or tingling
	  – Skeletal abnormalities
	  – Abnormal resting and exercise electrocardiograms

Table 6.1 (continued)

Diagnosis and classification	Treatment and relevant clinical features: cardiovascular conditions
	• *Aortic valve stenosis:* Narrowing of the aortic valve orifice. Normal aortic valve area is 3.0–4.0 cm². Assessment of the degree of aortic stenosis entails: – Measurement of the transvalvular flow – Determination of the transvalvular pressure gradient – Calculation of the aortic valve area • *Aortic regurgitation* (AR), or aortic insufficiency, is caused by inadequate closure of the aortic valve leaflets. It may result from disease of the aortic valve leaflets or by distortion or dilation of the aortic root and ascending aorta • *Tricuspid valve stenosis* (TS) is an uncommon valvular abnormality that most commonly occurs in association with other valvular lesions, particularly in patients with rheumatic heart disease • *Pulmonary valve regurgitation:* physiologic trace to mild pulmonic valve regurgitation (also known as pulmonic regurgitation or PR) commonly occurs in normal individuals. Greater degrees of PR are caused by various disorders and can lead to right ventricular volume overload and right heart failure • *Rheumatic carditis:* includes a spectrum of lesions ranging from pericarditis, myocarditis, and valvulitis during ARF; there is a transition from rheumatic carditis to rheumatic heart disease (RHD), with chronic valvular lesions that evolve over years following one or more episodes of ARF (algorithm 1A-B). RHD is defined as permanent heart valve damage subsequent to ARF • *Acute rheumatic fever (ARF)* is a nonsuppurative sequela that occurs 2–4 weeks following group A *Streptococcus* pharyngitis and may consist of – Arthritis – Carditis – Chorea – Erythema marginatum – Subcutaneous nodules

Contents

7.1   **History: Questions to Ask** 73

7.2   **Physical Examination** 74

7.3   **Cardinal Paramedical Respiratory System Examinations** 74

7.4   **Respiratory System Red Flags** 74

Respiratory diseases are disorders that affect the lungs and other parts of the respiratory system (Fig. 7.1). They may be caused by infection, by allergies, by smoking tobacco, or other forms of air pollution.

The major respiratory pathologies are infections of the airways. By convention, the airways are divided into upper airways and lower airways. Anatomic entities of the upper airways consist of the nose and its mucosal lining, the sinuses, the pharyngo-laryngeal complex, the trachea, and the bronchi. The bronchiole and the lung parenchyma constitute the lower airways (Table 7.1).

Most airway infections are caused by a self-limiting viral invasion of the mucosal lining of the upper airway. However, the initial viral infection may be complicated with a secondary bacterial infection. This benign condition may also be complicated by a life-threatening bacterial superinfection. The predilecting conditions for bacterial superinfection include poor nutritional condition, poor ENT hygiene, immunodeficiency, diabetes, and senescence. The clinician should make reasonable efforts to obtain a good history and do physical and paramedical investigations, which will allow good clinical risk stratification.

Allergy is the underlying pathophysiologic basis of a series of airway diseases. Specific diagnoses may include rhinitis, sinusitis, conjunctivitis, and asthma.

Further etiologic factors include chronic exposure to toxic fumes and dust. Malformation of the chest wall should be considered in the differential diagnosis of airway afflictions. Examples include pectus carenum, pectus excavatum, sternal dysgeneses, scoliosis, hiatus hernia, and gastro-esophageal reflux diseases.

7.1   History: Questions to Ask

- Do you have chest pain?
- Do you cough?
- Do you produce sputum?

M. Touray, A. Touray, *Clinical Work and General Management of a Standard Minimal-Resource Facility*, Sustainable Development Goals Series, https://doi.org/10.1007/978-3-030-71032-3_7

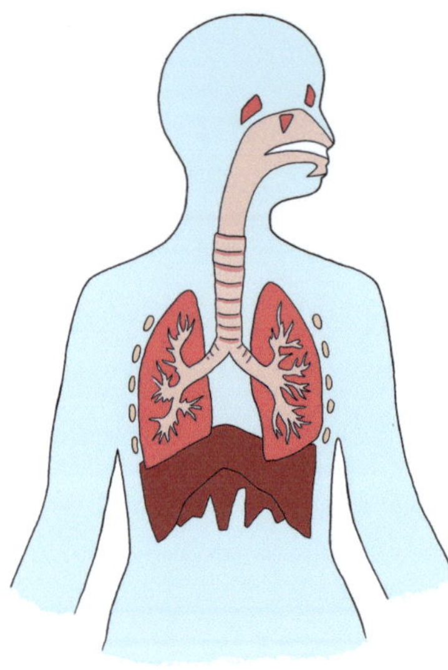

Fig. 7.1 Respiratory system: A mnemonic illustration representing main respiratory anatomic structures and their corresponding pathologies

- Did you ever spit blood?
- Did you live with or care for somebody who was coughing a lot?
- Do you have fever or night sweats?
- Do you have labored breathing during light effort, for example, walking on a flat surface at a slow pace?

7.2   Physical Examination

- Inform the morphology of the lung: antero-posterior diameter, etc.
- Appreciate the breathing pattern: Harmonious? Labored? Kussmaul? Whispering?
- Count the number of breaths per minute.
- Auscultate all lung fields: Crepitations? Wheezing? Stridor? Silent?
- Perform lung percussion to detect tenderness.

7.3   Cardinal Paramedical Respiratory System Examinations

- Full blood count
- Chest X-ray
- AFB sputum analysis
- Tuberculin test

7.4   Respiratory System Red Flags

- Diminishing level of consciousness
- Poorly tolerated dyspnea
- High fever >38.5°C
- Hypoxemia or hypercapnia
- Age over 65
- Elevated respiratory rate >25 resp per minute
- Signs of right-sided heart failure
- Poor response to routine treatment regime
- Cardiac arrhythmia

Table 7.1 Respiratory conditions and their treatment

Diagnosis and classification	Treatment and relevant clinical features: respiratory conditions
Acute respiratory distress syndrome in adults An acute, diffuse, inflammatory form of lung injury that may follow a wide variety of clinical events *Signs and symptoms* • Tachypnea • Use of accessory muscles, and/or retractions • Head bobbing • Nasal flaring • Grunting *Clinical diagnosis (Berlin definition)* • Respiratory symptoms begin within one week of a known clinical insult • Bilateral opacities present on a chest radiograph • Respiratory failure not explained by cardiac failure or fluid overload • Presence of severe to moderate impairment of oxygenation	*Treatment* Supportive care • Evaluation and treatment of underlying cause *General clinical management principles* • Wise use of sedatives • Hemodynamic management • Nutritional support • Control of blood glucose levels • Prophylaxis against deep venous thrombosis and gastrointestinal bleeding *Pathophysiology* • Physiologically, lungs regulate the movement of fluid to maintain a small amount of interstitial to avoid fluid retention in the alveoli • This regulatory mechanism is interrupted by lung injury, causing excess fluid in both the interstitial and alveoli • This fluid retention leads to impaired gas exchange, decreased compliance, and increased pulmonary arterial pressure *Etiologies and predisposing conditions* • Trauma • Sepsis • Pancreatitis • Shock • Multiple transfusions • Drug overdose • Pulmonary insults • Tuberculosis • Airway obstruction • Near drowning • Transfusion-related acute lung injury • Toxic gas inhalation • Oxygen toxicity • Lung contusion • High-altitude exposure • Drug toxicity, for example, Amiodarone *Clinical features* • Dyspnea • Reduction in arterial oxygen saturation • Tachypnea • Tachycardia • Diffuse crackles • Acute confusion, cyanosis • Diaphoresis • Cough • Chest pain • Wheezing • Hemoptysis • Fever

(continued)

Table 7.1 (continued)

Diagnosis and classification	Treatment and relevant clinical features: respiratory conditions
	Differential diagnostics • *Respiratory tract:* infections, asthma, anaphylaxis, foreign bodies, trauma, smoke inhalation • *Cardiovascular:* congenital heart disease, acute decompensated heart failure, arrhythmia, shock, pericarditis • *Nervous system:* ingestion, CNS trauma, seizures, or CNS infection, hypotonia • *Gastrointestinal:* intra-abdominal trauma, small-bowel obstruction, bowel perforation • *Metabolic and endocrine diseases:* diabetic ketoacidosis, severe dehydration, sepsis, toxic ingestions, inborn errors of metabolism • *Hematologic:* acute chest syndrome (patients with sickle cell disease), acute severe anemia from blood loss or hemolysis, hemoglobin variants
Asthma Reversible obstruction of the airway characterized by variable airway obstruction, sensitivity, and inflammation *Classifications* • Allergic • Intrinsic • Iatrogenic	*Treatment* • Eviction of allergen *Acute phase* • Hydrocortisone, ampoule 100 mg, 1 amp diluted in 250 ml 0.9% NaCl, infused iv immediately. Hydrocortisone ampoule 100 mg may also be delivered iv without dilution in normal saline Inhaled short-acting beta mimetic: • Salbutamol 2 puffs by spacer *or* • Salbutamol 2.5 mcg diluted in 3 ml of normal saline; nebulize every 20 min for 1 h • Prednisolone 1−2 mg/kg po stat *and* • Oxygen 6−8 L/min where available *Chronic treatment* • Prednisolone, tab, 5 mg, 2, tab, every morning for 5 d after crisis *Maintenance oral treatment* • Short-acting beta agonist receptor: salbutamol when needed, and adapt according to stage of asthma *Essential clinical notes* • Episodic chronic symptoms of wheezing, dyspnea, and cough • Symptoms frequently worst at night or in the early mornings • Prolonged expiration and diffuse wheezing on physical examination • Limitation of airflow on pulmonary function testing and or positive bronchoprovocation challenge • Reversibility of airflow obstruction, either spontaneously or following bronchodilator therapy *Signs and symptoms* • Shortness of breath • Severe respiratory distress • Tachycardia • Wheezing • Reduced breath sounds • Inability to speak, cannot count up to five • Excess of beta agonist may cause: • Tremor • Tachycardia • Hypokalemia *Note:* Ensure compliance with a good inhalation technique

Table 7.1 (continued)

Diagnosis and classification	Treatment and relevant clinical features: respiratory conditions
Bronchiectasis A congenital or acquired disorder of the large bronchi characterized by permanent, abnormal dilation and destruction of the bronchial walls. It may be caused by chronic inflammation or infection of the airways and may be localized or diffuse	*Treatment* • Identify and treat underlying cause • Elective referral to appropriate tertiary *Pathophysiology* Initiation of the disease process requires two factors • An infectious insult • Impaired drainage, airway obstruction, or a defect in host defense • The initiated cascade of host immune and inflammatory response causes permanent morphologic changes such as dilatation and destruction of the bronchi and bronchiole walls *Etiology* • Tobacco-cigarette smoking • Airway obstruction (e.g., foreign body aspiration) • Defective host defenses • Rheumatic and systemic diseases • Dyskinetic cilia • Pulmonary infections • Cystic fibrosis *Clinical features* • Chronic productive cough with dyspnea and wheezing • Radiographic findings of dilated thickened airways with scattered irregular opacities
Bronchopneumonia Infection of the lung tissue caused by various bacterial species, viruses, fungi, or parasites *Classification* Classified in terms of infecting organism *1. Community-acquired pneumonia* occurs outside the hospital or within 48 h of hospital admission • *Streptococcus pneumoniae* • *Streptococcus pyogenes* • *Mycoplasma pneumonia* • *Hemophilus influenza* • *Staphylococcus aureus* • *Staphylococcus* • Aspiratory as in CVA	*Treatment* • Uncomplicated community-acquired: • Amoxicillin, tab, 500 mg, 3× tab/d, 5 d *or* • Doxycycline, tab, 100 mg, 2 × 1 tab/d, 5 d *or* • Cephalexin, tab, 500, 3 × 1 tab/d, 5 d *Second-line antibiotherapy* • Erythromycin, tab, 500 mg, 4 × 1 tab/d, 5 d • Complicated community-acquired pneumonia: • Penicillin G, ampoule 1.2 million units, 4 × 1 amp/24 h *or* • Ceftriazone amp 500 mg, 3 × 1 amp/24 h, *then* • Co-amoxicillin, tab, 1 g, 2 × 1 tab/d, 10 d *or* • Ciproxin, tab, 500 mg, 2 × 1 tab/d, 10 d *or* • Azithromycin, 500 mg tab, 1 tab/d, 7 d • When empyema suspected, add: Metronidazole, tab, 500 mg, 3 × 1 tab/d, 7 d *To cover atypical or CPC* • Cotrimoxazole, tab, (Sulfamethoxazole 800/ Trimethoprim160), 2 × 1 tab/d, 7 d *or* • Azithromycin, tab, 500 mg, 1 tab/d, 3 d *Possible cause of no response to treatment* • Noncompliance • Emesis • Parapneumonic effusion • Pulmonary abscess • Empyema • Resistant germ or unusual germ *Symptomatic relief* Bromhexine: adjunct mucolytic (leave 2 h of interval from taking the antibiotic) Paracetamol NSAID

(continued)

Table 7.1 (continued)

Diagnosis and classification	Treatment and relevant clinical features: respiratory conditions
2. Hospital-acquired pneumonia or nosocomial pneumonia: pneumonia contracted by a patient in a hospital at least 48–72 h after being admitted	*Signs and symptoms* • Fever • Cough productive or nonproductive • Sputum production, rusty or blood stained, yellowish green • Pleuritic chest pain—worse on deep breathing or coughing • Fast breathing • Fast pulse rate *Diagnostic features* • Fever or hypothermia • Tachypnea • Cough with or without sputum • Dyspnea, chest discomfort • Sweats and/or rigors • Bronchial breath sounds or inspiratory crackles upon chest auscultation • Parenchymal opacity on chest X-ray
Chronic cough A cough that lasts eight weeks or longer in adults, or four weeks in children *Classifications* • Acute cough, lasting less than 3 weeks • Subacute cough, lasting between 3 and 8 weeks • Chronic cough, lasting more than 8 weeks	*Treatment* • Identify cause and treat accordingly • Thoroughly interrogate allergic etiology • Tobacco cessation • If gastroesophageal reflux disease is suspected: Omeprazole, tab, 20 mg, 2 × 1 tab/d *Etiologies* • Upper airway cough syndrome: due to postnasal drip • Asthma • Gastroesophageal reflux • ACE inhibitor • Airway affections: non-asthmatic eosinophilic bronchitis, chronic bronchitis, bronchiectasis, neoplasm, foreign body pulmonary parenchyma: interstitial lung disease, lung abscess • Laryngopharyngeal reflux: • Lung cancer • Tobacco smoking *Clinical evaluation* • History: post infectious? Recent ACE inhibitor use? • Chest X-ray • Methacholine challenge *Complication* • Exhaustion, self-consciousness • Insomnia • Headache, dizziness, musculoskeletal pain • Hoarseness • Excessive perspiration • Urinary incontinence

Table 7.1 (continued)

Diagnosis and classification	Treatment and relevant clinical features: respiratory conditions
Chronic obstructive pulmonary disease (COPD) Chronic inflammation of the bronchial mucosa due to irritants such as tobacco smoke Limited expiratory flow (forced expiratory volume [FEV] >70%) *Classification* • Chronic bronchitis • Emphysema *Diagnostic features* • History of cigarette smoking • Chronic cough, dyspnea, and sputum production • Ronchi, decreased intensity of breath sounds • Prolonged expiration on physical exam • Airflow limitation on pulmonary function testing that is not fully reversible is mostly progressive	*Treatment* • Exacerbation is often due to viral respiratory tract infection Exacerbations: • Inhaled short-acting beta mimetic: Salbutamol 2 puffs every 20 min for 1 h • Inhaled anticholinergic: Atrovent every 4–6 h • When severe dyspnea: • Prednisolone, tab, 5 mg, 5 tabs/morning, 5 d • Mucolytics: Bromhexine, tab, 4 mg, 2 × 1 tab/d, 5 d • Oxygen 2 L/min (with frequent monitoring) • Antibiotics if associated infection suspected: yellowish-greenish abundant mucous: Doxycycline 100 mg, 2× daily for 5 d *Long-term treatment* • Patient education • Counseling on quitting cigarette smoking • Professional reconversion • Short-acting beta mimetics: Ventolin (Albuterol) Aerosol/spray, 1 puff as needed • Inhalation corticoid therapy: Symbicort (Budesonide/formoterol), 1 puff/d • Inhaled anticholinergic: Atrovent (ipratropium) *Clinical considerations for managing BPCO* • The WHO GOLD grading system may be applied to scale the management • Proper management improves life expectancy • Stop smoking • Seasonal vaccinations • Oxygen therapy • GOLD staging *Aggravating criteria* • Increasing dyspnea • Increasing sputum • Discolored sputum

Empyema thoracis
Collection of pus in the pleural cavity; develops when pyogenic bacteria invade the pleural space, from an adjacent pneumonia, or iatrogenic inoculation
 	
Nomenclature
Parapneumonic pleural effusion
	Treatment
	• Metronidazole, bag for iv infusion, 500 mg 3 × 1 bag iv/ d, 5 d
	  and
	• Ceftriaxone ampoule, 1 g, 2 × 1 amp/d, for 5 d
	• Total duration of treatment depends on the monitored clinical improvement of the patient
	• Refer to tertiary center if hemodynamically unstable (BP >90/60)
	• Assure adequate follow-up
	• Provide balance diet-nutrition
	• Consider drainage (refer to adequate center)
	  – Complications
	  – Residual pleural thickening on chest X-ray
	  – Fibrothorax and pleural calcification
	  – A thickened pleura as it may progress to pleural fibrosis

(continued)

Table 7.1 (continued)

Diagnosis and classification	Treatment and relevant clinical features: respiratory conditions
Hyperventilation syndrome Inappropriate increase in alveolar ventilation that leads to hypocapnia *Psychopathology* Associated with psychological pathologies such as panic disorder	*Treatment* • Identify and address cause of the condition • Provide adequate, individualized and adapted psychological support *Etiology* • Anxiety • Pregnancy • Hypoxemia • Obstructive pulmonary disease • Sepsis • Hepatic dysfunction • Fever or pain *Signs and symptoms of hyperventilation:* the presenting clinical characteristics may differ depending on whether the hyperventilation is acute or chronic *Acute hyperventilation* • Tachycardia • Hyperpnea • Paresthesia • Chest pain or tightness • Carpopedal spasms • Tetany • Anxiety and fear *Chronic hyperventilation* Nonspecific symptoms including • Fatigue • Dyspnea • Anxiety • Palpitation • Dizziness
Obstructive sleep apnea syndrome Passive collapse of upper airway during sleep as a result of loss of normal pharyngeal muscle tone	*Treatment* • Lifestyle adaptation: weight loss or stabilization, regular physical exercise; for example, walk 1 h per day 7 days a week • Continuous positive airway pressure (CPAP) where available • Body weight reduction where applicable: target BMI is 25 kg/M^2 or less *Diagnostic features* • Daytime somnolence and fatigue • History of loud snoring with apneic events • Overnight polysomnography demonstrating apneic episodes and hypoxemia

Table 7.1   (continued)

Diagnosis and classification	Treatment and relevant clinical features: respiratory conditions
Pleural effusion Accumulation of fluid in the pleural space, meaning between the parietal pleura and the pulmonary pleura *Classification* • Transudate • Exudate	*Treatment* • Treat underlying cause • Prompt referral to tertiary center *Etiology* • Empyema • Malignancy • Tuberculosis • Esophageal rupture • Rheumatoid effusion *Diagnostic features* • May be asymptomatic • Chest pain frequently seen in the setting of pleuritis • Trauma or infection • Dyspnea is common with large infusions • Dullness to percussion and decreased breath sounds over the effusion • Radiographic evidence of effusion • Diagnostic findings on thoracentesis
Pneumothorax Collection of air in the pleural space, secondary to an underlying lung condition *Classification* • Spontaneous: occurs without a precipitating event in a person who does not have known lung disease • Traumatic	*Treatment* • Reassure, bedrest, monitor vital signs • If dyspnea refer to tertiary center *Risk factors* • Smoking • Positive family history • Marfan syndrome • Anorexia nervosa *Diagnostic features* • Acute onset of unilateral chest pain on dyspnea • Unilateral chest expansion • Decrease tactile fremitus • Hyper resonance • Diminished breath sounds • Mediastinal shift, cyanosis, and hypotension in tension pneumothorax
Pulmonary neoplasm malignancies *Good to know* Most common cancer worldwide Responsible for the most cancer deaths followed by liver and gastrointestinal cancers	*Treatment* • Provide adequate supportive care • Address to tertiary center *Risk factors* • Smoking • Radiotherapy • Environmental toxins • Pulmonary fibrosis • HIV infection • Genetic factors • Alcohol

(continued)

Table 7.1 (continued)

Diagnosis and classification	Treatment and relevant clinical features: respiratory conditions
	Clinical manifestations • Cough • Hemoptysis • Chest pain • Dyspnea • Dysphonia-hoarseness • Pleural changes • Superior vena cava syndrome • Pancoast syndrome *Classification* • *Adenocarcinoma* most common type of lung cancer • *Adenosquamous carcinomas* malignant glandular and squamous components • *Squamous cell carcinoma* presence of keratin production by tumor cells and/or intercellular desmosomes • *Large cell carcinoma* is a malignant epithelial neoplasm lacking both glandular and squamous • *Sarcomatoid* heterogeneous group of non-small-cell lung carcinomas • *Pleomorphic carcinoma* • *Spindle cell carcinoma* • *Giant cell carcinoma*
Sarcoidosis A systemic disease of unknown etiology characterized by granulomatous inflammation of the lung	*Treatment* • Corticoid therapy where clinically indicated: Prednisone, tab, 40 mg, 1 tab/d, with 5 mg decrease on weekly base *and* • Omeprazole 20 mg tab, 1 tab/d, 4 weeks *Clinical evaluation* • History, including occupational and environmental exposure • Full physical examination • Laboratory testing • Chest radiograph • Pulmonary function tests • Electrocardiogram • Ophthalmological examination *Diagnostic features* • Symptoms related to the lungs, skin, eyes, nerves, kidney, and other tissues • Demonstration of noncaseous granulomas in biopsy specimen • Exclusion of other granulomatous disorders • Bilateral hilar adenopathy • Pulmonary reticular opacities • Skin, joint, and/or eye lesions

Table 7.1 (continued)

Diagnosis and classification	Treatment and relevant clinical features: respiratory conditions
Sleep disorder A group of syndromes characterized by disturbance in one's amount of sleep, quality or timing of sleep, or in behaviors or physiological conditions associated with sleep. There are about 70 different sleep disorders	*Treatment* • Determine sleep disorder and treat underlying cause if any • In acute situation for insomnia: Diazepam 2 mg, tabs, 1 tab at bedtime, maximal 10 d • CPAP for obstructive sleep apnea *Non-pharmacological treatment* • Adequate behavior and cognitive counseling, and provide explication of sleep pattern • Encourage to adopt good sleep hygiene: • Suppress use of stimulants: glucocorticoids and certain antidepressant (e.g., SSRI), chronic use of opioids • Advice about maladaptive behavior: for example, use of alcohol to induce sleep *Cognitive behavioral therapy* • Arrange a stable bedtime and wake time 7 days per week • Sleep restriction: reduce time in bed to approximate the total hours of estimated sleep • Stimulus control: advice to use the bed only for sleep and sex; try to sleep only when sleepy; and get out of bed if anxiety occurs while unable to sleep • Adopt good sleep hygiene: avoidance of substances that interfere with sleep, avoidance of naps to maximize sleep drive, and optimization of the comfort of the sleep environment *Classification* • *Insomnia:* short-term insomnia disorder, chronic insomnia disorder, and other insomnia disorder • *Sleep-related breathing disorders*: central sleep apnea syndromes, obstructive sleep apnea disorders, sleep-related hypoventilation disorders, sleep-related hypoxemia disorder • *Central disorders of hypersomnolence:* narcolepsy type, idiopathic hypersomnia, hypersomnia due to a medical disorder, hypersomnia due to a medication or substance, hypersomnia associated with a psychiatric disorder, insufficient sleep syndrome • *Circadian rhythm sleep-wake disorders:* chronic/recurrent pattern of sleep-wake rhythm disruption caused by an alteration in the endogenous circadian timing system and the desired or required sleep-wake schedule • *Parasomnias:* undesirable physical events (complex movements, behaviors) or experiences (emotions, perceptions, dreams) that occur during entry into sleep, within sleep, or during arousals from sleep • *Sleep-related movement disorders*: restless legs syndrome, periodic limb movement disorder, sleep-related cramps, sleep-related bruxism (teeth grinding), sleep-related rhythmic movement disorder, benign sleep myoclonus of infancy, propriospinal myoclonus at sleep onset, sleep-related movement disorder due to a medical disorder, sleep-related movement disorder due to a medication or substance, sleep-related movement disorder, unspecified • *Other sleep disorders:* a myriad of other sleep disorders which are beyond the scope of this book

(continued)

Table 7.1 (continued)

Diagnosis and classification	Treatment and relevant clinical features: respiratory conditions
Tuberculosis Communicable disease caused by *Mycobacterium tuberculosis*. The bacilli usually attack the lungs, causing pulmonary TB *Terminology* • Latent tuberculosis infection • Primary tuberculosis • Active tuberculosis • Drug-resistant tuberculosis • Multidrug-resistant tuberculosis • Extensively drug-resistant tuberculosis	*Treatment* • Prompt referral to tertiary center taking reasonable anti-contagion measures, for example, nose-mouth mask on the patient • TB bacteria can also attack other parts of the body, such as the spine, lymph nodes, brain, and kidneys; this is known as extra-pulmonary TB • The common tab drugs are: Isoniazid tab: 5 mg/kg per day in a single dose, maximum daily dose 300 mg Pyrazinamide, tab, 400 mg, 500 mg or 750 mg: 25 mg/kg, Ethambutol (Myambutol) tab, 100 mg or 400 mg: 25 mg/kg Rifampin (Rifadin), tab, 300 mg: yy/kg *Risk factors for acquisition of infection* • Household exposure • Incarceration • Drug use • Residence in in endemic area • Chest radiograph: pulmonary opacities mostly of apical location • Acid fast bacilli on smear of sputum or sputum culture positive for *M. tuberculosis* *Signs and symptoms* • Chills, rigor, fever, and night sweats • Fatigue • Loss of appetite • Weight loss and weakness or tiring easily • Malaise (a feeling of general discomfort or illness) • Productive cough
Upper respiratory tract infection *Terminology* • The common cold • Influenza • Infectious mononucleosis • Pertussis • Pharyngitis • Sinusitis	*Treatment* • Paracetamol, 500 mg tabs, 3 × 2 tab/d as needed (max 4 g daily) • Mostly self-limiting *Prevention* • Preventing spread of infection (hand hygiene) • Adherence to local vaccination schemes *Signs and symptoms* • Fever • Cough • Runny nose • No fast breathing

Contents

8.1 **History: Questions to Ask** 87

8.2 **Physical Examination** 87

8.3 **Cardinal Paramedical Gastroenterology Examinations** 87

8.4 **Gastroenterology Red Flags** 87

Gastrointestinal disorders comprise any condition or disease that occurs within the gastrointestinal tract: namely mouth, esophagus, stomach, small intestine, large intestine, and anus (Fig. 8.1).

Afflictions of the gastroenterology system are common presentations among all age groups (Table 8.1). Most conditions are self-limiting entities. Specific diagnoses of self-limiting conditions include simple gastroenteritis, diet-induced constipation, and food intolerances (for example, lactose). Therapy entails eviction of the causative agent, increased fluid intake, and appropriate dietary advice.

Life-threatening gastroenterology pathologies are also encountered. In those circumstances, history and/or physical examinations reveal "red flags." These include fever, bloody diarrhea, mucous diarrhea, and signs of dehydration. Ingestion of food contaminated with salmonella or shigella may be revealed by a carefully taken history. The detection of red flags warrants prompt institution of antibiotherapy.

Esophageal and gastroduodenal affliction secondary to *H. pylori* infection has a high prevalence, estimated to be 80% in the general public. Good history and physical examination in the absence of available paramedical evaluation is sufficient to start the triple therapy to eradicate *H. pylori*.

Malformations such as Hirschsprung's disease, sigma-rectal volvulus, and vesicorectal fistulae are also encountered. Inflammatory GI conditions, such as Crohn's and ulcerative hemorrhagic rectocolitis are rare but should be borne in mind.

Infectious and oncologic hepatopathies are responsible for a significant incidence of mortality and morbidity. A clinical approach combined with a judicious use of pertinent laboratory tests and abdominal ultrasonography are sufficient to make the diagnosis and gauge the prognosis.

The risk of colorectal cancers should always be considered by the examining clinician. Do not shy away from proctology. Common symptoms are bleeding per rectum, perianal pruritus, and anal pain, which may be exacerbated during defecation.

© The Author(s), under exclusive license to Springer Nature Switzerland AG 2021
M. Touray, A. Touray, *Clinical Work and General Management of a Standard Minimal-Resource Facility*, Sustainable Development Goals Series, https://doi.org/10.1007/978-3-030-71032-3_8

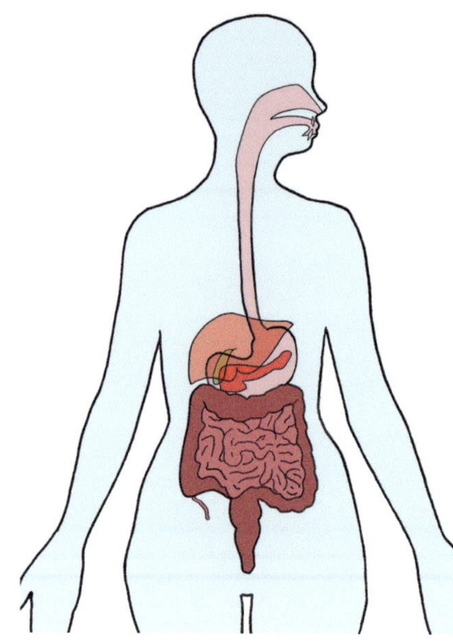

Gastroenterology

Abdominal pain (p88)
Anal fissure (pile) (p90)
Anorectal infections: Proctitis (p91)
Antibiotic-associated colitis (p91)
Ascites (p89)
Cholecystitis (p91)
Cholelithiasis (p92)
Chronic hepatic disease (p92)
Chronic pancreatitis (p92)
Common GI complaints (p98)
Constipation (p93)
Diabetic gastroparesis (p94)
Diarrhea (p94)
Diverticular disease of the colon (p95)
Gastric tumors (p95)
Gastritis and Gastropathies (p96)
Gastroenteritis (p96)
Gastroesophageal reflux diseases (p97)
Gastrointestinal gas (p97)
Halitosis (p98)
Helminthic infections (p99)
Hemorrhoids (p99)
Hepatocellular carcinoma (p99)
Hiatus hernia (p99)
Hiccups (p99)
Hirschsprung disease (p100)
Inflammatory bowel disease (p100)
Intestinal obstructions (p101)
Irritable bowel syndrome (p101)
Larva migrans (cutaneous hookworm) (p102)
Malnutrition (p102)
Mesenteric ischemia (p103)
Pancreatitis (p90)
Perianal pruritus (p103)
Perineal fistulas (p104)
Rectal prolapse (p104)
Schistosomiasis/Bilharziasis (p104)
Sigmoid volvulus (p106)
Spontaneous bacterial peritonitis (p105)
Ulcerative colitis (p105)

Fig. 8.1 Gastroenterology: A mnemonic illustration representing main gastrointestinal anatomic structures and their corresponding pathologies

8.1 History: Questions to Ask

- Do you have belly pain?
- Do have nausea, vomiting, or diarrhea?
- Has your appetite changed?
- Have you lost or gained weight?
- Has the color of your stool changed? Any blood and/or mucus?

8.2 Physical Examination

- Inspect the form of the abdomen: globulus, caput medusae, distended?
- Any scars?
- Palpate: any tenderness, any mass, organomegaly?
- Auscultate: frequency and quality of bowel noises?

8.3 Cardinal Paramedical Gastroenterology Examinations

- Full blood count
- Stool examination (macroscopy and microscopy)
- SS-Agar-based identification of shigella and salmonella in stool sample
- Urine sticks
- Pregnancy test (beta-hCG)
- Abdominal echography
- Plane abdominal X-ray

8.4 Gastroenterology Red Flags

- Nonintentional significant loss of weight (>10% of habitual weight)
- Progressive dysphagia and/or odynophagia
- More than 1 week of persistent vomiting
- Unexplained anemia
- Hematemesis, rectorrhagia, and/or melena
- Past history of gastric surgery
- Palpable abdominal mass or palpable adenopathy
- Flagrant jaundice
- Voluminous diarrhea or nocturnal diarrhea
- Positive family history for chronic inflammatory disease, and colorectal or ovarian cancer
- Recent prolonged antibiotherapy
- Associated high fever (>38.5°C)
- Gross abnormal laboratory findings: aspartate aminotransferase (ASAT) and alanine aminotransferase (ALAT) >5× upper limit, thrombocytopenia
- Evidence for the hepatic encephalopathy: jaundice, confusion, and flapping tremor
- Positive Murphy signs, known or documented esophageal varices
- Age >50

Table 8.1 Gastroenterology conditions and their treatment

Diagnosis and classification	Treatment and relevant clinical features: gastroenterology conditions
Abdominal pain Pain felt in the area between the chest and the pelvis *Classification* • *Acute abdominal pain:* onset less than 3 weeks • *Chronic abdominal pain*: onset more than 3 weeks • *Abdominal pain of unspecified origin*: pain in the abdomen after exclusion of most common gastrointestinal diseases using history, physical examination, and appropriate paramedical investigations • *Surgical abdomen* or acute abdomen: Acute onset of severe abdominal pain with clinical signs of peritonitis (rebound tenderness, and distended nondepressible abdomen, most likely needing immediate surgical attention) *Regional approach* • Right upper quadrant pain • Epigastric pain • Left upper quadrant pain • Lower abdominal pain • Diffuse abdominal pain	*Treatment* • Attempt to identify and treat underlying cause • In the absence of identified cause: counsel and provide psychological support • In sustained case: Amitriptyline, tab, 25 mg, 1 tab/d, 21 d, maximum daily dose 75 mg • If psychological support proves insufficient, consider an SRRI *Clinical evaluation* • Description: location and radiation, temporal elements, temporal elements, severity, precipitants or palliation, and associated symptoms • *Associated symptoms: other gastrointestinal symptoms* (nausea, vomiting, diarrhea, constipation, hematochezia, melena, and changes in transit) • *Genitourinary symptoms*: dysuria, frequency, and hematuria • *Constitutional symptoms*: fevers, chills, fatigue, weight loss, and anorexia would be concerning for infection, malignancy, or systemic illnesses • *Cardiopulmonary symptoms:* cough, dyspnea, orthopnea, and exercise intolerance may suggest a pulmonary or cardiac etiology. Orthostatic hypotension may indicate early shock or be associated with adrenal insufficiency • *Supplementary history*: past medical history • Alcohol, family history, travel history, sick contacts, and comprehensive medication history: NSAID and steroid use • *Physical examination*: vital signs, abdominal examination (inspection, auscultation, percussion, and palpation), rectal examination, pelvic examination, and eyes for scleral icterus • *Paramedical studies:* determined by history and physical examination *Red flags in the setting of abdominal pain* • Unstable vital signs • Signs of peritonitis on abdominal exam, for example, abdominal rigidity and rebound tenderness • Clinical suspicion that the abdominal pain is from a life-threatening condition (e.g., acute bowel obstruction, acute mesenteric ischemia, perforation, acute myocardial infarction, and ectopic pregnancy) *Judicious use of paramedical studies* • Blood urea nitrogen (BUN), creatinine, and blood glucose • Complete blood count with differential • Lipase and/or amylase • Pregnancy test in women of childbearing age • Aminotransferases, alkaline phosphatase, and bilirubin • Electrolytes (Na/K) when available • Abdominal echography • Thoracoabdominal computer tomography where available

Table 8.1 (continued)

Diagnosis and classification	Treatment and relevant clinical features: gastroenterology conditions
	Differential diagnosis • Right upper quadrant pain: acute hepatitis, perihepatitis, liver abscess, Budd-Chiari syndrome, portal vein thrombosis, biliary colic, acute cholecystitis, and acute cholangitis • *Epigastric pain*: acute myocardial infarction, acute pancreatitis, chronic pancreatitis, peptic ulcer disease, gastroesophageal reflux disease, gastritis/gastropathy, functional dyspepsia, and gastroparesis • *Left upper quadrant pain*: splenomegaly, splenic infarct, splenic abscess, and splenic rupture • *Lower abdominal pain:* appendicitis, diverticulitis, nephrolithiasis, pyelonephritis, acute urinary retention, cystitis, and infectious colitis • *Diffuse abdominal pain:* lactose intolerance, bowel obstruction, perforation of the gastrointestinal tract, acute mesenteric ischemia, inflammatory bowel disease (ulcerative colitis/Crohn's disease), viral gastroenteritis, spontaneous bacterial peritonitis, colorectal cancer, ketoacidosis, adrenal insufficiency, irritable bowel syndrome, blood-borne illness, constipation, and diverticulosis *Clinical tips* • Irritable bowel syndrome is common. It is proposed after excluding other causes
Ascites Accumulation of fluid in the abdominal cavity *Grading ascites* • Grade 1—mild ascites detectable only by ultrasound examination • Grade 2—moderate ascites manifested by moderate symmetrical distension of the abdomen • Grade 3—large or gross ascites with marked abdominal distension *Description of ascites* • Clear • Turbid or cloudy • Milky • Opalescent • Pink or hemorrhagic • Brown	*Treatment* • Determine and address underlying cause • Palliative ascites paracentesis *and/or* • Spironolactone, 25 mg tabs, 2 tabs/morning, as needing *and* • Torsemide tabs, 5 mg, 1 tab/morning *Etiology* • *Hepatic origin/portal hypertension:* cirrhosis, alcoholic hepatitis, acute liver failure, and hepatic veno-occlusive disease • *Cardiac origin:* heart failure and constrictive pericarditis • *Peritoneal disease:* malignant ascites, for example, ovarian cancer: infectious peritonitis, for example, tuberculosis or fungal infection, and eosinophilic gastroenteritis • *Hypoalbunemia*: severe malnutrition, nephrotic syndrome, and protein losing enteropathy • *Myxedema* • *Cancer* • *Tuberculosis* • *Pancreatic disease* *Clinical signs and symptoms* • Abdominal distension that may be painless or associated with abdominal discomfort • Weight gain • Early satiety, and dyspnea resulting from fluid accumulation and increased abdominal pressure • Fever, abdominal tenderness, and altered mental status

(continued)

Table 8.1 (continued)

Diagnosis and classification	Treatment and relevant clinical features: gastroenterology conditions
	Characterizing ascites • Tests for tuberculous peritonitis • Total protein concentration • Cell count • Culture • Glucose concentration • Lactate dehydrogenase concentration • Gram stain • Cytology • Carcinoembryonic antigen concentration (CAE)
Pancreatitis Inflammatory process of the pancreas *Classification based on time of onset* • *Acute:* onset less than 3 weeks • *Chronic:* onset more than 3 weeks *Classification based on intensity of pain and organ damage* • *Mild*: absence of organ failure and local or systemic complications • *Moderately severe*; transient organ failure (resolves within 48 h) and/or local or systemic complications without persistent organ failure (>48 h) • *Severe*: persistent organ failure that may involve one or multiple organs *Differential diagnosis* • Peptic ulcer disease • Choledocholithiasis or cholangitis • Cholecystitis • Perforated viscus • Intestinal obstruction • Mesenteric ischemia • Hepatitis	*Treatment* • Supportive treatment • Adequate pain control • Antibiotherapy if concomitant signs of infection • Ceftriaxone 500 mg ampoule, 3 × 1 amp/d, and then switch to oral after 24 h Co-amoxicillin, tab, 1 g, 1 tab/d, 7 d *Etiology* • Mechanical • Toxic • Metabolic • Infection • Trauma • Congenital • Vascular *Paramedical investigations* • Laboratory findings: elevated serum lipase or amylase • Imaging: abdominal and chest radiographs • Abdominal ultrasound • Abdominal computer tomography *Sign and symptoms of acute/chronic pancreatitis*: • *Acute pancreatitis:* upper abdominal pain, abdominal pain that radiates to the back, abdominal pain that feels worse after eating, fever, rapid pulse, nausea, vomiting, and tenderness when touching the abdomen • *Chronic pancreatitis*: upper abdominal pain, losing weight without trying, and oily, smelly stools (steatorrhea) *Clinical features of acute pancreatitis* • Abrupt onset of epigastric pain with radiation to the back • Often related to alcohol intake • Nausea, vomiting, sweating, and weakness • Abdominal tenderness and distention or fever • High white blood cell count • Elevated serum amylase • Elevated serum lipase
Anal fissure Linear-shaped ulcers that are usually less than 5 mm in length located in the perianal skin folds *Synonyms* • Pile • Intergluteal fissure	*Treatment* • Appropriate dietary advice to promote regular bowel movement • Proper perineal hygiene: wash regularly with neutral soap, apply hydrating creams to avoid xeroderma • Surgical treatment where available *Etiology* • Trauma to the anorectal wall during defecation caused by straining • Constipation • High internal sphincter muscular tone

Table 8.1 (continued)

Diagnosis and classification	Treatment and relevant clinical features: gastroenterology conditions
Pathogenesis • Starts with a tear to the anoderm within the anal canal • The tear then triggers cycles of recurring anal pain and bleeding • Results in the development of a chronic anal fissure • Common cause of anal pain and anal bleeding	*Management tips* Provide diets that promote regular bowel movement: • Five fruits per day • 3 L of clean water per day • Walk at least 30 min per day
Anorectal infections: Proctitis Inflammation of the anorectal area by infection	*Treatment* • Identify and treat the etiology • Advice to improve anogenital hygiene • For fungal infection: Clotrimazole cream 5%, apply 2× daily *Etiologic agents of proctitis* • *Neisseria gonorrhea* • *Treponema pallidum* • *Chlamydia trachomatis* • Herpes simplex type 2 *Signs and symptoms* • Anorectal discomfort • Tender anal sphincter • Constipation • Condylomata acuminata
Antibiotic-associated colitis A common complication of prolonged antibiotherapy, *Clostridium difficile,* is an anaerobic, gram-positive, spore-forming bacillus that colonizes the intestinal tract after alteration of the normal gastrointestinal flora	*Treatment* • Metronidazole tabs, 500 mg 3 × 1 tab/d, 10 d *Diagnostic features* • Most cases of antibiotic-associated diarrhea do not involve *Clostridium difficile*
Cholecystitis A syndrome of right upper quadrant pain, fever, and leukocytosis associated with gallbladder inflammation *Paramedical evaluation* Ultrasonographic is effective in diagnosing: Sonographic Murphy	*Treatment* • Cefalexin tabs, 500 mg, 3 × 500 mg, 7 d • Paracetamol, tab, 500 mg, 3 × 2 tab/d as needed *Pathogenesis* • Mostly occurs in the setting of cystic duct obstruction • Secondary infection of bile within the biliary system contributes to development of cholecystitis *Risk factors (6 Fs mnemonic)* • Female • Fat • Fair • Family • Fertile • Over 40 years *Clinical manifestation* • Abdominal pain: right upper quadrant or epigastrium • Fever • Nausea • Vomiting • Anorexia • Positive Murphy's sign • Leukocytosis with an increased number of band forms (i.e., a left shift)

(continued)

Table 8.1 (continued)

Diagnosis and classification	Treatment and relevant clinical features: gastroenterology conditions
Cholelithiasis Presence of gallstones in the gall bladder *Compositions* • Cholesterol stones • Black pigment stones • Brown pigment stones	*Treatment* • Advise diet rich in fiber • Regular physical exercise • Weight reduction • Cholecystectomy • Ursodeoxycholic acid, Urso Forte, tab, 300 mg, 2 × 1 tab/d, 2 weeks *Drugs implicated in gallstone formation* Fibrates Ceftriaxone Hormone replacement Oral contraceptive *Note* • Presence of gall stones in the gall bladder is highly prevalent • The majority of cases are asymptomatic
Chronic hepatic disease *Classification* • Infectious: viral, bacterial, and parasitic • Nonalcoholic fatty liver disease, alcoholic hepatitis, and primary biliary cholangitis • Primary sclerosing cholangitis	*Treatment* • Treat complications of disease • Ascites • Salt-restricted diet • Oral Torsemide tab, 5 mg, 1 tab/d *and* • Spironolacton tab, 25 mg, 1 tab/d, • If hyponatremia: <130 mmol/L liquid restriction Hepatic encephalopathy • Low-protein diet and laxatives *and* • Laxative, for example, Bisacodyl, tab, 5 mg/d, 5 d *Evaluation* • Conduct routine screening for Hepatitis B virus infection • Ultrasound • Alpha-fetoprotein dosage follow-up to know if it evolves to cirrhosis or hepatocellular carcinoma • Refer to appropriate tertiary center for hepatology unit for management and possible enrollment into cancer screening study *Etiology* • Viral hepatitis B, C, and D • Side effects of herbal treatment • Alcoholic hepatitis • Parasitic (helminth) • Toxic (Paracetamol, anti-TB treatment, etc.) • Metabolic • Traumatic *Complication* • Hepatocellular carcinoma; management mostly palliative • Refer to appropriate tertiary hepatology unit for management and possible enrollment into hepatic cancer study
Chronic pancreatitis (CP) A syndrome involving progressive inflammatory changes in the pancreas that result in permanent structural damage, which can lead to impairment of exocrine and endocrine function	*Treatment* • Identify the underlying etiology • Analgesia: Tramadol tabs, 100 mg, 3 × 1 tab/5 d *and* • Ibuprofen 400 mg tabs, 3 × 1 tab/d *and* • Omeprazole 20 mg tabs/1 tab/d 10 d • Creon Amylase (8000 U), and Lipase (10000 U), and Protease (600 U) tab, 1, tab, during or after a meal 2–3×/d • Refer to an appropriate tertiary center for tertiary care

Table 8.1 (continued)

Diagnosis and classification	Treatment and relevant clinical features: gastroenterology conditions
Complications • Pseudocyst formation • Bile duct or duodenal obstruction • Pancreatic ascites or pleural effusion • Splenic vein thrombosis • Pseudoaneurysm • Pancreatic cancer *Differential diagnosis* • Pancreatic cancer • Autoimmune pancreatitis • Lymphoma • Pancreatic endocrine tumors • Acute pancreatitis	*Pathogenesis* • Recurrent episodes of acute pancreatitis may lead to chronic pancreatitis over time *Chronic versus acute pancreatitis* • CP may be asymptomatic over long periods of time • The serum amylase and lipase concentrations tend to be normal in patients with CP • Morphologically, CP is a patchy focal disease characterized by a mononuclear infiltrate and fibrosis *Clinical features* • Chronic intermittent epigastric pain • Steatorrhea due to fat malabsorption • Pancreatic diabetes • Weight loss • Abnormal pancreatic imaging
Constipation A stool frequency of less than 3 per week. The condition is often treated on the basis of a patient's impression that there is a disturbance in bowel function	*Treatment* • Identify and treat underlying cause: In general, advice patient to eat and exercise well: eat five fruits a day, drink 3 L of water a day, and walk at least 30 min a day • Fiber-rich diet with adequate fluid intake • Bisacodyl, tab, 5 mg, 1 tab/d *Causes of constipation* • Inadequate fiber or fluid intake (dehydration) • Poor bowel movement, bowel obstruction • Systemic disease conditions: hypothyroidism, diabetes, uremia, and neurologic conditions • Medications: calcium channel blockers, psychotropics, and NSAIDs • Structural abnormalities, rectal prolapse, rectoceles, intussusception, and anal fissures • Slow colonic transit • Pelvic floor dyssynergia • Irritable bowel syndrome • Psychogenic *Diagnosis based upon the presence of the following* • Straining during defecations • Lumpy or hard stools • Sensation of incomplete evacuation • Sensation of anorectal obstruction • Manual maneuvers to facilitate (e.g., digital evacuation and support of the pelvic floor) • Fewer than three spontaneous bowel movements per week *Type of laxatives* • Mucilage • Osmotic (Movicol) • Stimulant enables peristalsis and lowers the reabsorption of water and electrolytes, for example, Bisacodyl

(continued)

Table 8.1 (continued)

Diagnosis and classification	Treatment and relevant clinical features: gastroenterology conditions
Diabetic gastroparesis A syndrome of objectively delayed gastric emptying in the absence of a mechanical obstruction	*Treatment* • Paracetamol, tab, 500 mg, 3 × 2 tab/d as needed (max 4 g daily) • Mostly self-limiting *Prevention* • Adequate long-term control of blood sugar level • Preventing spread of infection (hand hygiene) • Adherence to local vaccination schemes *Signs and symptoms* • Fever • Cough • Runny nose • No fast breathing
Diarrhea Passage of loose or watery stools, at least three times in a 24-h period *Classification* • *Acute diarrhea:* ≤14 d in duration • *Persistent diarrhea*: >14 d and ≤30 d • *Chronic diarrhea*: >30 d of diarrhea • *Invasive diarrhea or dysentery*: diarrhea with visible blood • *Watery diarrhea*: also termed rice water diarrhea	*Treatment* • Determine underlying cause: watery diarrhea usually does not need antibiotherapy; treat with oral rehydration and watchful waiting • Rehydration: adequate fluid intake, ORS, syrup, soup, tea (up to 3 L in 24 h), assure good urine output • Azithromycin, tab, 500 mg, 1 tab/d, 3 d *or* • Ciproxin tabs, 500 mg, 2 × 1 tab/d, 5 d *Prevention* • Regular hand washing with soap • Provision of safe drinking water • Adequate disposal of human waste • Breastfeeding of infants and young children • Regularization of safe handling and processing of food • Control of flies and other vectors *Risk factors* • Crowding and poor sanitation • Immune suppression, for example, HIV infection *Microbiology* • Epidemic diarrhea: *Shigella dysenteriae, Vibrio cholerae*, and *Campylobacter* • Norwalk-like viruses • Enteroaggregative *E. coli* • Enterotoxigenic *Bacteroides fragilis* *Clinical features and complications* • Hypovolemia of various severity • Sunken eyes, dry mouth and tongue, thirst, and decreased skin turgor • Decreased consciousness, inability to drink, and a weak pulse • Acute kidney insufficiency • Bacteremia • Hemolytic uremic syndrome • Guillain-Barré syndrome *Clinical signs of diarrhea-induced hypovolemia* • Early hypovolemia—signs and symptoms may be absent • Moderate hypovolemia—thirst, restless or irritable behavior, decreased skin turgor, and sunken eyes • Severe hypovolemia—diminished consciousness, lack of urine output, cool moist extremities, rapid and week pulse, low or undetectable blood pressure, and peripheral cyanosis

Table 8.1 (continued)

Diagnosis and classification	Treatment and relevant clinical features: gastroenterology conditions
Diverticular disease of the colon Presence of diverticula particularly. The sigmoid is the part of the colon exposed to the highest pressure *Diagnostic features of diverticulitis* • Acute abdominal pain and fever • Left lower abdominal tenderness and mass • High white blood cell count *Risk factors* • Diet: low fiber, high fat, and red meat • Physical inactivity • Obesity • Cigarette smoking • Drugs: chronic overuse of NSAIDs, steroids, and opiates	*Treatment* • Symptomatic relief with adequate pain control: Paracetamol tab, 500 mg, 3 × 2 tabs/d, 5 d Where antibiotherapy indicated • Ciproxin tabs, 500 mg, 3 × 1 tab/, 10 d *Pathogenesis* • Diverticula develop at weak spots • Mucosa and submucosa to herniate through the muscle layer • Abnormal colonic motility is an important predisposing factor *Nomenclature* • *Diverticulum* is a sac-like protrusion of the colonic wall • *Diverticulosis* is the presence of diverticula and may be asymptomatic or symptomatic • *Diverticular disease* is clinically significant; symptomatic diverticulosis due to diverticular bleeding, diverticulitis, or segmental colitis • *Diverticulitis* inflammation, and focal necrosis ensues, resulting in perforation • *Diverticular bleeding:* as a diverticulum herniates, over time, the vasa recta and artery are exposed to injury, predisposing them to rupture into the lumen • *Segmental colitis* associated with diverticula • Symptomatic uncomplicated diverticular disease
Gastric tumors A mass in the gastric mucosal lining detected by clinical examination or paramedical investigation *Nomenclature* • *Early gastric cancer* is invasive gastric cancer that invades no more deeply than the submucosa • *Gastric adenocarcinoma* • *Gastrointestinal stromal tumors* • *Gastric polyps* • *Lymphomas* may be primary or secondary *Clinical features* • Weight loss • Abdominal pain tends to be epigastric, vague, and mild early in the disease • Dysphagia • *Diagnostic tools* • Abdominopelvic CT scan • Endoscopic ultrasonography • Chest imaging	*Treatment* • Characterize clinically • Abdominal echography followed by prompt referral to a tertiary center Protective factors • Fruits, vegetables, and fiber • Reproductive hormones *Serological tumor markers* • Serum levels of carcinoembryonic antigen (CEA) • The glycoprotein CA 125 antigen (CA 125), • Carbohydrate antigen 19–9 (CA 19–9) • Cancer antigen 72–4 (CA72 4) may be elevated in patients with gastric cancer *Red flags suggestive of a gastrointestinal malignancy* • New onset of dyspepsia in patient ≥ 60 years • Evidence of gastrointestinal bleeding (hematemesis, melena, hematochezia, and occult blood in stool) • Iron deficiency anemia • Anorexia • Unexplained weight loss • Dysphagia • Odynophagia • Persistent vomiting • Gastrointestinal cancer in a first-degree relative *Signs and symptoms* • Dull epigastric pains • Vomiting blood • Black tarry stools • Anemia • Palpable epigastric mass

(continued)

Table 8.1 (continued)

Diagnosis and classification	Treatment and relevant clinical features: gastroenterology conditions
	Risk factors • Diet: salt and salt-preserved foods • Low folate levels • Obesity • Smoking • Occupational exposures • *Helicobacter pylori* • Alcohol • Socioeconomic status • Gastric surgery
Gastritis and Gastropathies *Gastritis* is an inflammatory process involving the gastric mucosa *Gastropathy* is a gastric mucosal disorder with minimal to no inflammation *Nomenclature* • Nonerosive gastritis: *Helicobacter pylori* or stress-induced gastritis, nonerosive • Erosive gastritis • Hemorrhagic gastritis • NSAID-induced gastritis • Alcoholic gastritis • Portal hypertensive gastropathy	*Treatment* • Triple therapy if *Helicobacter pylori*: • Doxycycline, tab, 100 mg, 1 tab/d, 10 d *or* • Amoxicillin, tab, 500 mg, 3 × 1 tab/d, 10 d *and* • Metronidazole, tab, 500 mg, 3 × 1 tab/d, 10 d *and* • Omeprazole, tab, 40 mg, 1 tab/d, 10 d *Clinical management* • Comprehensive patient education • When clinical suspicion is high, presumptive diagnosis can be made and treated: *Helicobacter pylori* • Avoid spicy foods and very hot beverages, as it has been shown that these increase the incidence of esophageal metaplasia • Long-term reflux can cause metaplasia of the esophageal epithelium, called Barrett's esophagus *Complications of ulcer disease* • Gastrointestinal hemorrhage • Perforation • Gastric outlet obstruction *Management tips* • Advise weight loss if obese • Eat small, frequent, regular meals, and avoid fatty foods • Smoking and alcohol cessation • Avoid stooping/bending down from the waist, especially after eating • Avoid tight clothes • Elevate head of bed or use a pillow
Gastroenteritis Diarrheal disease (three or more times per day) of rapid onset that lasts less than 2 weeks and may be accompanied by nausea, vomiting, fever, or abdominal pain *Classification* Acute watery diarrhea • Cholera • Dysentery • Antibiotic induced *Etiology* • Viral (norovirus) • Bacterial infections • Food intolerance	*Treatment* • Mostly self-limiting: advise on high fluid intake (>3L/24 h) Antibiotherapy: indicated when fever, bloody diarrhea, and duration more than 3 weeks • Ciproxin, tab, 500 mg, 2 × 1 tab/d, 5 d *or* • Doxycycline, tab, 100 mg, 2 × 1 tab/hourly, 5 d • In pregnancy: Erythromycin tab, 500 mg, 4 × 1-tab/d, 5 d • Oral rehydration solution (ORS), sachet, 3 × 1 sachets/d, 3 d *and* • NaCl 0.9%, iv infusion bag, 2 bags iv, in case of severe dehydration • Domperidone (Motilium), tab, 10 mg, 3 × 1 tab/d, 5 d *Clinical management* • Improved personal and food hygiene • Often viral with spontaneous resolution • Treat with antibiotics when signs of dysentery: bloody stool, mucopurulent stool, fever > 38°C, and pain

Table 8.1 (continued)

Diagnosis and classification	Treatment and relevant clinical features: gastroenterology conditions
	Criteria for hospitalization • Volume depletion/dehydration • Intractable vomiting • Abnormal electrolytes or renal function • Excessive bloody stool or rectal bleeding • Severe abdominal pain • Symptoms more than 1 week • Age 65 or older with signs of hypovolemia • Comorbidities (e.g., diabetes mellitus and immunocompromise) • Pregnancy *Clinical manifestation* • Diarrhea, nausea, vomiting, fever, or abdominal pain • Diffuse abdominal tenderness on palpation • Signs of dehydration: dry mucous membranes, decreased skin turgor, tachycardia, and hypotension • Altered mental status *Management tips* • Encourage high fluid intake: chicken soup, tea, syrups, etc. • For every professional food handler, perform stool test (searching for salmonella and shigella). If test positive, treat food handlers even when asymptomatic • A 5-d course of oral Ciproxin: 500 mg 2×/d • Discourage the use of loperamide, tab, 4 mg
Gastroesophageal reflux diseases (GERD) Upward passage of gastric contents into the esophagus is a normal, physiologic process. Gastroesophageal reflux disease (GERD) is present when reflux is associated with symptoms or complications	*Treatment* • Diet advice: frequent small meals • Omeprazole, tab, 40 mg, 1 tab/d • Advice to go to bed minimum 3 h after food ingestion • Adequate use of pillows to raise the head when in decubitus *Clinical features* • Heartburn (pyrosis) • Regurgitation • Dysphagia • Chest pain • Hypersalivation • Globus sensation is the almost constant perception of a lump in the throat • Nausea *Terminology* • Erosive esophagitis • Nonerosive reflux disease
Gastrointestinal gas Subjective feeling of excessive intestinal gas which may be due to excessive air swallowing, increased intraluminal production from malabsorbed nutrients, decreased gas absorption due to obstruction or dysfunctional gas clearance, or expansion of intraluminal gas	*Treatment* • Identify underlying cause • Treat accordingly • Provide ample education • Advice to improve eating habit: eat slowly, chew adequately, swallow with closed mouth, and avoid talking when chewing • If lactose intolerance suspected, advice milk eviction *Belching:* involuntary or voluntary expulsion of air from the stomach or esophagus *Flatus and bloating:* passing per anus of air swallowed or of gas derived from bacterial fermentation of undigested carbohydrates

(continued)

Table 8.1 (continued)

Diagnosis and classification	Treatment and relevant clinical features: gastroenterology conditions
Common GI complaints • Belching • Bloating • Abdominal pain • Flatulence *Sources of GI gas* • Air swallowing • Intraluminal production • Diffusion from the blood	*Etiology/differential diagnosis* • Dietary: gas-producing foods • Excessive air swallowing • Increased intraluminal production from malabsorbed nutrients • Intestinal obstruction: adhesions and malignancies • Motility disorder: diabetes and medication • Irritable bowel syndrome • Malabsorption: lactose intolerance • Decreased gas absorption due to obstruction • Expansion of intraluminal gas due to changes in atmospheric pressure • Infectious: small intestinal bacterial overgrowth and giardiasis *Red flags in patients with flatulence* • Nocturnal abdominal pain • Weight loss • Hematochezia • Systemic symptoms including weight loss or fever • Diarrhea or steatorrhea • Vomiting • Severe abdominal tenderness, organomegaly
Halitosis Bad breath, malodor with intensity beyond a socially acceptable level perceived *Terminology* • Physiologic halitosis • Pathologic halitosis • Pseudohalitosis *Subjective halitosis (pseudohalitosis)* is complaint of bad breath without objective confirmation. It is classified as psychologic or neurologic *Management tips* Patients need ensured confidentiality and an appropriate history taking constellation to talk about this humiliating and debilitating symptom	*Treatment* • Identify the cause and treat it When no identified cause: • Proper hydration • Good oral hygiene • Omeprazole, tab, 40 mg, 2 × 1 tab/d, 21 d *Etiology:* cause may be multifactorial, originating from any of the many organic components *Intraoral causes* • Poor oral hygiene • Gingivitis and periodontitis caused by gram-negative anaerobes • Dental caries and food rest • Excessive tongue covering • Xerostomia as in salivary gland dysfunction • Tonsillar pathologies • Oral tumors with necrosis *Nasal causes* • Acute or chronic sinusitis • Postnasal drip • Foreign bodies in the nose *Respiratory causes* • Pulmonary infections • Gastroesophageal reflux • Zenker's diverticulum • Gastrocolic fistulae • *Helicobacter pylori* infection • GERD *Systemic diseases* • Advanced renal disease • Advanced liver disease (fetor hepaticus) • Diabetic ketoacidosis *Advice* If no specific cause for the halitosis is found, advise on improving dental and oral hygiene

Table 8.1 (continued)

Diagnosis and classification	Treatment and relevant clinical features: gastroenterology conditions
Helminthic infections (worm infection) Infestation of the abdominal lumen and mucosal lining with worms *Classification* • Flatworms such as trematodes and cestodes • Thorny headed worms • Roundworms or nematodes: *Taenia saginata, Taenia solium,* and *Hymenolepsis nana* • Hookworm • It is common and causes anemia	*Treatment* • Mebendazole, tab, 100 mg, 2 × 1 tab/d, 3 d *or* • Mebendazole, tab, 500 mg start dose • To be repeated in 10 d *or* • Albendazole, 400 mg single dose • To be repeated after 10 d *Note:* Helminthicides are directed against hatched worms and have no effect on eggs. If treatment is not repeated in 10 d, a reinfection cycle will persist *Management tips* Repeat course after 10 d: explain to the patient why *Signs and symptoms* • Anal itching • Cough • Worms in stool • Abdominal distension • Skin itching • Weight loss • Anemic symptoms: fatigue, pallor, dizziness, and headache • Abdominal cramps and pain • Vomiting and constipation
Hemorrhoids Normal vascular structures in the anal canal arising from a channel of arteriovenous connective tissues that drains into the superior and inferior hemorrhoidal veins	*Treatment* • Laxative if constipation: Lactulose 10–20 g (15–30 mL) every other day *or* • Bisacodyl tab, 5 mg, 1 tab/d 5 d • Paracetamol, 500 mg tabs, 3 × 2 tab/d as needed (max 4 g daily) • Mostly self-limiting *Prevention* Advice to avoid constipation: eat five fruits a day, drink 2–3 liters of water a day, and walk at least 1 h a day
Hepatocellular carcinoma (HCC) An aggressive tumor of hepatocellular origin that often occurs in the setting of chronic liver disease and cirrhosis	*Treatment* • Management mainly palliative • Refer to MRC hepatology unit for management and possible enrollment into hepatic cancer study • Refer to MRC Hepatology Unit
Hiatus hernia Herniation of elements of the abdominal cavity through the esophageal hiatus of the diaphragm	*Treatment* • Treat as GERD when symptomatic: Omeprazole tab, 20 mg 1 tab/d, 6 weeks • Advise on dietary hygiene (eat and exercise well) • Use of cushions when in decubitus position • Eat at least 2–3 h before going to bed
Hiccups "Gasping" due to an involuntary, intermittent, spasmodic contraction of the diaphragm and intercostal muscles. Hiccups represent a reflex arc made up of several neural pathways	*Treatment* • Identify and treat underlying cause. In most cases, prokinetics (e.g., Domperidone) or muscle relaxants (e.g., Diazepam) or proton pump inhibitor (e.g., Omeprazole) may be prescribed • Omeprazole 20 mg tab, 2 × 1 tab/d 10 d *and/or* • Domperidone (Motilium) 10 mg, tab, 3 × 1 tab/d, as needed *or* • Diazepam 5 mg tabs, 2 × 1 tab/d as needed

(continued)

Table 8.1 (continued)

Diagnosis and classification	Treatment and relevant clinical features: gastroenterology conditions
	Causes of hiccups • Gastric distention, carbonated beverages, swallowing air, and overeating • Sudden temperature changes, hot liquids, and then cold showers • Alcohol ingestion • States of heightened emotion, excitement, stress, and laughing *Clinical features* • Usually benign and self-limited • May be persistent and distressful • Could be a sign of serious underlying illness
Hirschsprung's disease A congenital motor disorder of the gut caused by a developmental failure during fetal life. Results in noninnervated segment of the colon which fails to relax, causing a functional obstruction	*Treatment* • Refer to tertiary center for surgical care *Pathophysiology* • Think when newborn has no meconium • Defect in the craniocaudal migration of neuroblasts • Preponderant in males • Male-to-female ratio is 3:1
Inflammatory bowel disease This includes ulcerative colitis and Crohn's disease *Complications of Crohn's disease* • Abscess • Intestinal obstruction • Abdominal and rectovaginal fistulas • Perianal disease • Carcinoma • Hemorrhage • Malabsorption	*Treatment* • Salofalk (5 amino salicylic acid 5-ASA), tab, 500 mg, 3 × 1 tab/d *or* • Corticosteroid (Prednisolone 0.5 mg/kg, 1× daily) *or* • Immunomodulators and drugs, for example, methotrexate tab, 2.5 mg, 1 tab/w • Biologic therapies: anti-TNF need referral to tertiary center *Diagnostic features of Crohn's disease* • Insidious onset • Intermittent bouts of low-grade fever, diarrhea, and right lower quadrant pain • Right lower quadrant mass and tenderness • Perianal disease with abscess and fistulas • Radiographic or endoscopic evidence of ulceration, fissuring, or fistulas of the small intestine or colon *Pathophysiology* Red blood in stool caused by changes in the structure of the mucosa and submucosa of the wall of the colon, with widespread inflammation and superficial ulceration *Clinical manifestations* • Colitis • Fulminant colitis and toxic megacolon • Perforation • Musculoskeletal • Eye: uveitis and episcleritis • Skin: erythema nodosum and pyoderma gangrenosum • Hepatobiliary: primary sclerosing cholangitis and fatty liver

Table 8.1 (continued)

Diagnosis and classification	Treatment and relevant clinical features: gastroenterology conditions
Intestinal obstructions Perturbed physiologic peristaltic movement of the intestine leading to intraluminal retention of fecal material *Small bowel obstruction* Bowel obstruction occurs when the normal flow of intraluminal contents is interrupted. Obstruction can be • Functional (due to abnormal intestinal physiology) • Mechanical obstruction *Differential diagnosis* • Adynamic (paralytic) ileus • Large bowel obstruction	*Treatment* • Evaluate to determine underlying cause • Prompt referral to tertiary center for surgical review *Etiology* • Postoperative adhesions and hernias • Tumors • Stricture • Intramural hematoma • Intussusception • Gallstones • Foreign bodies *Risk factors* • Prior abdominal or pelvic surgery • Abdominal wall or groin hernia • Intestinal inflammation • History of or increased risk for neoplasm • Prior irradiation • History of foreign body ingestion *Diagnostic tools* • Plain radiography • Abdominal CT • Abdominal ultrasonography • Small bowel contrast enema *Signs and symptoms* • Dull epigastric pains • Hematemesis • Melena • Anemia *Clinical presentation* • Nausea • Vomiting • Cramping abdominal pain • Obstipation, that is, inability to pass flatus or stool • Signs of dehydration: tachycardia, orthostatic hypotension, reduced urine output, and dry mucus membrane • Abdominal distention • Hyperresonance or tympany to percussion • Abnormal masses on palpation • Gross or occult blood • Digital rectal examination (DRE): fecal impaction or rectal mass
Irritable bowel syndrome An idiopathic clinical entity characterized by chronic (>6 months) abdominal pain that occurs in association with altered bowel habits *Diagnostic features* • Chronic functional disorder characterized by abdominal pain with alterations in bowel habits • Symptoms usually begin in late teens, early 20s • Limited evaluation to exclude organic causes of symptoms	*Treatment* • Empathic psychologic support • Symptomatic treatment • Amitriptylin tab, 25 mg, 2 × 1 tab/d *Associated clinical conditions* • Fibromyalgia • Chronic fatigue syndrome • Gastroesophageal reflux disease • Functional dyspepsia and noncardiac • Chest pain • Psychiatric disorders: major depression, anxiety, and somatization

(continued)

Table 8.1 (continued)

Diagnosis and classification	Treatment and relevant clinical features: gastroenterology conditions
Classification • IBS with predominant constipation • IBS with predominant diarrhea • IBS with mixed bowel habits • IBS unclassified	*Red flags in irritable bowel syndrome (IBS)* • Age of onset after 50 years • Rectal bleeding or melena • Nocturnal diarrhea • Progressive abdominal pain • Unexplained weight loss • Laboratory abnormalities (iron deficiency anemia, elevated C-reactive protein, or fecal calprotectin) • Family history of irritable bowel disease (IBD) or colorectal cancer *Clinical features* • Chronic abdominal pain • Both somatic and psychological complaints • Changed bowel habits: constipation or diarrhea • Dyspepsia • Heartburn • Chest pain • Headaches • Fatigue • Neurologic dysfunction • Gynecologic symptoms • Anxiety or depression
Larva (cutaneous) migrans (hookworm) Cutaneous larva migrans is a clinical syndrome consisting of an erythematous migrating linear or serpiginous cutaneous track *Classification* • Cutaneous disease • Pulmonary disease	*Treatment* • Local treatment: Thiabendazole, tab, 400 mg, 2 tablets crushed in soft paraffin and applied topically by occlusive dressings • Systemic treatment: Albendazole, tab, 400 mg, 2 × 1 tab/d, 3 d *Etiology* • Human skin infection with the larvae of the dog or cat hookworms *Ancylostoma braziliense* or *Ancylostoma caninum* • Hematogenous spread to lungs causing dry cough for 1–2 weeks *Signs and symptoms* • Usually, a history of spending long hours on sandy beaches prior to appearance of scaly and highly itchy skin lesions
Malnutrition Deficiencies, excesses, or imbalances in a person's intake of energy and/or nutrients (WHO 2016) *Classifications:* two main categories *Undernutrition:* • Stunting: low height for age • Wasting: low weight for height • Underweight: low weight for age • Micronutrient deficiencies or insufficiencies: a lack of important vitamins and minerals *Obesity and diet-related noncommunicable diseases:* such as heart disease, stroke, diabetes, and cancer	*Treatment* • Identify and treat underlying cause • Provide balanced diet: fruits, vegetables, grains, dairy, and protein foods *Diagnostic criteria* (two or more of the following): • Insufficient energy intake • Weight loss • Loss of muscle mass • Loss of subcutaneous fat • Localized or generalized fluid accumulation that may mask weight loss • Diminished functional status as measured by handgrip strength *Etiology of involuntary loss of weight* • Inadequate dietary intake: social factors, financial limitation, medical and psychiatric factors, and physiologic factors • Anorexia: loss of appetite • Sarcopenia: disuse or muscle atrophy • Cachexia: inflammatory effects of disease

Table 8.1 (continued)

Diagnosis and classification	Treatment and relevant clinical features: gastroenterology conditions
	Causes of weight loss in geriatric age The Mnemonic: *MEALS ON WHEELS*: *M*edication (e.g., Digoxin, Theophylline, and SSRI) *E*motional *A*lcoholism *L*ate-life paranoia *O*ral factors *N*osocomial infection *W*andering and other dementia-related factors *H*yperthyroidism *E*nteral problems *E*ating problems *L*ow salt, low cholesterol, and other therapeutic diets *S*ocial factors, stones (chronic cholecystitis)
Mesenteric ischemia Reduction in blood flow to any part of the intestine. Usually caused by any process that reduces intestinal blood flow, such as arterial occlusion, venous occlusion, or arterial vasospasm *Acute mesenteric* The sudden onset of small intestinal hypoperfusion due to occlusive or nonocclusive obstruction of the arterial blood supply or obstruction of venous outflow *Chronic mesenteric* Develops in patients with mesenteric atherosclerosis causing episodic intestinal hypoperfusion related to eating	*Treatment (acute)* • Fluid resuscitation • Ciproxin, tab, 500 mg, 2 × 1 tab/d, 10 d • Paracetamol, 500 mg, tabs, 3 × 1 g/d, as needed • Aspirin, tab, 100 mg, 1 tab/d • Address cardiovascular risk factors: high blood pressure, obesity, high cholesterol level, and sedentarity *Clinical features* • Personal and family history • Abdominal pain • Abdominal distension • Rebound tenderness and guarding • Occult blood may be present in the stool • Think of this diagnostic entity when pain is chronic and mainly postprandial
Perianal pruritus Perianal itching and discomfort Pruritus ani	*Treatment* • Identify and treat etiology • Mebendazole 400 mg single dose to be repeated in 2 weeks *or* • Mebendazole, tab, 100 mg, 2 × 1 tab/d, during 3 d, to be repeated in 2 weeks • Clotrimazole crème, 2× daily *Etiology* • Worm infestations: *Enterobius vermicularis* (pinworm) and *Trichuris trichiura* (whipworm) are common nematode infections causing pruritus ani. Diagnose by Tape test • Poor perineal hygiene • Fistulas • Fissures • Prolapsed hemorrhoids • Skin tags • Mild incontinence and fecal soilage • Contact dermatitis • Bacterial and viral infections: staphylococcus and streptococcus, condyloma, herpes, and syphilis • Molluscum contagiosum • Parasitic infestations, for example, oxyuria • Candida infection • Systemic disease: diabetes, cholestasis, lymphoma, leukemia, pellagra, renal failure, thyrotoxicosis, hypothyroidism, HIV disease, and deficiencies in vitamin A, D, and iron • Dietary factors: spicy foods, chocolate, and tomatoes may cause irritation and should be eliminated

(continued)

Table 8.1 (continued)

Diagnosis and classification	Treatment and relevant clinical features: gastroenterology conditions
Perineal fistulas The chronic manifestation of the acute perirectal process that may form an anal abscess *Terminology* • Enteric fistula • Arteriovenous fistula • Vesicovaginal fistula	*Treatment* • Thorough clinical assessment • Provide analgesia • Advise about healthy lifestyle with the view of providing good bowel movement (diet rich in fiber, regular physical exercise, and 2–3 L of fluid intake daily) • Refer to tertiary center for surgical care where indicated *Etiology* • Crohn's disease • Lymphogranuloma venereum is a chronic infection in the lymphatic system caused by *C. trachomatis* and can cause inflammatory perirectal masses • Radiation proctitis • Rectal foreign bodies • Primary perianal actinomycosis can cause a simple fistula-in-ano or an inflamed perirectal mass in immunocompromised individuals • Obstetric injury *Pathogenesis* • Ten anal crypt glands are arranged circumferentially within the anal canal at the level of the dentate line • Anatomically, the glands penetrate the internal sphincter and end in the intersphincteric plane • An anorectal fistula is the connection between two epithelial structures and connects the anal abscess from the infected anal crypt glands to the perirectal skin and sometimes to other pelvic organs • Anorectal fistulas may originate from one of the infected glands *Note:* Fistula formation may constitute a complication of female genital mutilation
Rectal prolapse Protrusion of all layers of the rectum through the anus, manifesting as concentric rings of rectal mucosa	*Treatment* • Conservative: fiber-rich diet • Surgical: rectopexy • Push prolapsed rectum back inside if protruding • Ensure good anal hygiene *Risk factor* Childbirth increases risk of rectal prolapse
Schistosomiasis (Bilharziasis) A disease caused by infection with parasitic blood flukes *Microbiology* • Five schistosome species can cause infection in humans • Three major species are *Schistosoma mansoni* (Africa and South America), *S. haematobium* (Africa and the Middle East), and *S. japonicum* (China, Taiwan, the Philippines, and Southeast Asia)	*Treatment* • Praziquantel, tab, 600 mg, 1 tab/d, 5 d *Clinical tips* • If treated promptly, full functional recovery is possible • Squamous carcinoma of the urinary bladder can occur with *Schistosoma haematobium* infection *Clinical manifestations* • Swimmer's itch: rash • Acute schistomiasis syndrome: a systemic hypersensitivity reaction to schistosome antigens • Chronic infection • Intestinal schistosomiasis: chronic or intermittent abdominal pain, poor appetite, and diarrhea. In heavy infection, chronic colonic ulceration may lead to intestinal bleeding and iron deficiency anemia • Hepatosplenic schistosomiasis

Table 8.1 (continued)

Diagnosis and classification	Treatment and relevant clinical features: gastroenterology conditions
The life cycle of schistosomiasis • Requires intermediate (snail) and definitive (human) hosts • Infection of human occurs in freshwater ponds and rivers	• Genitourinary schistosomiasis • Glomerular disease • Neuroschistosomiasis *Schistosoma haematobium main symptoms:* • Hematuria • Diarrhea may be bloody *Schistosoma mansoni:* may infiltrate the paravertebral plexus, leading to spinal cord compression or cauda equina lesion, causing paralysis
Spontaneous bacterial peritonitis Ascitic fluid infection without an evident intraabdominal surgically treatable source *Microbiology* • *Escherichia coli* • *Klebsiella* spp. • Bacteroides	*Treatment* • Salt and water restriction • Empiric antibiotherapy • Ciproxin, tabs, 500 mg 2 × 1 tab/d, 10 d *or* • Ceftriaxone, ampoule 1 g • 2 amp/d, 3 d and • Spironolactone, 25 mg tabs, 1 tab/morning, 5 d *and* • Furosemide, 40 mg tab, 1 tab/morning *Diagnostic features* • A history of chronic liver disease and ascites • Fever and abdominal pain • Paralytic ileus • Altered mental status • Peritoneal signs (guarding and rebound tenderness) commonly encountered on examination • Ascitic fluid neutrophil count greater than 250 white blood cells common
Ulcerative colitis (UC) Recurring episodes of inflammation limited to the mucosal layer of the colon. It commonly involves the rectum and may extend in a proximal and continuous fashion to involve other parts of the colon *Classification of UC* *Mild:* four or fewer stools per day with or without blood, no signs of systemic toxicity, and a normal erythrocyte sedimentation rate (ESR) *Moderate:* frequent loose, bloody stools (>4 per d), mild anemia, and mild abdominal pain *Severe:* ≥ 6 per d of loose bloody stools, with severe cramps, fever, tachycardia, anemia, or an elevated ESR (≥30 mm/h). Patients may have rapid weight loss	*Treatment* • Salofalk, 5-aminosalicylic acid (5-ASA), and rectal application (suppositories or enemas) *or* • Sulfasalazine, tab, 500 mg, 3 × 1 tab/d *or* • Prednisone, 50 mg, 1 tab/d, 5 d *and* • Omeprazole, 40 mg, 1 tab/d, 10 d *Extraintestinal manifestation of UC* • Musculoskeletal: arthritis • *Eye:* uveitis and episcleritis • *Skin:* erythema nodosum and pyoderma gangrenosum • *Hepatobiliary:* primary sclerosing cholangitis, fatty liver, and autoimmune liver disease • *Hematopoietic/coagulation:* an increased risk for both venous and arterial thromboembolism • *Pulmonary:* airway inflammation, parenchymal lung disease, serositis, thromboembolic disease, and drug-induced lung toxicity *Complications of UC* • Severe bleeding • Fulminant colitis and toxic megacolon • Perforation *Diagnostic features of UC* • Bloody diarrhea • Lower abdominal cramps on the fecal urgency • Anemia and low serum albumin • Sigmoidoscopy may lead to diagnosis

(continued)

Table 8.1 (continued)

Diagnosis and classification	Treatment and relevant clinical features: gastroenterology conditions
	Differential diagnosis • Crohn's disease • Infectious colitis • Radiation colitis • Diversion colitis • Solitary rectal ulcer syndrome • Graft versus host disease • Diverticular colitis • Medication-associated colitis
Sigmoid volvulus Torsion of a segment of the alimentary tract, often leading to bowel obstruction. The most common sites of volvulus are the sigmoid colon and cecum	*Treatment* • Appropriate analgesia • Refer to surgeon *Pathogenesis* Occurs when an air-filled loop of the sigmoid colon twists about its mesentery. Obstruction of the intestinal lumen and impairment of vascular perfusion ensues *Risk factors* • Anatomic factors • Because of a relatively long sigmoid, Africans are more prone to volvulus • Colonic dysmotility *Diagnostic evaluation* • Good history and physical examination • Abdominal radiographs • Abdominal CT scan

Urology and Nephrology

9

Contents

9.1   **History: Questions to Ask** 108

9.2   **Physical Examination** 108

9.3   **Cardinal Paramedical Urology and Nephrology Examinations** 109

9.4   **Urology and Nephrology Red Flags** 109

Urology is the field of medicine that focuses on the urinary tract and the male genital organs (Fig. 9.1). The organs covered by urology include the kidneys, ureters, urinary bladder, urethra, and male reproductive organs: testes, epididymis, vas deferens, seminal vesicles, prostate, and penis.

The urinary tract consists of the kidneys, bladder, ureters, and urethra.

Disease conditions of the urogenital system are common in both males and females in BMC's ambulatory setting.

Infection is the major pathophysiological basis. Infectious agents are bacterial (*E. coli*, *Bacteroides*, etc.), protozoal (*Gardnerella*), and fungal (*Candida albicans*). When basic first-line urinary tract infection (UTI) treatments fail, in subsequent visits, the clinician should consider other etiologies including chlamydia, gonorrhea, and syphilis.

Recurrent UTIs and inadequately managed infections may lead to pelvic inflammatory disease (PID). This multimicrobial infection is commonly encountered in women of childbearing age. PID, which affects the quality of life of a significant number of women, is the major cause of female infertility. PID is essentially a clinical diagnosis, and when it is suspected in the history, therapy should promptly be instituted.

Structural anomalies of the urogenital system should be recognized and adequately addressed. This category of urogenital pathologies includes phimosis, rectovaginal fistulas, and functional effects of female genital mutilation.

Oncologic conditions may present as scrotal masses, pelvic masses, macroscopic hematuria, bone pain, progressive prostatism, urinary retention, and unexplained loss of weight.

In this chapter, we address common disorders of the urogenital system that are encountered in a standard minimal-resource facility (Table 9.1).

© The Author(s), under exclusive license to Springer Nature Switzerland AG 2021

M. Touray, A. Touray, *Clinical Work and General Management of a Standard Minimal-Resource Facility*, Sustainable Development Goals Series, https://doi.org/10.1007/978-3-030-71032-3_9

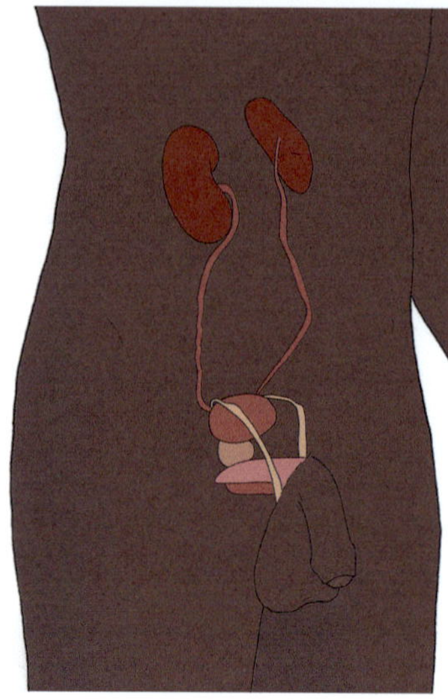

Fig. 9.1 Urology and nephrology: A mnemonic illustration representing main uronephrologic anatomic structures and their corresponding pathologies

9.1   History: Questions to Ask

- Does it hurt/burn when urinating?
- Does your bladder feel empty after urinating?
- Do you see blood or pus in your urine?
- Evaluate episodes of at-risk sexual intercourse: multiple partners, unprotected, and promiscuity?
- Do you have pain during intercourse?
- Any contraceptive devices inserted?
- Any past history of UTI?
- Evaluate menstruation: date of last menstruation, duration, painfulness, and estimated quantity of bleeding?
- Mnemonic: The five Ps for urogenital treatment are as follows: partners, prevention of pregnancy, protection from sexually transmitted diseases (STDs), practices, and past history of STDs.

9.2   Physical Examination

- Inspect external genitalia.
- Palpate suprapubic region.
- Palpate the renal lodges.
- Perform rectal examination if needed.

9.3 Cardinal Paramedical Urology and Nephrology Examinations

- Full blood count
- Pregnancy test (beta-hCG)
- Urine sticks and urine microscopy
- Uterosalpingography
- X-ray (exclude or confirm bone metastasis)
- Ultrasonography of relevant organ systems

9.4 Urology and Nephrology Red Flags

- Clinical and/or historic suspicion of extrauterine gestation
- Pelvic mass with associated pain
- Hematuria
- Recurrent urinary tract infection (>4 episodes per year)
- Associated fecal incontinence
- Visible vaginal bleeding
- History of pelvic surgery

Table 9.1 Urology and nephrology conditions and their treatment

Diagnosis and classification	Treatment and relevant clinical features: urology and nephrology conditions
Acute renal failure (ARF) Deterioration of kidney function (within hours to days) resulting in azotemia (raised creatininemia) and failure of the kidney to maintain fluid electrolyte and acid-base homeostasis *Assessment of ARF* • Determine disease duration • Urinalysis: proteinuria and hematuria • Estimation of the glomerular filtration rate (GFR)	*Treatment of fluid losses* • Evaluate to determine etiology • Correct fluid loss replacement: 0.9% NaCl iv in cases of diarrhea or vomiting • ORS for oral intake *Etiology* • Nephrotoxic agents • Infections • Urinary tract obstructions • Immunologic insult to renal structures *Classifications* • Prerenal • Functional • Intrinsic (intrarenal) • Postrenal
Balanitis Inflammation of the glans penis. When the prepuce (foreskin) also becomes involved, the condition is known as balanoposthitis *Dermatologic conditions* • Eczema • Lichen planus • Lichen sclerosus • Contact dermatitis • Bowenoid papulosis • Carcinoma in situ	*Treatment* • Ketoconazole cream, 2×/d until symptoms subside • Advise on groin hygiene: keep clean and dry and avoid underwear made of synthetic material *Etiology/pathogenesis* Inadequate hygiene in uncircumcised men; buildup of sweat, debris, exfoliated skin, and bacteria or fungi can occur, resulting in inflammation *Risk factors* • Diabetes mellitus • Trauma (e.g., zipper injury) • Obesity • Edematous conditions (e.g., congestive heart failure, cirrhosis, and nephrotic syndrome) *Management tips* • Patient education on hygiene • Partner treatment • Improved perineal hygiene *Clinical manifestations* • Pain, tenderness, or pruritus of the glans and/or foreskin • Erythema and a purulent exudate • Ulcerations • Candidal balanitis has a white, curd-like exudate • Anaerobic bacterial infections present a thick, foul-smelling purulent exudate

(continued)

Table 9.1 (continued)

Diagnosis and classification	Treatment and relevant clinical features: urology and nephrology conditions
Benign prostatic hypertrophy (BPH) *Diagnostic features* • Obstructive or irritative voiding symptoms • May have enlarged prostate on rectal examination • Absence of urinary tract infection, neurologic disorder, stricture disease, prostatic, or bladder malignancy *Nomenclature* *Benign prostatic hyperplasia* *Complications* • Acute urinary retention • Recurrent urinary tract infections • Hydronephrosis • Renal failure *Differential diagnosis* • Urethral stricture • Bladder neck contracture • Prostate cancer • Urinary tract infection and acute prostatitis • Neurogenic bladder • Bladder calculi • Bladder cancer *Good to know* BPH is not believed to be a risk factor for prostate cancer. However, currently debatable	*Treatment* • Patient education • Watchful waiting: biannual office consultation • Surgical therapy: transurethral resection of the prostate (TURP) • Alpha blockers: Tamsulosin tab, 0.4 mg, 1 tab/d daily • 5-alpareductase inhibitors • Alfuzosin (Xatral), tab, 10 mg, 1 tab/d *or* • Tamsulosin (Pradif), tab, 0.4 mg, 1 tab/d • Intermittent catheterization if urinary retention *Clinical assessment:* a comprehensive clinical assessment consisting of history, physical examination, and paramedical investigation • *History:* urethral trauma, urethritis, or urethral instrumentation that could lead to urethral stricture, and cigarette smoking • *Physical examination:* DRE • *Paramedical:* urinalysis, serum creatinine, PSA • Genitourinary ultrasonography, postvoid residual urine volume, and urethrocystoscopy *Clinical findings* *Obstructive symptoms* • Hesitancy • Decreased force and caliber of urine stream • Sensation of incomplete bladder emptying • Double voiding, meaning urinating a second time within 2 h • Straining to urinate • Postvoid urgency *Irritative symptoms* • Increased frequency or nocturia • Enlarged prostate on digital rectal examination
Candidiasis Disease caused by the yeast *Candida albicans. Candida albicans* can cause vaginal yeast infections, diaper rash, and skin rashes that emerge in moist, warm folds of skin, and thrush (white patches inside the mouth and throat) *Diagnostic entities* • Balanitis, balanoposthitis • Cheilitis • Folliculitis • Intertrigo • Migrating cheilitis • Onyxis and perionyxes • Oral thrush • Septicemia (immunosuppressed patients) • Vulvovaginitis	*Treatment* Oral and esophageal candidiasis: • Fluconazole tabs, 100 mg, 1×/d, 10 d Vaginal candidiasis: • Fluconazole, vaginal ovule, 1×/d, 3 d • Canesten ovules, 2× daily, 3 d • Most females may have vaginal candidiasis after antibiotherapy. Hence, anticipate and explain at the time of prescribing antibiotherapy to a female patient *Preventive health advice* • Maintain good skin hygiene: shower daily with a nonaggressive soap; dry skin, and especially skin folds, with cotton towel • Avoid tight synthetic underwear • Keep interdigital spaces clean and dry as often as possible

Table 9.1 (continued)

Diagnosis and classification	Treatment and relevant clinical features: urology and nephrology conditions
Chronic renal failure (CRF) The presence of kidney damage *or* decreased kidney function for 3 or more months, irrespective of the cause. *Note:* CRF constitutes a heterogeneous group of disorders characterized by alterations in kidney structure and function, which manifest in various ways depending upon the underlying cause or causes and the severity of disease	*Treatment* • Treat underlying cause • Enalapril tabs, 10 mg, 1 × 1 tab/d • Refer to tertiary center when creatinine exceeds 300 μmol/L • Patient education *Assessing kidney damage and function* • Albuminuria • Urinary sediment abnormalities • Imaging abnormalities • Pathologic abnormalities • Glomerular filtration rate (GFR) and serum creatinine. The GFR is considered the best index of overall kidney function • Declining GFR indicates progressive kidney disease
Cryptochidia Undescended testis *Complications* • Inguinal hernia • Testicular torsion • Testicular trauma • Subfertility • Testicular cancer	*Treatment* • Elective surgical referral • Evaluate by repeated complete abdominal echography *Terminology* • *Cryptorchidism:* a testis that is not within the scrotum and does not descend spontaneously into the scrotum by 4 months of age • *Absent testis:* an absent testis due to agenesis or atrophy secondary to intrauterine vascular compromise • *Undescended testes:* undescended testes have stopped short along their normal path of descent into the scrotum. They may remain in the abdominal cavity or may be palpable in the inguinal canal or just outside the external ring • *Retractile testes:* normal testes that have been pulled into a suprascrotal position by the cremasteric reflex • *Ascending testes:* descending in a scrotal position in early childhood and then "ascend" and become undescended *Note:* Increased risk for malignant transformations
Epididymitis Inflammation of the epididymis and its surrounding structures, namely testis, tunica vaginalis, spermatic cord, appendix testis, and appendix	*Treatment* • Ciproxin, tab, 500 mg, 2 × 1 tab/d, 10 d *and* • Ibuprofen, tab, 500 mg, 2 × 2 tab/d, 5 d *Etiology* • Infection mainly by *N. gonorrhoeae* and *C. trachomatis* *Pathogenesis of scrotal pain* • *Testis* (testicle) is the male gonad responsible for production of sperm and androgens, mainly testosterone • *Tunica vaginalis* is a fascial layer encapsulating a potential space that encompasses the anterior two thirds of the testis • *Epididymis* is a tightly coiled tubular structure located on the posterior aspect of the testes running from its superior to inferior poles • *Spermatic cord*, which consists of the testicular blood vessels and the vas deferens, is connected to the base of the epididymis • *Appendix testis* is a small vestigial structure on the anterosuperior aspect of the testis *Diagnostic features* • Fever • Irritative voiding symptoms • Pain and enlargement of epididymis

(continued)

Table 9.1 (continued)

Diagnosis and classification	Treatment and relevant clinical features: urology and nephrology conditions
Erectile dysfunction Consistent or recurrent inability to acquire or sustain an erection of sufficient rigidity and duration for sexual intercourse *Note:* Cardiovascular risk factors: on average, erectile dysfunction occurs 3 years prior to a cardiovascular event	*Treatment* • Identify underlying cause • Provide psychological support • Phosphodiesterase-5 inhibitors (PDE5): Sildenafil, tab, 50 mg, as needed *Physical examination* • Blood pressure • Secondary sex characteristic • Genital organs • Prostate (>50 years old) *Laboratory evaluation* • Fasting blood sugar • Testosterone • Cholesterol
Fever of unknown origin (FUO): a clinical diagnosis with determined criteria shown below *Defining criteria* • Fever higher than 38.3 °C on several occasions • Duration of fever for at least 3 weeks • Uncertain diagnosis after 1 week of study in the hospital	*Treatment* • Symptomatic treatment as efforts are made to determine underlying course • Refer to tertiary center for tertiary care *Etiology* • Infections: tuberculosis and endocarditis • Malignancies • Systemic rheumatic diseases, for example, vasculitis and rheumatoid arthritis • Gallbladder disease • Primary HIV infections or opportunistic infections *Clinical evaluation* • History • Physical examination • FBC including differential and platelet count • Blood cultures where available • Routine blood chemistry, including liver enzymes and bilirubin • If liver tests are abnormal, hepatitis A, B, and C serologies • Urinalysis, including microscopic examination, and urine culture • Chest radiograph

Table 9.1 (continued)

Diagnosis and classification	Treatment and relevant clinical features: urology and nephrology conditions
Genital ulcers and STDs (male and female) Discontinuation of the skin of external genitalia due to infectious conditions *Diagnostic entities* • Chancroid • Chlamydia • Genital herpes • Gonorrhea • Hepatitis B and C • Syphilis	*Treatment* *Chancroid* • Azithromycin, tab, 250 mg, 4, tab, orally in a single dose *or* • Ciprofloxacin, tab, 500 mg, 2 × 1 tab/d, 5 d *or* • Erythromycin, tab, 500 mg, 4 × 1 tab/d, 7 d *Chlamydia* • Azithromycin, tab, 250 mg, 4, tab, single dose (to be taken under direct observation) *or* • Doxycycline, 100 mg tabs, 2 × 1 tab/d, 7 d *Genital herpes* • Acyclovir, tab, 200 mg, 4 × 1 tab/d, 7 d for first attack • Acyclovir, tab, 200 mg, 4× daily, 5 d for recurrent episodes • Acyclovir cream to apply twice daily *Gonorrhea* • Ceftriaxone ampoule, 250 mg, IM in a single dose *and* • Azithromycin, tab, 250 mg, 4, tab, orally in a single dose • If ceftriaxone is not available: • Cefixime 400 mg orally in a single dose *and* • Azithromycin, tab, 250 mg, 4, tab, orally in a single dose *Hepatitis B and C (see Table 8.1)* *Syphilis* • Benzathine penicillin ampoule, IM 2.4 million unit: 1-amp IM single dose *or* • Procaine Penicillin, ampoule 1.2 million units, 1-amp, IM, daily for 10 d *or* • Doxycyclin, tab, 100 mg, 2 × 1 tab/d, 10 d *For pregnant women or those allergic to penicillin* • Erythromycin, tab, 500 mg, 4 × 1 tab/d, 10 d
Genital warts (venereal) Human papillomavirus (HPV) is a common cause of cutaneous and mucosal infection. Condylomata acuminata (anogenital) warts are manifestations of HPV and manifest as soft papules or plaques on the external genitalia, perianal skin, perineum, or groin *Good to know* Male circumcision may reduce risk for HPV infection	*Treatment* • Podophyllin 10−25% apply carefully to external genital, perianal, vaginal, and rectal warts while avoiding normal tissue. Wash thoroughly 4 h after application • Consider HPV vaccination: for example, Gardasil, scheme: shots 0 M, 1 M, and 6 M *Transmission of HPV* • Transmitted through contact with infected skin or mucosa • The virus invades the cells of the epidermal basal layer through microabrasions • Anogenital HPV infection is almost always acquired through sexual contact • Warts are not required for transmission but are highly infectious because of their high viral load *Risk factors* • Promiscuous sexual activity • Immunosuppression • Smoking

(continued)

Table 9.1 (continued)

Diagnosis and classification	Treatment and relevant clinical features: urology and nephrology conditions
Hematuria Presence of blood in urine and is a symptom of an underlying disease *Laboratory definition* 3 or more red blood cells (RBCs) per high-power field in a spun urine sediment *Classification* • *Macroscopic hematuria:* visualization of red-brown urine • *Microscopic hematuria:* blood detectable only on examination of the urine sediment by microscopy	*Treatment* • Identify and address underlying cause • Facilitate follow-ups where indicated *Etiology:* bleeding may originate from any of the various structures of the urine collecting system • *Renal:* benign or malignancy renal mass, glomerular bleeding, structural disease, for example, polycystic kidney disease, pyelonephritis, malignant hypertension, arteriovenous malformation, and papillary necrosis • *Ureter:* malignances, stone, strictures, polyps, or postsurgical conditions • *Bladder:* malignancy, radiation, cystitis, bladder stone, and polyps • *Prostate/Urethra:* benign prostate hypertrophy, prostate cancer, prostatic procedures, traumatic catherization, urethritis, and urethral diverticulum *Clinical evaluation:* comprehensive clinical assessment consisting of history, physical, and paramedical investigations • *History:* current pyuria, symptoms of URTI, positive family history of renal disease, unilateral flank pain, symptoms of prostatic obstruction in elder men, recent vigorous exercise or trauma, history of bleeding disorder, medication, and history of sickle cell disease or trait • *Physical examination* • *Laboratory:* dipstick and sediment microscopy to visualize red cell casts (glomerular versus non-glomerular etiology) • *Imaging:* lower abdominal ultrasonography, computed tomography where available. Other imaging modalities include: CT urography, intravenous pyelography, MRI urography, retrograde pyelography, and cystoscopy *Risk factors for associated malignancy* • Male gender • Age >35 years • Past or current heavy smoking history • Occupational exposure to chemicals or dyes (benzenes or aromatic amines), such as printers, painters, and chemical plant workers • History of gross hematuria • History of irritative voiding symptoms • History of chronic urinary tract infection • History of pelvic irradiation • History of exposure to cyclophosphamide • History of a chronic indwelling foreign body • History of analgesic abuse, which is also associated with an increased incidence of carcinoma of the kidney

Table 9.1 (continued)

Diagnosis and classification	Treatment and relevant clinical features: urology and nephrology conditions
Infertility "a disease of the reproductive system defined by the failure to achieve a clinical pregnancy after 12 months or more of regular unprotected sexual intercourse." *Alternative definition* *Infertility* is the inability of a sexually active, non-contracepting couple to achieve pregnancy in one year	*Treatment* • After evaluation, refer for specialized care with adequate documentation *Evaluation and assessment* • Medical history • Physical examination • Semen analysis • Assess ovulatory function • Rule out tubal occlusion and assess the uterine cavity • A test or tests of ovarian reserve such as cycle day 3 follicle-stimulating hormone (FSH) or estradiol • Anti-Mullerian hormone (AMH) • Assessment of fallopian tube patency: hysterosalpingogram
Male infertility The inability of a couple to conceive a child after 1 year of sexual intercourse without contraceptive use, *or* pregnancy does not result after 1 year of normal sexual activity without contraceptives	*Treatment* • Extensively assess and educate • If failure to conceive persists, refer to appropriate tertiary center for specialized urology evaluation *Evaluation of male infertility* • Semen analysis • Hormone testing: testosterone, prolactin, TSH • Genetic testing • Testicular biopsy • Imaging *Etiology* • Prior testicular insults: torsion, cryptochidia, and trauma • Infections: mumps orchitis, epididymitis, and sexually transmitted infections (STIs) • Environmental factors: excessive heat, radiation, and chemotherapy • Prolonged pesticide exposure • Medication: testosterone, cimetidine, SSRI spironolactone, and phenytoin • Drugs: alcohol, tobacco, and marijuana • Sexual dysfunction • Frequency and timing of intercourse • Use of lubricants • Past medical or surgical history • Diabetes mellitus with decreased spermatogenesis, retrograde, or anejaculation *Clinical assessment* • Medical history • Sexual history • Physical examination • Semen analysis • Determine serum testosterone level

(continued)

Table 9.1 (continued)

Diagnosis and classification	Treatment and relevant clinical features: urology and nephrology conditions
Molluscum contagiosum A chronic localized infection by pox virus, consisting of flesh-colored, dome-shaped papules on the skin of an infected individual	*Treatment* • Podophyllin 10–25% in tinct, apply very carefully to external genital, perianal, vaginal, and rectal warts while avoiding normal tissue. Wash thoroughly 4 h after application • Cryotherapy • Curettage *Transmission* The poxvirus family, *molluscum contagiosum*, is spread by direct skin-to-skin contact and thus can occur anywhere on the body. The virus can be transmitted via autoinoculation by scratching or touching a lesion *When and why to treat* • Limitation of lesion spread to other sites • Reduction in the risk of transmission to others • Resolution of pruritus • Prevention of scarring that can result from lesions that become inflamed, traumatized, or secondarily infected • Reduction in patient or parental psychological stress over the appearance of lesions
Nephrotic and nephritic syndromes Diseases of the glomerulus can result in two different urinary and clinical patterns: nephritic and nephrotic *Nephritic syndrome* Heavy proteinuria (which may be in the nephrotic range), edema, hypertension, and/or renal insufficiency may be observed *Nephrotic syndrome* Clinical and laboratory features of renal disease defined by the presence of heavy proteinuria (protein excretion greater than 3.5 g/24 h), hypoalbuminemia (less than 3 g/dL), and peripheral edema	*Treatment* • Refer for specialized treatment • Corticoid therapy is indicated in most cases: Hydrocortisone ampoule 100 mg, 3 amps iv in the morning for 3 d Due to absence of specific treatment for underlying disease, treatment may be purely symptomatic: • *Proteinuria:* low-dose ACE or ARBs and protein restriction also may slow disease progression • *Edema:* both peripheral and ascitis are due to sodium retention. Treated with dietary sodium restriction (to approximately 2 g of sodium per day) and diuretics • *Hyperlipidemia:* reverses with disease remission • *Hypercoagulability:* Warfarin where needed *Etiology* • Diabetes mellitus • Amyloidosis • Systemic lupus erythematosus • Minimal change disease • Focal segmental glomerulosclerosis • Membranous nephropathy *Complication* • Proteinuria • Periorbital edema • Protein malnutrition • Hypovolemia • Acute kidney injury • Thromboembolism • Infection • Proximal renal tubular acidosis: glucosuria, aminoaciduria, phosphaturia, bicarbonaturia, and vitamin D deficiency
Orchitis Infection/inflammation of the testes	*Treatment* • Ciproxin, tab, 500 mg, 2 × 1 tab/ d, 10 d • Paracetamol, tab, 500 mg, 3 × 2 tab/d, 5 d *and/or* • Naproxen, tab, 500 mg, 2 × 1 tab/d, 5 d • For more detail see Epididymitis

Table 9.1 (continued)

Diagnosis and classification	Treatment and relevant clinical features: urology and nephrology conditions
Phimosis Tight foreskin that cannot be retracted to expose the glans penis *Paraphimosis* is a retracted foreskin in an uncircumcised or partially circumcised male that cannot be returned to normal	*Treatment* • Surgical circumcision • Analgesia • Antibiotherapy where indicated: Ciproxine tab, 500 mg, 2 × 1 tab/d, 5 d *Pathophysiology* • Paraphimosis is caused by foreskin entrapment behind the coronal sulcus • Impairment of lymphatic and venous flow from the constricting ring of foreskin causes venous engorgement of the glans penis with swelling. Arterial flow to the glans penis becomes compromised over a period of hours to days • Educate on perineal hygiene *Signs and symptoms* • Swelling of the penis and penile pain • Edema and tenderness of the glans penis • Painful swelling of the distal retracted foreskin • A constricting band of tissue proximal to the head of the penis at the coronal sulcus • The penile shaft appears flaccid and unaffected
Prostatitis Infection of the prostate, usually caused by gram-negative organisms *Microbes involved* • *E. coli* • *Proteus* • *Klebsiella, Enterobacter*, and *Serratia* • *Pseudomonas aeruginosa* *Complications* • Bacteremia • Epididymitis • Chronic bacterial prostatitis • Prostatic abscesses • Metastatic infection (e.g., spinal or sacroiliac infection) • Valvular heart disease or a valvular prosthesis is at risk for endocarditis with prostatitis	*Treatment* • Acute: Ciproxin, tab, 500 mg, 2 × 1 tab/d, 10 d • Chronic: Ciproxin, tab, 500 mg, 2 × 1 tab/d, 21 d • Based on clinical evolution, antibiotherapy may be extended to 6 weeks *Pathogenesis* • Entry of microorganisms into the prostate gland almost always occurs via the urethra. In most cases, bacteria migrate from the urethra or bladder through the prostatic ducts, with intraprostatic reflux of urine • There may be concomitant infection in the bladder or epididymis • NSAID and/or PCM for pain control *Risk factors* • Cystitis • Urethritis • Other urogenital tract infections • Urethral strictures • Urogenital instrumentation *Clinical manifestation* • Fever and chills • Malaise, myalgia, and dysuria • Irritative urinary symptoms: frequency, urgency, and urge incontinence • Pelvic or perineal pain • Cloudy urine • Pain at the tip of the penis • Swelling of the acutely inflamed prostate can cause voiding symptoms, ranging from dribbling and hesitancy to acute urinary retention

(continued)

Table 9.1 (continued)

Diagnosis and classification	Treatment and relevant clinical features: urology and nephrology conditions
Pubic lice (pediculosis pubis) Infestation by one of three varieties of lice that specifically infest humans *Phthirus pubis* *Classification* • Pediculosis pubis • Pediculosis corporis • Pediculosis capitis	*Treatment* • Shave off pubic hair • Apply permethrin 1% cream to affected area and wash after 10 min or • Benzyl benzoate 25% over affected area and wash off after 24 h • Repeat after 3 d if indicated or • Ivermectin, tab, 3 mg, 0.250 g/kg orally, repeated on the tenth day (for example, for a 70 kg patient, give 6, tab, of the 3 mg tablet per mouth on day 0 and repeat the same dosage at day 10) *Signs and symptoms* • Itching in pubic and perianal areas • Compromised personal and household hygiene • Positive history of contagiosity
Pyelonephritis Infectious inflammatory disease involving the kidney parenchyma and renal pelvis	*Treatment* • Ceftriaxone, ampoule 2 g, 1 amp single dose iv, then • Ciprofloxacin, tab, 500 mg 2 × 1 tab/d, 7 d or • Cotrimoxazole, tab, 800/160, 2 × 1 tab/d, 10 d *Complications* • Sepsis and shock • Abscess formation • Acute bacterial prostatitis *Clinical features* • Fever • Perineal or suprapubic pain and tenderness are common on rectal examination flank pain • Irritative avoiding symptoms • Positive urine culture
Scrotal hernia The presence of abdominal content in the scrotum	*Treatment* • Elective surgical referral • Patient education
Sexually acquired acute inguinal lymphadenitis Localized enlargements of the lymph nodes in the groin area, which are painful and may be fluctuant	*Treatment* • Erythromycin, tab, 500 mg, 4 × 1 tab/d, 14 d (for pregnant women) *or* • Doxycyclin, tab, 100 mg, 2 × 1 tab/d, 14 d • Incision and drainage where needed *Clinical features* • Very painful inguinal lymph nodes (bubo) • Valley in the groin (groove sign) • There may be transient genital ulcers
Sexually transmitted diseases (STDs) A series of contagious infectious diseases transmitted from an infected person to a non-infected person through biological fluids (blood, semen, and saliva)	*Treatment* • Diagnostic assessment • Empiric treatment, common drug regiments are as follows: Amoxicillin, tab, 500 mg, 3 × 1 tab/d, 5 d *or* Co-trimoxazole 800/160, 2× tab/d, 5 d *or* Doxycycline, tab, 100 mg, 2 × 1 tab/d, 5 d • Etiologic treatment where urine culture and antibiotic sensitivity analysis are available

Table 9.1 (continued)

Diagnosis and classification	Treatment and relevant clinical features: urology and nephrology conditions
Microbiology and etiology • *C. trachomatis* • *N. gonorrhoeae* • Syphilis • HIV • Herpes simplex • Chancroid • Pubic lice • *Trichomonas vaginalis* • *Condylomata acuminata* • *Mycoplasma genitalium* • Lymphogranuloma venereum • Hepatitis B and C virus	*Risk factors* • Behavioral • Sexual activity within early and middle adolescence • Multiple partners • Inconsistent use of condoms • Alcohol and other drug consumption • Residing in a detention facility • Mood disorders *Clinical notes* • All STDs have a subclinical or latent period, and patients may be asymptomatic • Simultaneous infections with several organisms are common • All patients who seek STD testing should be screened for syphilis and HIV. Partner notification and treatment are important to prevent transmission and the "ping-pong" effect • Genital ulcers may be present • Herpes simplex virus • Primary syphilis and chancroid • Lymphogranuloma venerum
Syphilis An STD caused by the spirochete *Treponema pallidum* *Diagnostic tests* Serologic tests provide a presumptive diagnosis of syphilis • Nontreponemal tests: based upon the reactivity of serum from infected patients to a cardiolipin-cholesterol-lecithin antigen, for example, Venereal Disease Research Laboratory (VDRL) • Treponemal: used as confirmatory tests for syphilis when the nontreponemal tests are reactive, for example, *T. pallidum* particle agglutination assay (TPPA)	*Treatment* • Benzathine penicillin ampoule, 2.4 million units, 1 amp, IM single dose or • Doxycyclin, tab, 100 mg, 2 × 1 tab/d, 10 d *Syphilis in pregnancy* Treat with penicillin or erythromycin if allergic to penicillin *Congenital syphilis* Treat with procaine penicillin 50,000 units/kg body weight *Classification of syphilis* *Primary syphilis* • Localized infection. Characteristic genital or extragenital painless ulcer (chancre) • Locoregional adenopathy Secondary syphilis • Generalized infection • Syphilitic roseola: erythematous macules on trunk, and hypopigmented squamous papules on torso, limbs, and face • Condyloma lata: soft papules or nodules in the anogenital and buccal mucosa • Fever • Adenopathy • Headache *Tertiary syphilis* • *Chronic complications* involving the skin and neurologic and cardiovascular systems • *Skin:* soft nodule and nonitchy palmoplantar nodules • *Neurology:* meningeal and meningovascular inflammation, and dementia • *Cardiovascular:* aortic aneurysm and aortic valve insufficiency

(continued)

Table 9.1 (continued)

Diagnosis and classification	Treatment and relevant clinical features: urology and nephrology conditions
Testicular mass (seminoma, etc.) Is either germ cell seminoma or nongerm cell seminomas	*Treatment* • Evaluate clinically and by echography • Prompt referral
Testicular torsion Torsion of the testicle, mostly traumatic	*Treatment* • Urgent surgical referral For pain control • Paracetamol, tab, 500 mg, 3 × 2 tab/d *and* • Ibuprofen 400 mg, 2 × 1 tab/d 5 d
Urinary infection, low and high Infection of the urogenital system ranging from the urethra, bladder, and ureter to the kidney	*Treatment* • Cotrimoxazole, tab, (Sulfamethoxazole 800 mg Trimethoprim 160 mg) 2 × 1 tab/d, 5 d *or* • Amoxicillin, 500 mg tab, 3 × 1 tab/d, 5 d *and* For pain control • Paracetamol tab, 500 mg. 3 × 2 tab/d 5 d *and* • Ibuprofen, tab, 400 mg, 2 × 1 tab/d
Urinary incontinence in men Involuntary leakage of urine *Urine analysis* Infection Blood	*Treatment* • Determine and address underlying cause • Protective pads and undergarments • External catheters • Pelvic floor muscle exercises • Lifestyle modification, particularly weight loss and fluid consumption • Bladder training • Biofeedback to supplement pelvic muscle exercises *Classification* • Urge urinary incontinence: a sense of urgency • Stress urinary incontinence: incontinence with physical exertion, coughing, sneezing, laughing, or lifting or with gravitational change (arising from bed) • Mixed incontinence • Overflow incontinence: a sense of incomplete emptying, pelvic discomfort, and bedwetting • Postvoid dribbling: limited to the postvoid setting and without symptoms of UUI • Functional incontinence • Incontinence after prostate treatment *Etiology* • Benign prostate hypertrophy (BPH) • Neurologic conditions, for example, stroke, and normal pressure hydrocephalus • Medications that can increase bladder contractility or exacerbate obstructive effects: antihistamines, decongestants, and benzodiazepines • Prostate surgery (TURP and radical prostatectomy) • Urethral stricture disease • Urinary tract infection (UTI)—burning, frequency, and/or fever • Constipation that could contribute or be comorbid with urinary incontinence • Caffeine and alcohol consumption • Obesity

Table 9.1   (continued)

Diagnosis and classification	Treatment and relevant clinical features: urology and nephrology conditions
Urinary stone disease Formation of crystalline precipitates in the kidney, ureter, or urinary bladder *Nomenclature* • Nephrolithiasis • Urinary calculi • Renal stone • Ureteral stone	*Treatment* • Paracetamol, tab, 500 mg, 3 × 2 tab/d, 5 d • Naproxen, tab, 500 mg, 2 × 1 tab/d, 5 d *and* • Tramadol, tab, 100 mg, 1 tab/d, 5 d *Etiology* • Calcium oxalate • Calcium phosphate • Cystine • Uric acid *Risk factors* • History of prior nephrolithiasis • Positive family history of stones • Enhanced enteric oxalate absorption, often in the setting of malabsorption, for example, gastric bypass procedures, bariatric surgery, and short bowel syndrome • Upper urinary tract infections • Diabetes, obesity, gout, and hypertension • Low fluid intake *Differential diagnosis* • Bleeding within the kidney (glomerular bleeding) • Pyelonephritis • Ectopic pregnancy • Rupture or torsion of an ovarian cyst • Dysmenorrhea • Abdominal aortic aneurysm • Acute intestinal obstruction, diverticulitis, or appendicitis • Biliary colic and cholecystitis • Acute mesenteric ischemia • Herpes zoster • Individuals seeking attention or narcotics may pretend to have renal colic *Diagnostic features* • Severe flank pain • Nausea and vomiting • Hematuria • Identification and localization on noncontrast CT or ultrasonography *Complications* • Persistent renal obstruction leading to permanent renal damage if left untreated

Contents

10.1 **Common Gynecology Diagnostic Procedures** 123

10.2 **Pregnancy Diagnosis** 125

10.3 **Antenatal Visits** 125

10.4 **Laboratory Tests to Be Done During Routine Antenatal Visits** 125

10.5 **Guidelines for Referral to Specialized Care** 125

Obstetrics and gynecology encompasses the two subspecialties attending to women's health. Obstetrics covers pregnancy, childbirth, and the postpartum period, whereas gynecology covers the health of the female reproductive system—the breast, vagina, uterus, the adnexa, ovaries, and the external genital organs (Table 10.1).

Obstetrics-antenatal care is an important specialty that greatly affects the well-being of the community. At BMC, a specific day is preserved for this significant clinical activity: Thursday mornings from 8:00 to 14:00. Every pregnant woman goes through BMC's routine medical consultation procedure before being referred to a trained midwife for specific antenatal care (Fig. 10.1).

Pregnant women are cared for from diagnosis to delivery, as outlined below. An example of a delivery record chart is included in Appendix B.

10.1 Common Gynecology Diagnostic Procedures

- Colposcopy: visualization of the cervical, vaginal, or vulva epithelia at 5–50× magnification.
- Dilation and curettage (D & C): dilation of the cervix and curettage of the entire endometrial cavity using correct metal curette or suction cannula.
- Hysterosalpingography: injection of radiopaque dye through the cervix to visualize the uterine cavity and oviducts, often used to investigate infertility.
- Hysteroscopy: visual examination of the uterine cavity with a small fiber-optic endoscope passed through the cervix.
- Laparoscopy visualization of the abdominal and pelvic cavity through a small fiber-optic endoscope passed through a sub-umbilical incision.

M. Touray, A. Touray, *Clinical Work and General Management of a Standard Minimal-Resource Facility*, Sustainable Development Goals Series, https://doi.org/10.1007/978-3-030-71032-3_10

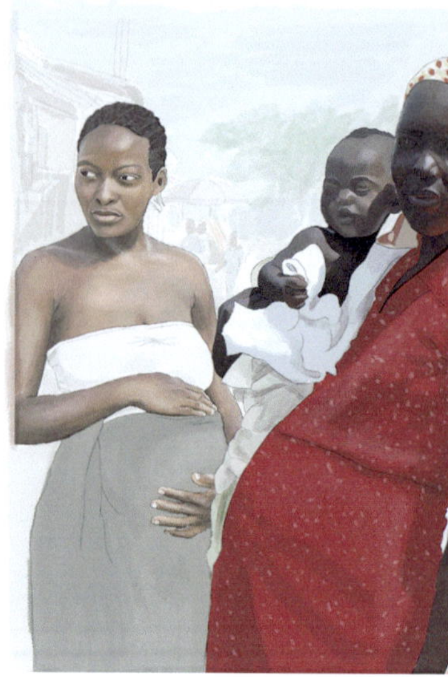

OB, Gyn, Antenatal care

List of obstetrics, gynecology and antenatal care disorders that are described in the text. For easy reference, the corresponding page on which the disease condition is described is in brackets.

Abdominal pain in pregnancy (p126)
Acute renal failure (p127)
Amenorrhea (primary and secondary) (p127)
Anemia in pregnancy (p127)
Bartholin duct cysts and abscess (p128)
Bleeding in pregnancy (p128)
Candidiasis (p129)
Carcinoma of the cervix (p129)
Care of mother and baby immediately after delivery (p130)
Chronic renal failure (p130)
Eclampsia (p130)
Ectopic pregnancy (p131)
Emergency contraception (p131)
Endometriosis (p131)
Female genital mutilation (p132)
Female genital prolapse (p132)
Female Infertility (p137)
Female sexual dysfunction (p133)
Fever of unknown origin (p133)
Genital ulcers and STDs (p133)
Genital warts (venereal) (p134)
Gestational diabetes (p134)
Gestational trophoblastic neoplasia (p135)
Hydatiform mole pregnancy (p135)
Hypertension in pregnancy (p136)
Leiomyoma uteri (p137)
Malaria in pregnancy (p138)
Medication to facilitate delivery (p138)
Menometrorrhagia (p138)
Menopause (p139)
Molluscum contagiosum (p139)
Non-progression of fetus (p139)
Pelvic inflammatory disease (PID) (p140)
Pelvic pain syndrome (p140)
Polycystic ovary syndrome (p141)
Postpartum hemorrhage (p141)
Preeclampsia (p142)
Prelabor rupture of membrane (p142)
Premenopausal abnormal uterine bleeding (p143)
Preterm labor (p143)
Pubic lice (pediculosis pus) (p143)
Puerperal fever sepsis (p144)
Pyelonephritis (p144)
Sexually acquired acute inguinal lymphadenitis (p144)
Sexually transmitted diseases (p145)
Syphilis in pregnancy (p145)
Urinary stone disease (p146)
Urinary tract infection (p146)
Vaginal discharge (p146)
Vaginitis, vulvovaginitis (p146)
Vaginosis (p147)

Fig. 10.1 Gynecology-Obstetrics: A mnemonic illustration representing main anatomic Gynecology-Obstetrics structures and their correspond pathologies

10.2   Pregnancy Diagnosis

- History: amenorrhea, tender and enlarged breasts, morning emesis, enlarged abdomen, fetal movements.
- Laboratory: urinary beta human chorionic gonadotropin (HCG).
- Visual confirmation of fetus in uterus at ultrasonography.

10.3   Antenatal Visits

- Routine antenatal care
  - Monthly antenatal visit from pregnancy diagnosis until 28 weeks, then twice-monthly visits until birth.
  - In high-risk pregnancies (such as hypertension and diabetes in pregnancy; previous history of spontaneous abortion; or higher-order gestations [twins, triplets]), more frequent visits are appropriate.
- Focused antenatal care
  - Total of four elective visits after pregnancy diagnosis, at 12, 26, and 32 weeks, and then once between 36 and 38 weeks.
  - The goal is to maximize good quality over quantity of visits.
  - This timetable is suitable for low-risk or uncomplicated pregnancies as well as for centers with facilities for good pregnancy supervision.

10.4   Laboratory Tests to Be Done During Routine Antenatal Visits

- First antenatal visit
  - Weight and height, BMI
  - Blood pressure
  - Urine dipstick: proteinuria, leukocyturia, bacteriuria
  - Simple blood count: hemoglobin
  - Blood group (ABO & Rhesus)
  - HIV counseling and testing, provider-initiated counseling and testing (PICT)
  - Venereal Disease Research Laboratory
  - Sickling test
  - Thick blood film: malaria blood film
  - Hepatitis B surface antigen
  - Ultrasound scan
- Subsequent antenatal visits
  - Blood pressure (every visit)
  - Urinalysis (every visit)
  - Hemoglobin (Hb) (at first, second, and third trimester)
  - Ultrasound (at diagnosis, second, and third trimesters)

10.5   Guidelines for Referral to Specialized Care

- At pregnancy diagnosis, a history of:
  - Poor obstetric outcomes: two or more consecutive spontaneous abortions: miscarriages or stillbirths
  - Two or more Caesarean sections
  - Higher-order pregnancies (twins, triplets, etc.)
  - Sickle cell disease
  - Asthma
  - Diabetes
  - Chronic kidney disease
  - Heart failure
- During the course of pregnancy:
  - Severe preeclampsia
  - Severe anemia (Hb < 6.0 g/dL)
  - Premature rupture of membranes (PROM)
  - Incessant bleeding, miscarriage
  - Placenta previa
  - Abruptio placentae
  - Intrauterine fetal death (IUFD)
  - Active genital herpes infection
- During labor
  - Prolonged labor (>12 h) irrespective of cause
  - Fetal distress

Table 10.1 Pregnancy and obstetrics conditions and their treatment

Diagnosis and classification	Treatment and relevant clinical features: pregnancy and obstetrics conditions
Abdominal pain in pregnancy Discomfort felt in the abdominoperineal region during pregnancy	*Treatment* • Patient education and reassurance • Identify and treat treatable underlying cause • Locate pregnancy and rule out extrauterine pregnancy (EUP) • Paracetamol, tab, 500 mg, 3 × 2 tab/d, 5 d *Etiology* • *Round ligament*: early in pregnancy, unilateral mild pelvic pain related to modification of one of the round ligaments • *Miscarriage*: defined as the loss of a pregnancy before 20 weeks of gestation • *Placental abruption*: acute placental abruption (i.e., decidual hemorrhage leading to the premature separation of the placenta prior to delivery) • *Pregnancy-related liver disease*: preeclampsia syndrome characterized by the new onset of hypertension and usually proteinuria after 20 weeks of gestation in a previously normotensive woman; right upper quadrant or epigastric pain is a sign of liver involvement and signifies the severe spectrum of the disease • *HELLP syndrome*: *H*emolysis with a microangiopathic blood smear, *el*evated *l*iver enzymes, and a *l*ow *p*latelet count are the findings in HELLP syndrome • *Acute fatty liver:* occurs in the second half of pregnancy, usually in the third trimester • *Uterine rupture:* caused by labor, intra-amniotic infection, fetal position or movement, or uterine incarceration • Fibroid degeneration or torsion • Bleeding ovarian cyst • *Constipation:* common in pregnancy and may cause considerable abdominal discomfort • Torsion of ovary, fallopian tube, or uterus • Pelvic inflammatory disease (PID) • Gastroesophageal reflux, gastritis • Gallbladder disease • Pneumonia involving the lower lobes • Pancreatic disease • Rectus sheath hematoma • Adrenal hemorrhage • Hiatal hernia • Acute appendicitis • Nephrolithiasis • Inflammatory bowel disease • Diverticulitis • Urinary tract infection • Pyelonephritis • Gastroenteritis • Extrauterine pregnancy • Sickle cell crisis *Life-threatening causes of abdominal pain* • Trauma • Spontaneous hemoperitoneum • Aneurysm: dissection and rupture of arterial aneurysms (e.g., splenic, renal, uterine, ovarian, aorta) • Mesenteric venous thrombosis *Note: Drugs are generally contraindicated in pregnancy except when the benefits outweigh the risks*

Table 10.1 (continued)

Diagnosis and classification	Treatment and relevant clinical features: pregnancy and obstetrics conditions
Acute renal failure Deterioration of kidney function (within hours to days) resulting in azotemia (as measured by creatinine) and failure of the kidney to maintain fluid electrolyte and acid–base homeostasis *Classifications* • Prerenal • Functional • Intrinsic (intrarenal) • Post-renal	*Treatment of fluid losses* • Correct underlying • Correct fluid loss replacement as follows: • Sodium chloride 0.9%, 500 ml bag for iv infusion, 1–2 bags/d iv, in cases of diarrhea and vomiting • ORS for oral intake *Etiology* • Nephrotoxic agents • Infections • Urinary tract obstructions • Immunologic insult to renal structures *Clinical assessment* • Disease duration • Urinalysis: proteinuria, hematuria • Estimation of the GFR
Anemia in pregnancy HB of 8–10 g/dl	*Treatment/prophylaxis* • Fefol (ferrous sulfate 200 mg/folic acid 0.5 mg) tab, 1 tb/d after food, possible with citrus juice *and* • Multivitamin, tab, 3 1 tabx/d *and* • Antimalarial prophylaxis *and* • Mebendazole tab, 500 mg, 1, tab, single dose after first trimester *Investigations* FBC • Blood film for malaria parasites • Sickling and Hb electrophoresis • Serum iron and ferritin • Stool analysis for hookworm ova • Urinalysis for schistosome ova and urobilinogen
Amenorrhea The absence of menses may be a transient, intermittent, or permanent condition resulting from dysfunction of the hypothalamus, pituitary, ovaries, uterus, or vagina	*Treatment* • Identify and treat underlying pathology (hyperprolactinemia, primary ovarian insufficiency (premature ovarian failure), intrauterine adhesions, polycystic ovary syndrome, thyroid disease) where possible • Refer for gynecologic management were needed *General management tips* • Lifestyle changes • Cognitive behavioral therapy • Management of low bone density *Etiology* • *Structural abnormalities*: congenital abnormality in Mullerian development, congenital defect of urogenital sinus development, intrauterine adhesions • *Hypothalamic dysfunction*: isolated GnRH deficiency, functional hypothalamic amenorrhea (weight loss, eating disorders, excessive exercise, stress, severe or prolonged illness, inflammatory or infiltrative diseases, brain tumors, cranial irradiation, traumatic brain injury • *Pituitary dysfunction*: Hyperprolactinemia, pituitary tumors, empty sella syndrome, pituitary infarct, or apoplexy • *Ovarian dysfunction*: primary ovarian insufficiency, polycystic ovary syndrome • *Other*: Hyperthyroidism, hypothyroidism, uncontrolled diabetes mellitus types 1 and 2, exogenous androgen use

(continued)

Table 10.1 (continued)

Diagnosis and classification	Treatment and relevant clinical features: pregnancy and obstetrics conditions
Classification • *Primary amenorrhea*: The absence of menses at age 15 years in the presence of normal growth and secondary sexual characteristics. Usually of genetic origin • *Secondary amenorrhea*: The absence of menses for more than 3 months in girls or women who previously had regular menstrual cycles or 6 months in girls or women who had irregular menses	*Clinical evaluation*: comprehensive clinical evaluation consisting of history, physical examination, and paramedical investigations • *History*: – Interrogate on the presence of stress, change in weight, diet, or exercise habits, or is there an eating disorder or illness (that might result in functional hypothalamic amenorrhea), drugs that might cause or be associated with amenorrhea, hirsutism, acne, and a history of irregular menses (suggestive of hyperandrogenism) – Symptoms of hypothalamic-pituitary disease, including headaches, visual field defects, fatigue, or polyuria and polydipsia? Any symptoms of estrogen deficiency, including hot flashes, vaginal dryness, poor sleep, or decreased libido suggesting primary ovarian insufficiency? Had galactorrhea, which suggests hyperprolactinemia? – History of obstetrical catastrophe, severe bleeding, dilatation and curettage, or endometritis or other infection that might have caused scarring of the endometrial lining (Ascherman's syndrome)? • *Physical examination:* – Height and weight. A body mass index (BMI) greater than 30 kg/m^2 is observed in 50% or more of women with PCOS – Parotid gland swelling and/or erosion of dental enamel would suggest an eating disorder – Examination for evidence of galactorrhea – Vulvovaginal exam • *Paramedical evaluation*: rule out pregnancy (urinary Beta HCG, , FSH, serum PRL, TSH)
Bartholin duct cysts and abscess The Bartholin glands are located in the vulva. Blockage of the Bartholin ducts is a common cause of a vulvar mass. The most common Bartholin masses are cysts or abscesses; Bartholin benign and malignant tumors are rare *Synonym* • Greater vestibular glands	*Treatment* • Appropriate perineal hygiene • Incision and drainage • Co-amoxicillin tab, 1 g, 2 × 1 tab/d, 5 d *Pathophysiology* • The Bartholin glands are located in the vulva • The gland drains to the vulva openings • The draining system of the gland may be locked leading to liquid collection, abscess and cyst formation
Bleeding in pregnancy Bleeding from the vagina, a common event at all stages of pregnancy	*Treatment* • Abdominopelvic ultrasound scan • Reassurance • Strict bed rest if threatened abortion • Give antibiotics if signs of infection are present • Refer to Ob-Gyn if threatened or inevitable abortion *Etiology* • Ectopic pregnancy • Miscarriage (threatened, inevitable, incomplete, complete) • Implantation of the pregnancy • Cervical, vaginal, or uterine pathology (e.g., polyps, inflammation/infection, trophoblastic disease) *Differential diagnosis* • Based on the gestational age, a variety of differential diagnoses should be evoked *First trimester* • Physiological due to implantation • Ectopic pregnancy • Molar pregnancy • Fetal loss/miscarriage

Table 10.1 (continued)

Diagnosis and classification	Treatment and relevant clinical features: pregnancy and obstetrics conditions
	Second–third trimester • Placenta previa • Placental abruption • Idiopathic *Management tips* • Patient education • Avoid speculum • Digital vaginal examination in the acute phase
Candidiasis Superficial/deep skin or mucosal infection caused by fungi (e.g., *Candida albicans*)	*Treatment* Oral and esophageal candidiasis: • Fluconazol, tab, 50 mg, 1×/d, 10 d Vaginal candidiasis: • Fluconazole vaginal ovule, 1×/d, 3 d • Canesten vaginal ovules, 2 × 1 ovule/d, 3 d *Diagnostic entities* • Cheilitis • Folliculitis • Intertrigo • Migrating cheilitis • Onyxis and perionyxes • Oral thrush • Septicemia (immunosuppressed patients) • Vulvovaginitis *Note:* Most women may have vaginal candidiasis after antibiotherapy. Hence, anticipate and explain at the time of prescribing antibiotherapy to a female patient
Carcinoma of the cervix Cancer of the uterine cervix Human Papilloma Virus is central to the development of cervical neoplasia *Histopathology* • Squamous cell carcinoma • Adenocarcinoma • Adenosquamous • Rare histologic forms	*Prevention* • HPV vaccination • Regular pap smear • Visual inspection of cervix with acetic acid *Risk factors* • Early onset of sexual activity • Multiple sexual partners • A high-risk sexual partner (e.g., a partner with multiple sexual partners or known HPV infection) • History of vulvar or vaginal squamous intraepithelial neoplasia • Immunosuppression (e.g., HIV infection) *Signs and symptoms* • Postcoital bleeding • Excessive prolonged vaginal bleeding • Postmenopausal bleeding • Foul smelling vaginal discharge • Lower abdominal pain • Weight loss • Urinary symptoms, for example, dysuria, frequency, incontinence • Rectal pain

(continued)

Table 10.1 (continued)

Diagnosis and classification	Treatment and relevant clinical features: pregnancy and obstetrics conditions
Care of mother and baby immediately after delivery (see also 17.2, Initial care after birth)	*After-birth care for the normal child without risk factors* • *Cord clamping: delayed umbilical cord clamping (≥ 1 min) is recommended to prevent anemia* • *Temperature: to prevent hypothermia, the newborn is immediately dried with warmed cotton towel and placed on the mother's chest/belly* • *Airways: Be aware of baby positioning to ensure opening of the airways* • *Breathing: respiratory rate 30–60/min* • *Circulation: heart rate >100/min* • *The Apgar score is assessed at 1, 5, and 10 min post delivery* • *Encourage breastfeeding shortly after delivery and skin-to-skin contact* • *First exam should be performed about 2 h after delivery (under radiant warmer and good light)* • *Thermoregulation: rectal temperature 36.5–37.5 °C* • *Measurements: weight, length, and head circumference* • *Respiration: normal range 30–60/min, signs of respiratory distress?* • *Circulation: normal range 100–160/min, periphery is warm and well perfused* • *Malformation?* • *The vitamin K prophylaxis and the active and passive hepatitis B vaccination, according to guidelines* • *Prophylactic eye drops (Azithromycin or tetracycline eye drop) to prevent neonatal gonococcal and chlamydial ophthalmia are no longer recommended*
Chronic renal failure Defined as the presence of kidney damage (usually detected as urinary albumin excretion of 30 mg/d or more, or equivalent) or decreased kidney function (defined as an estimated glomerular filtration rate [eGFR] <60 mL/min/1.73 m^2) for three or more months, irrespective of the cause	*Treatment* • Treat underlying cause • Enalapril, tab, 10 mg, 2 × 1 tab/d or • Perindopril, tab, 5 mg, 1 tb/d • Treatment concept: treat reversible causes of renal failure to prevent or slow the progression of renal disease *Treatment of the complications of renal failure* • Adjusting drug doses when appropriate for the level of estimated glomerular filtration rate (eGFR) • Identification and adequate preparation of the patient in whom renal replacement therapy will be required • Refer to tertiary center when creatinine exceeds 300 μmol/L • Patient education *Etiology (children and adults confounded)* • Congenital anomalies of the kidney and urinary tract • Primary glomerular disease • Cystic/hereditary/congenital diseases • Secondary glomerular disease/vasculitis • Interstitial nephritis/pyelonephritis • Diabetes • Transplant complications • Neoplasms/tumors • Miscellaneous conditions • Etiology uncertain
Eclampsia New onset, generalized, tonic-clonic seizures or coma in a woman with preeclampsia *Note* Eclampsia is the convulsive manifestation of preeclampsia and one of several clinical manifestations at the severe end of the preeclampsia spectrum	*Treatment* • Stop and prevent further seizures • Control the elevated blood pressure • Deliver baby as promptly as possible • Monitor closely for the onset of multiple organ failure • Magnesium sulfate: iv 0.5 g/ml in 2 ml ampoule (equivalent to 1 g in 2 ml; 50% weight/volume); 0.5 g/ml in 10 ml ampoule (equivalent to 5 g in 10 ml; 50% weight/volume)

Table 10.1 (continued)

Diagnosis and classification	Treatment and relevant clinical features: pregnancy and obstetrics conditions
Ectopic pregnancy Implantation of conceived fetus in the tubal lining or in the peritoneum. Also known as extrauterine pregnancy 96% occur in the fallopian tube	*Treatment* • Evaluate appropriately (history, laboratory work-up, ultrasound) • Prompt referral to tertiary care with proper documentation for gynecological-surgical extraction *Risk factors* • Previous ectopic pregnancy • PID and other genital infections, for example, pelvic tuberculosis • Infertility • In vitro fertilization • Tubal reconstructive surgery • Smoking • Increasing age *Diagnostic features* • Menorrhagia or irregular vaginal bleeding and spotting • Pelvic pain, usually adnexal • Adnexal mass by clinical examination or ultrasound • Failure of serum Beta HCG to double every 48 h • No intrauterine pregnancy seen on the transvaginal ultrasound *Clinical presentation* • First-trimester vaginal bleeding and/or abdominal pain • Classic clinical triad: • Pelvic pain • Metrorrhagia • Amenorrhea *Note:* Pelvic pain occurring among women of childbearing age: evoke or rule out ectopic pregnancy
Emergency contraception (EC) Entails products that prevent pregnancy from occurring after an episode of unprotected intercourse which may happen as a result of contraception non-use or imperfect use or from forced sexual activity. EC does not interrupt an existing pregnancy. It does *not* cause abortion	*Treatment* • Levonorgestrel, tab, 1.5 mg, 1 tab to be taken orally within 24 h of event, note if high BMI *or* • Ethinyl estradiol tab, 100 mcg plus Norgestrel, tab, 1 mg, 2 × 1 tab/d, 1 d Consider STD prophylaxis • Ciprofloxacin oral, tab, 500 mg, 2 × 1 tab/d, 5 d *and* • Metronidazole tab, 500 mg, 4, tab, orally immediately as a single dose or 500 mg tabs, 3 × 1 tab/d, 5 d • Adequate counseling • Inform about possible contraceptive methods
Endometriosis An abnormal growth of endometrium outside the uterus, mainly in the dependent parts of the pelvis and in the ovaries, causing chronic pain and infertility	*Treatment* • Rule out PID; refer to tertiary center with adequate documentation Pain control: • Paracetamol 500 mg, 3 × 2 tab/d • Ibuprofen 400 mg, 2 × 1 tab/d *Diagnostic features* • Dysmenorrhea • Dyspareunia • Chronic pelvic pain • Increased frequency among infertile women • Abnormal uterine bleeding

(continued)

Table 10.1 (continued)

Diagnosis and classification	Treatment and relevant clinical features: pregnancy and obstetrics conditions
Female genital mutilation Surgical removal of parts of the female external genitalia motivated by cultural, religious, or motives other than medical *Procedures* • Clitoridectomy • Excision • Infibulation • Other non-medical procedures	*Treatment* • Psychological support • Surgical repair where indicated • Primary prevention • Education • Preservation of young women's integrity *Secondary and tertiary prevention* • Awareness • Corrective surgery *Acute complications* • Contention injuries • Death • Gangrene • Hemorrhage • Pain • Painful miction • Urinary retention • Septicemia • Shock • Tetanus *Long-term complications (vary according to social context)* • Dyspareunia • Infertility • Menstrual dysfunction • Obstetrical complications • Scarring: infected fistula, keloid • Urinary dysfunction: incontinence, infections
Female genital prolapse When the muscles of the female pelvis floor weaken, organs such as the uterus, urethra, bladder, or rectum may protrude down into the vagina *Classification* With the vaginal wall a reference: • Anterior • Middle • Posterior *Pelvic organ prolapse nomenclature:* Various organs may protrude or prolapse into the vaginal canal *Cystocele:* A hernia of the bladder wall into the vagina *Ureterocele:* Sagging of the urethra after its detachment from the symphysis pubis during childbirth *Rectocele:* Herniation of the terminal rectum into the posterior vagina *Enterocele:* A vaginal vault hernia containing small intestine mostly in the posterior vagina	*Treatment* • High-fiber diet and laxatives • Weight reduction when obese • Evaluate associated incontinence • Surgical measures • Refer promptly to tertiary center for gynecological review *Signs and symptoms* • Usually, asymptomatic • Anterior prolapse: urinary incontinence, miction dysfunction, urinary retention • Middle prolapse: feeling of pelvic pressure/heaviness, bulge • Posterior prolapse: fecal incontinence, incomplete stool evacuation (hand pressure may be needed) • Sensation of motion or protrusion in the vagina • Urinary or fecal incontinence • Constipation • A sense of incomplete bladder emptying • Dyspareunia *Risk factors* • Age • Childbirth • Hysterectomy • Menopause • Obesity • Multiparity • Pregnancy

Table 10.1 (continued)

Diagnosis and classification	Treatment and relevant clinical features: pregnancy and obstetrics conditions
Female sexual dysfunction Includes lack of sexual desire, impaired arousal, inability to achieve orgasm, pain with sexual activity, or a combination of these issues *Classification* • Disorders of sexual desire • Sexual arousal disorder • Orgasmic disorder • Sexual pain disorder	*Treatment* • Adopt a multidisciplinary and multimodal approach • Counseling • Couples' therapy and sex therapy • Psychotherapy and psychopharmacology • Lifestyle changes, fatigue, stress, and lack of privacy contribute significantly to low libido and sexual problems for women *Clinical approach* Complete the evaluation and diagnosis Assess patient goals Counsel the patient Address partner issues Treat associated conditions
Fever of unknown origin (FUO) Fever of 38.3 °C for at least three weeks' duration Fever over 38.3 °C on several occasions Diagnosis has not been made for three outpatient visits or 3 d of hospitalization Fever is defined as a measured body temperature of 37.4 °C or more	*Treatment* • Assess according to available resources • Refer to tertiary center with proper documentation *Etiology* • *Infections:* Tuberculosis, endocarditis, primary HIV infections or opportunistic infections, gallbladder disease • *Systemic rheumatic diseases:* Vasculitis, rheumatoid arthritis, systemic lupus erythematosus, polymyalgia rheumatica, neutropenia • *Malignancies*: Lymphoma *Diagnostic tools* *Laboratory:* ESR, CRP, tuberculin skin test, HIV immunoassay, blood cultures where available, LFT, creatinine, rheumatoid factor *Imaging:* Abdominal and chest ultrasound, chest radiograph, CT scan of chest and abdomen and brain *Biopsy:* Skin, bone marrow, pleural fluid *Clinical assessment* • History and physical examination • FBC • Blood cultures where available • Routine blood chemistry, including liver enzymes and bilirubin • If liver tests are abnormal, hepatitis B serology • Urinalysis, including microscopic examination, and urine culture • Chest radiograph
Genital ulcers and STDs Infections (viral, bacterial, fungal, and ectoparasitic) that are acquired primarily by sexual intercourse *Diagnostic entities* • Chancroid • Chlamydia • Genital herpes • Gonorrhea • Hepatitis B, C • Syphilis	*Treatment* *Chancroid* • Azithromycin, tab, 250 mg, 4 tab orally in a single dose *or* • Ciprofloxacin tab, 500 mg, 2 × 1 tab/d, 3 d *or* • Erythromycin tab, 500 mg, 4 × 1 tab/d, 7 d *Chlamydia* • Azithromycin tab, 250 mg, 4, tab, single dose (preferably to be taken under direct observation) *or* • Doxycycline, tab,100 mg, 2 × 1 tab/d, 7 d *Genital herpes* • Acyclovir, tab, 200 mg, 4 × 1 tab/d, 7 d for first attack • Acyclovir, tab, 200 mg, 4× daily, 5 d for recurrent episodes • Acyclovir cream to apply twice daily

(continued)

Table 10.1 (continued)

Diagnosis and classification	Treatment and relevant clinical features: pregnancy and obstetrics conditions
	Gonorrhea • Ceftriaxone ampoule 250 mg, IM in a single dose *and* • Azithromycin, tab, 250 mg, 4, tab, orally in a single dose If Ceftriaxone is not available: • Cefixime, tab, 400 mg, 1 tab/d in a single dose *and* • Azithromycin, tab, 250 mg, 4, tab, orally in a single dose *Hepatitis B, C* • Refer to appropriate tertiary center to enquire availability of pegylated gamma interferon-based treatment *or* • A combination of interferon and antiviral treatment. This may not be readily available • *Lamivudine, tab,* 100 mg 1 tab/d, eight weeks followed by combination therapy with lamivudine plus *interferon alfa-2b* (10 MU SQ three times weekly) for 16 weeks *or* • *Lamivudine*, tab, 100 mg, 1 tab/d for 52 weeks *Syphilis* • Benzathine penicillin, ampoule, IM 2.4 million units, 1 ampoule IM single dose *or* • Procaine Penicillin, ampoule 1.2 million units, 1 amp IM/d, 10 d *or* • Doxycycline, tab, 100 mg, 2 × 1 tab/d, 10 d For pregnant women or those allergic to penicillin • Erythromycin tab, 500 mg, 4 × 1 tab/d, 14 d
Genital warts (venereal) Maculo squamous skin lesion mainly in the anogenital region often induced by Human Papiloma Virus infection	*Treatment* • Podophyllin 10–25%, apply in tinct carefully to external genital, perianal, vaginal, and rectal warts while avoiding normal tissue • Wash thoroughly 4 h after application
Gestational diabetes (GD) Defined as onset or first recognition of abnormal glucose tolerance during pregnancy GD is equally considered a development of diabetes mellitus during pregnancy in women whose pancreatic function is insufficient to overcome the insulin resistance associated with the pregnant state *Nomenclature* Hyperglycemia in pregnancy can be due to: • Diabetes in pregnancy, that is, preexisting diabetes complicating pregnancy *or* • Gestational diabetes mellitus (GDM)	*Treatment* • When available, use insulin for all diabetics in pregnancy • Adjust insulin doses accordingly • Folate supplementation 5 mg daily • Deliver after 38 weeks • Give parenteral corticosteroids to boost fetal lung maturity if delivery is imminent before 37 weeks of gestation • Benefits of adequate treatment are reduction of preeclampsia, a birth weight > 4000 g, shoulder dystocia *Maternal risks for contracting GD* • Personal history of impaired glucose tolerance • Ethnicity: African origin • Family history of diabetes • Pre-pregnancy weight ≥110% of ideal body weight or BMI > 30 kg/m^2 • Older maternal age (>25 or 30 years of age) • Previous unexplained perinatal loss or birth of a malformed infant • Glycosuria at the first prenatal visit • Previous birth of an infant ≥4000 or 4500 g (approximately 9 or 10 pounds) • Medical condition associated with development of diabetes: metabolic syndrome, polycystic ovary syndrome, current use of glucocorticoids, hypertension, or cardiovascular disease, acanthosis nigricans • Multiple gestation

Table 10.1 (continued)

Diagnosis and classification	Treatment and relevant clinical features: pregnancy and obstetrics conditions
	Adverse factors associated with GD • Preeclampsia, gestational hypertension • Hydramnios • Macrosomia and large for gestational age infant • Maternal and infant birth trauma • Operative delivery (cesarean, instrumental) • Perinatal mortality • Fetal/neonatal hypertrophic cardiomyopathy • Neonatal respiratory problems and metabolic complications (hypoglycemia, hyperbilirubinemia, jaundice hypocalcemia, polycythemia) • Neonatal hypoglycemia (<2.5 mmol/L) *Management tips* • Determine the specific type of diabetes: pregestational (Type I; Type II) or gestational by history • Admit patients • Ultrasound scan (to monitor well-being) and macrosomia • Urine dipstick: proteinuria and asymptomatic bacteriuria • Preexisting diabetes can lead to fetal malformations during pregnancy • Africans are more prone to develop gestational diabetes
Gestational trophoblastic neoplasia (GTN) Abnormal proliferation of trophoblastic tissue mostly following a hydatidform mole or a nonmolar pregnancy	*Treatment* • Evaluate appropriately • Refer to tertiary center with proper documentation *Clinical features* • Intermittent vaginal bleeding • Cough and hemoptysis • Weight loss • Pelvic examination may show an enlarged uterus or no abnormal findings • Positive pregnancy test (Beta HCG) • Chest X-ray: Cannonball metastases *Risk factors* • Hydatidiform mole • Positive family history • Positive personal history *GTN* comprises the following histologic types: • Invasive mole • Choriocarcinoma • Placental site trophoblastic tumor • Epithelioid trophoblastic tumor
Hydatidform mole pregnancy A gestational trophoblastic disease, which originates in the placenta and has the potential to locally invade the uterus and metastasize. A unique maternal tumor arising from gestational rather than maternal tissue *Classification* Malignant disease is referred to as *gestational trophoblastic neoplasia.* The histologic entities included in this group are: • Invasive mole • Choriocarcinoma • Placental site trophoblastic tumor • Epithelioid trophoblastic tumor	*Treatment* • Evaluate adequately • Refer for specialized gynecological management with proper documentation Risk factors • Prior molar pregnancy • Extremes of maternal age (≤15 and >35 years) • History of prior spontaneous abortion and infertility *Clinical features* • Amenorrhea, a positive pregnancy test • Signs of early pregnancy complications: bleeding, pelvic discomfort, hyperemesis gravidarum • Unusually high human chorionic gonadotropin (hCG)

(continued)

Table 10.1 (continued)

Diagnosis and classification	Treatment and relevant clinical features: pregnancy and obstetrics conditions
Hypertension in pregnancy Gestational hypertension is a clinical diagnosis defined by the new onset of hypertension (defined as systolic blood pressure $\geq$ 140 mmHg and/or diastolic blood pressure $\geq$ 90 mmHg) at $\geq$ 20 weeks of gestation in the absence of proteinuria or new signs of end-organ dysfunction	*Treatment* Hypertension only: • Alpha-methyl dopa (Aldomet), tab, 250 mg 2–3× 1 tab/d, increase gradually if needed (maximum dose 3 g/d) *or* • Hydralazine tab, 25 mg, 2 × 1 tab/d *or* • Nifedipin, tab, 20 mg, 2 × 1 tab/d • Refer to tertiary center if hypertension + proteinuria is present *Nomenclature* *Gestational hypertension:* a temporary (provisional) diagnosis for hypertensive pregnant women who do not meet criteria for preeclampsia Diagnosis changes to • *Preeclampsia*, if proteinuria, severe hypertension, or new signs of end-organ dysfunction develop • *Chronic hypertension*, if blood pressure elevation persists $\geq$12 weeks postpartum. Normal BP: Systolic <120 mmHg and diastolic <80 mmHg; Elevated BP: Systolic 120–129 mmHg and diastolic <80 mmHg • *Transient hypertension* of pregnancy, if BP returns to normal by 12 weeks postpartum *Risk factors* • History of preeclampsia • Pregestational diabetes • Chronic hypertension • Systemic lupus erythematosus • Pre-pregnancy BMI >25 • Antiphospholipid syndrome • Chronic kidney disease • Multifetal pregnancy • First pregnancy • Family history of preeclampsia • Prior pregnancy complications associated with placental insufficiency • Advanced maternal age • Use of assisted reproductive technology *Management tips* • Nifedipine may delay labor • Patient education to ensure patient comes for routine antenatal visits • Do urine dipstick checking for protein to rule in/out preeclampsia

Table 10.1 (continued)

Diagnosis and classification	Treatment and relevant clinical features: pregnancy and obstetrics conditions
Female infertility Pregnancy does not result after 1 year of normal sexual activity without contraceptives	*Treatment* • Evaluate adequately • Provide primary general medical care • Refer to tertiary center for gynecologic review and management *Evaluation and assessment* *History* • Duration of infertility • Menstrual history (cycle length and characteristics) • Medical, surgical, and gynecological history (including STIs, PID) • Obstetrical history • Sexual history • Family history • Personal and lifestyle history, including age, occupation, exercise, stress, dieting/changes in weight, smoking, and alcohol use, all of which can affect fertility *Physical examination* • BMI • Abnormalities of the thyroid gland • Galactorrhea • Signs of androgen excess (hirsutism, acne, male pattern baldness, virilization) *Diagnostic tests* • Documentation of normal ovulatory function • Perform a test to rule out tubal occlusion and assess the uterine cavity hysterosalpingogram • Assessment of ovulatory function: clomiphene citrate challenge test *Semen analysis* • Constitutes the cornerstone of the assessment of the male partner of an infertile couple • Semen sample should be collected after 2–7 d of abstinence • Semen sample should be submitted to the laboratory within 1 h of collection
Leiomyoma uteri Benign soft muscle tumor along with reactive fibrous tissue proliferation of the uterine mucosa *Nomenclature* • Leiomyoma • Fibroma • Fibroleiomyoma	*Treatment* • Watchful waiting: periodic office consultation • Address to gynecology if complications present *Complications* • Intermenstrual bleeding • Hypermenorrhea • Anemia • Impaired conception • Recurrent fetal loss • Dyspareunia *Signs and symptoms* • Typical age of onset: 40–50 years old • Common in women of African descent • Menorrhagia • Pain • Anemia • Abdominal bulge • Urinary dysfunction (mass effect)

(continued)

Table 10.1 (continued)

Diagnosis and classification	Treatment and relevant clinical features: pregnancy and obstetrics conditions
Malaria in pregnancy Infection of the present woman with one of the malaria-causing plasmodia species	*Treatment:Mild/uncomplicated* • Coartem (Artemether 20 mg and lumefantrin 120 mg), tab, 2 × 4 tab/d, 3 d *or* • Quinine, tab, 300 mg, 2 × 2 tab/d, 5 d *Severe/complicated* • Quinine, ampoule 600 mg, 1 amp in 500 ml of 5% dextrose to be infused iv during 2–4 h followed by oral Quinine, tab, 300 mg, 2 × 2 tab/d 5 d *or* • Coartem, tab, 2 × 4 tab/d, 3 d • Adequate fluid intake *Prevention* • Mosquito avoidance • Advocate for good communal hygiene
Medication to facilitate delivery Uncomplicated term child birth is a sequential multi-stage process including labor, delivery, recovery, and postpartum stages (LDRP). Several medication are used at the various stages. Based on the stage of the child birth, the medication may be analgesic, uterotonic, anti-infectious or supportive	*Analgesic* Tramadol 100mg in 500ml NaCl 0.0% infusion *Uterotonic* Oxytocin (Pitocin): 10 units/mL (1 mL, 10 mL, 50 mL): 100 Units infusion in 500ml NaCl 0.9 infusion *Anti-infectious* Optional, Benzylpenicillin 500mg im, followed by, Amoxicillin 500mg tabs, 3x 1 tab/day 3 days based on clinical judgement *Supportive* Sodium Chloride 0.9%, 3x 500ml within 12 hours
Menometrorrhagia Abnormally heavy, prolonged, and irregular uterine bleeding	*Treatment* Determine and manage underlying cause Refer to gynecology as needed *Etiology* • Structural abnormalities: uterine leiomyomas, endometrial polyps, adenomyosis, Cesarean scar defect, enhanced myometrial vascularity, for example, arteriovenous malformation • Ovulatory dysfunction • Bleeding disorders • Iatrogenic: for example, anticoagulants, hormonal contraceptives, intrauterine device • Neoplastic: endometrial hyperplasia or carcinoma, or uterino sarcoma • Infection and inflammation—endometritis, pelvic inflammatory disease • Disorders of local endometrial hemostasis *Clinical evaluation* • *History:* Menstrual history, sexual history, contraceptive history, precise questions to determine source of bleeding, premenarchal or postmenopausal? Is the patient pregnant? What is the bleeding pattern? Does the pattern suggest regular and ovulatory bleeding or irregular and possibly anovulatory bleeding? • *Physical examination*: abdominal and/or bimanual pelvic examination; inspection of the urethra may reveal a urethral caruncle, anorectal lesion (e.g., hemorrhoid or rectal mass), or positive fecal occult blood testing suggests non-genital source *Normal menstrual history* • Frequency every 24–38 d • Occurs at fairly regular intervals, with a variation from the interval from first day of bleeding of one cycle to the first day of the next of less than 7–9 d across cycles • Volume of blood ≥ 5–≤ 80 mL; clinically, excessive blood loss is defined as a volume that interferes with the woman's physical, emotional, social, and/or material quality of life • Duration is 4.5–8 d

Table 10.1 (continued)

Diagnosis and classification	Treatment and relevant clinical features: pregnancy and obstetrics conditions
	Paramedical work-up • Human chorionic gonadotropin (hCG) to exclude pregnancy • Complete blood count, hemoglobin, and/or hematocrit along with a ferritin level to assess for anemia • Urine analysis • Imaging by hysteroscopy • Lower abdominal sonography
Menopause Permanent cessation of menstruation occurs usually due to loss of ovarian function 45–55 years *Menopausal syndrome* Hormonal changes around menopause with associated physical, emotional, and psychological disorders of varying intensity: • Mood changes • Depression • Anxiety • Nervousness • Irritability • Loss of libido • Sleep impairment • Joint pain	*Treatment* • Address associated emotional and clinical syndromes • Discuss hormone replacement • Refer for gynecology assessment if needed *Complications* Atrophic changes in the genital tract may be complicated by: • Increased frequency of micturition and dysuria • Stress incontinence (urinary incontinence with coughing or straining) • Vaginal dryness and dyspareunia *Menopause and menopausal syndrome* Permanent cessation of menstrual periods determined retrospectively after a woman has experienced 12 months of amenorrhea without any other obvious pathological or physiological cause. It occurs at around age of 51 years in normal women *Note*: Final cessation of menstruation, either as a normal part of aging or as a result of surgical removal of both ovaries *Clinical manifestations and diagnostic features* • Irregular menstrual cycles • The cessation of menstruation • Elevated follicle-stimulating hormone • Marked hormonal fluctuations • Hot flashes and night sweats, vasopressor symptoms • Sleep disturbances • Mood symptoms: depression and irritability • Vaginal dryness and dyspareunia • Cognitive changes • Joint pain • Vaginal atrophy • Osteoporosis *Signs and symptoms* • Hot flushes (heat or burning in the face, neck, and chest with resultant sweating) • Nonspecific signs and symptoms: palpitations, faintness, dizziness, fatigue, weakness
Molluscum contagiosum Causative agent: pox virus	*Treatment* Apply 10–25% podophyllin in tinct very carefully to external genital, perianal, vaginal, and rectal warts while avoiding normal tissue. Wash thoroughly 4 h after application
Nonprogression of fetus No fetal heart activity can be detected by transabdominal echography	*Treatment* • Dilatation and curettage • Psychological support for mother • Exclude potential causes

(continued)

Table 10.1 (continued)

Diagnosis and classification	Treatment and relevant clinical features: pregnancy and obstetrics conditions
Pelvic inflammatory disease (PID) An ascending infection of the female reproductive organs A polymicrobial infection of the upper genital tract associated with STDs as well as endogenous organisms *Classification* • Acute PID • Chronic PID	*Treatment* *First line* • Ceftriaxone, ampoule, 1 g, 1 amp im as unique dose (where available) *and* • Metronidazole (Flagyl), tab, 500 mg, 3 × 1 tab/d, 10 d • Doxycycline, tab, 100 mg, 2 × 1 tab/d, 10 d *and* • Fluconazole, tab, 100 mg, 1, tab, single dose *Second line* • Azithromycin, tab, 500 mg 1×/d, 3 d *and* • Metronidazole (Flagyl), tab, 500 mg, 3 × 1 tab/d, 10 d *and* • Fluconazole, tab, 100 mg 1× tab, single dose • Consider gynecological referral for PAP smear • Educate about modes of transmission *Common etiologies are infections by:* • *N. gonorrhoeae* • *C. trachomatis* • *Mycoplasma hominis* *Diagnostic features* • Uterine, adnexal, or cervical motion tenderness • Abnormal discharge from the vagina or cervix • Absence of a competing diagnosis *Signs and symptoms* • Lower abdominal pain • Lower abdominal tenderness • Vaginal examination: tenderness over uterus, both fornices, and on moving the cervix • Fever • Purulent vaginal discharge
Pelvic pain syndrome Myofascial pelvic pain syndrome is a non-articular musculoskeletal pain disorder characterized by contracted bands of skeletal muscle that contain discrete, painful nodules, also called trigger *Primary dysmenorrhea* Menstrual pain associated with menstrual cycles in the absence of pathologic findings	*Treatment* • Rigorous etiologic evaluation • Directed etiologic treatment • Ibuprofen, tab, 400 mg, 2 × 1 tab/d, 5 d • Paracetamol, tab, 500 mg, 3 × 2 tab/d, 5 d *Differential diagnosis* • Gynecologic • Urologic • Musculoskeletal • Gastrointestinal • Vascular • Metabolic *Clinical presentation* • Pain in the pelvis, vagina, vulva, rectum, or bladder, or in more distant referral areas such as the thighs, buttocks, hips, or lower abdomen • Often associated symptoms include a sense of aching, heaviness, or burning in these areas and/or symptoms of overactive bladder, constipation, or dyspareunia

Table 10.1 (continued)

Diagnosis and classification	Treatment and relevant clinical features: pregnancy and obstetrics conditions
	Etiology • PID and tubo-ovarian abscess • Hemorrhage, rupture, or torsion of an ovarian neoplasm • Torsion or degeneration of a uterine leiomyoma • Endometriosis, especially rupture of endometrium • Endometritis • Ovarian hyperstimulation syndrome in women undergoing gonadotropin treatment for infertility • Ectopic pregnancy • Miscarriage • Appendicitis • Acute cystitis • Diverticulitis • Urinary tract calculi • Abdominal wall trauma
Polycystic ovary syndrome Endocrine disorder of unknown etiology that causes chronic anovulation, polycystic ovaries, and hyperandrogenism	*Treatment* • Weight reduction • Regular physical exercise • Refer to tertiary center for specialized gynecological care *Clinical findings* Menstrual disorders ranging from amenorrhea to menorrhagia Infertility Hirsutism and/or acne Increased risk of gestational diabetes and preeclampsia
Postpartum hemorrhage Postpartum women with bleeding that is greater than expected and results in signs and/or symptoms of hypovolemia: low BP, drowsiness	*Treatment* Strive to answer the three major questions: • Is the uterus empty? • Is the uterus ruptured? • Is the uterus atonic? *Etiology* • Placenta retention • Incomplete delivery • Obstetrical trauma: vaginal or cervical lacerations • Diffuse or focal uterine atony • Uterine inversion • Maternal coagulopathy or other bleeding diasthesis *Note: Primary cause of maternal death worldwide*

(continued)

Table 10.1 (continued)

Diagnosis and classification	Treatment and relevant clinical features: pregnancy and obstetrics conditions
Preeclampsia Blood pressure of 140 mmHg or higher systolic, or 90 mm or higher diastolic after 20 weeks of gestation Multisystemic progressive disorder due to new onset of hypertension and proteinuria or hypertension and significant end-organ dysfunction with or without proteinuria, in the last half of pregnancy or postpartum *Eclampsia* *Definition:* Seizures in the patient with evidence of preeclampsia *Diagnostic specifications* Defined as BP $\geq$ 140/90 mmHg with Proteinuria $\geq$1+	*Treatment* • Manage expectantly • Weekly antenatal visits • Weekly BP and dipstick measurement • Refer to tertiary center • Control BP with 20 mg Nifedipine; Aldomet • Give seizure prophylaxis with magnesium sulfate ($MgSO_4$) • *Injection:* 0.5 g/ml in 2 ml ampoule, (equivalent to 1 g in 2 ml; 50% weight/volume); 0.5 g/ml in 10 ml ampoule (equivalent to 5 g in 10 ml; 50% weight/volume) • Consent for pregnancy termination within 24–48 h *Diagnostic features* • Proteinuria of 0.3 g or more in 24 h • Progressive kidney injury • Thrombocytopenia • Elevated liver enzymes, low platelet count (HELLP) • Pulmonary edema • Vision changes or headache *Classification of preeclampsia*: mild or severe • *Mild:* BP < 160/100 mmHg and proteinuria <2+ with no signs of severity: headache, visual blurring, vomiting, epigastric pain, pedal edema • *Severe:* BP $\geq$ 150/100 mmHg and proteinuria $\geq$2+ and/or signs of severity
Prelabor rupture of membrane (PROM) Rupture of the membranes before the onset of labor	*Treatment* • PROM at term: induction of labor and delivery within 24 h • PPROM (less than 34 weeks) manage as premature labor *Note*: Prolonged PROM for more than 12 h is a risk for ascending infection resulting to chorioamnionitis *Clinical signs of chorioamnionitis* • Fever • Purulent vaginal discharge • Maternal tachycardia • Uterine tenderness *Signs and symptoms* • Leakage of fluid from the vagina • Sterile speculum examination reveals a clear fluid issuing from the cervical os or pool of fluid in the posterior vaginal fornix

Table 10.1 (continued)

Diagnosis and classification	Treatment and relevant clinical features: pregnancy and obstetrics conditions
Premenopausal abnormal uterine bleeding Average normal menstrual bleeding 5 d, a range of 3–7 d with mean blood loss of 40 ml	*Treatment* • Initial clinical evaluation • Consider tranexamic acid (Cyclokapron), 1 g tab, 3 × 1 tab/d *Terminology* • *Menorrhagia:* Blood loss of over 8 ml bleeding between periods • *Hypermenorrhea:* Bleeding that occurs more often than every 21 d • *Hypomenorrhea:* Bleeding that occurs less frequently than every 35 d *Etiology* • Structural abnormalities: uterine leiomyomas, endometrial polyps, adenomyosis, cesarean scar defect • Ovulatory dysfunction • Bleeding disorders • Neoplastic (endometrial hyperplasia or carcinoma, or uterino sarcoma) • Infection and inflammation: endometritis, PID • Disorders of local endometrial hemostasis
Preterm labor Preterm: <37 weeks' gestation Preterm is defined as babies born alive before 37 weeks of pregnancy are completed *Classification* Subcategories of preterm birth, based on gestational age: • Extremely preterm (less than 28 weeks) • Very preterm (28–32 weeks) • Moderate to late preterm (32–37 weeks)	*Treatment* If gestation <34 weeks: • Rehydrate before administration of tocolytic (e.g., Nifedipine) • Sodium chloride 0.9%, iv, 200 ml and • Nifedipine, tab, 20 mg, 2, tab, single dose *and* • Betamethasone ampoule, 6 mg, 2 amp IM, single dose *or* • Dexamethasone ampoule for injection, 2 mg, 2 ampoules IM single dose, *then* • Refer with adequate transport and medical personal to tertiary center • Induction or cesarean birth should not be planned before 39 completed weeks unless medically indicated *Etiology* • Infections: malaria, UTI • Hypertension • Drugs *Note:* Premature birth is the leading cause of neonatal death
Pubic lice (pediculosis pubis) Sexually transmitted infestation. *Phthirus pubis*, the crab louse, is the causative organism. Involves the pubic and perianal regions	*Treatment* • Shave off pubic hair • Apply permethrin 1% cream to affected area and wash after 10 min *or* • Benzyl benzoate 25% over affected area and wash off after 24 h • Repeat after 3 d if indicated *or* • Ivermectin, tab, 3 mg. 0.25 mg/kg orally, repeated in 2 weeks *Signs and symptoms* • Itching in pubic and perianal areas • Compromised personal and household hygiene • Positive history of contagiosity

(continued)

Table 10.1 (continued)

Diagnosis and classification	Treatment and relevant clinical features: pregnancy and obstetrics conditions
Puerperal fever sepsis A disease condition that results from infection of the placental site following delivery or abortion and is characterized in mild form by fever, but in serious cases, the infection may spread through the uterine wall or pass into the bloodstream (sepsis).	*Treatment* • Pen G, ampoule 500 mg, 4 × 1 amp, iv/d, 1 d *or* • Ceftriaxone, ampoule 1 g, 2 × 1 amp/d, 1 d *and* • Metronidazole, tab, 500 mg, 3 × 1 tab/d, 7 d • Oral maintenance with broad-spectrum antibiotics: amoxicillin *or* • Co-amoxicillin, tab, 1 g, 2 × 1tab/ 7 d *or* • Cephalexin tab, 500 mg, 2 × 1 tab/d, 7 d *and* • Metronidazole tab, 500 mg, 3 × 1 tab/d 7 d *Management tips* • Adequate hygiene from birth attendants • Adequate postpartum hygiene of perineum
Pyelonephritis Infectious inflammatory disease involving the kidney parenchyma and renal pelvis	*Treatment* • Ceftriaxone, ampoule for injection 2 g, 1 amp single dose, *then* • Ciprofloxacin, tab, 500 mg 2 × 1 tab/d, 7 d *or* • Cotrimoxazole, 800/160, 2 × 1 tab/d, 10 d *and* • Ibuprofen, 400 mg tabs, 3× tab/d, 5 d *and* • Paracetamol, 500 mg, 3 × 2 tab/d, 5 d *Complications* • Sepsis and shock • Abscess formation • Acute bacterial prostatitis *Clinical features* • Fever • Perineal or suprapubic pain and tenderness are common on rectal examination; flank pain • Irritative voiding symptoms • Positive urine culture *Management tips* • Increase fluid intake • Renal ultrasound to exclude renal abscess, a rare but insidious complication
Sexually acquired acute inguinal lymphadenitis Acute swelling of inguinal lymph nodes caused by lower extremity infection and sexually transmitted diseases such as chancroid, lymphogranuloma venereum, genital herpes, or syphilis	*Treatment* • Erythromycin, tab, 500 mg, 4 × 1 tab/d, 7 d (for pregnant women) *or* • Amoxicillin, tab, 500 mg, 3 × 1 tab/d, 7 d *Clinical features* • Very painful inguinal lymph nodes (bubo) • Valley in the groin (groove sign) • May be transient genital ulcers

Table 10.1 (continued)

Diagnosis and classification	Treatment and relevant clinical features: pregnancy and obstetrics conditions
Sexually transmitted diseases Viral, bacterial or fungal infection acquired through proximity and exchanges of biological fluid during sexual intercourse. Contagious ectoparasitic infestation is included	Also see Table 9.1: Urology and nephrology conditions and their treatment *Clinical notes* • All STDs have a subclinical or latent period, and patients may be asymptomatic • Simultaneous infections with several organisms are common • All patients who seek STD testing should be screened for syphilis and HIV. Partner notification and treatment are important to prevent transmission and "ping-pong" effect *Complications of untreated sexually transmitted infections* • Upper genital tract infections • Secondary infertility • Chronic pelvic pain • Cervical cancer • Chronic infection with hepatitis viruses and HIV *Genital ulcers may be present in:* • Herpes simplex virus • Primary syphilis and chancroid • *Lymphogranuloma venereum* *The STD list* • Chlamydia • Gonorrhea • Genital herpes • Bacterial vaginosis • Hepatitis • Human papilloma virus • Pelvic inflammatory disease • Syphilis • Trichomoniasis
Syphilis in pregnancy	*Treatment* • Benzathine penicillin, ampoule for injection 2.4 million units, 1 amp IM single dose • Treat with penicillin or erythromycin if allergic to penicillin Classification: based on chronicity and constellation of clinical signs and symptoms *Primary syphilis* • Localized infection. Characteristic genital, extragenital painless ulcer (chancre) • Locoregional adenopathy *Secondary syphilis* • Generalized infection • Syphilitic roseola: erythematous macules on trunk, hypopigmented squamous papules on trunk, limbs, and face • Condyloma lata: Soft papules or nodules in the anogenital and buccal mucosa • Fever • Adenopathy • Headache *Tertiary syphilis* • Chronic complications involving the skin, neurologic, and cardiovascular systems • Skin: Soft nodule, non-itchy palmoplantar nodules • Neurology: meningeal and meningovascular inflammation, dementia • Cardiovascular: aortic aneurysm and aortic valve insufficiency

(continued)

Table 10.1 (continued)

Diagnosis and classification	Treatment and relevant clinical features: pregnancy and obstetrics conditions
Urinary tract infection Common in pregnant women. By convention, UTI is defined either as a lower tract (acute cystitis) or upper tract (acute pyelonephritis) infection *Classifications* • Low UTIs • Acute cystitis • High UTI • Pyelonephritis • Asymptomatic bacteriuria	*Treatment* Simple UTI • Amoxicillin, tab, 500 mg, 3 × 1 tab/d, 5 d *or* • Nitrofurantoin, tab, 100 mg, 2 × 1 tab/d, 5 d *or* • Erythromycin, 500 mg tabs, 4 × 1 tab/d, 5 d *or* • Azithromycin, 500 mg single dose followed by 250 mg, tab, 1×/d, 4 d • Increase fluid intake *Signs and symptoms* • Lower abdominal pain • Fever • Rigors • If renal angle pain/tenderness, then suspect pyelonephritis • Dysuria • Frequency of micturition
Urinary stone disease	*Diagnostic features* • Severe flank pain • Nausea and vomiting • Identification and localization on non-contrast CT or ultrasonography
Vaginal discharge Infection-inflammation of the kidney, ureter, urinary bladder, or urethra and vulva	*Treatment* • Patient evaluation to determine etiology • Institute appropriate etiologic treatment *Etiology* • Bacterial vaginosis: overgrowth of anaerobes such as *Gardnerella vaginalis* • Candidiasis • Trichomonas vaginalis infection • HPV associated condyloma acuminata • Physiologic changes related to menstrual cycle irritants • Lichen planus *Note: N. gonorrhoeae and C. trachomatis* are common causes of cervicitis, but often they do not cause a vaginal discharge
Vaginitis, vulvovaginitis Disorders of the vagina caused by infection, inflammation, or changes in the normal vaginal flora	*Treatment* • Topical fluconazole, 2×/d, 10 d • Metronidazol, tab, 500 mg tabs, 3 × 1 tab/d, 5 d • Nystatin vaginal ovule, 2×/d, 5 d *Etiologic classifications* • Vulvovaginal candidiasis • *Trichomonas vaginalis* vaginitis • Bacterial vaginosis *Diagnostic features* • General irritation • Pruritus • Vaginal discharge • Odor • Discomfort • Abnormal or malodorous discharge

Table 10.1 (continued)

Diagnosis and classification	Treatment and relevant clinical features: pregnancy and obstetrics conditions
Vaginosis Vaginal bacteria and pH balance disruption	*Treatment* • Metronidazol, tab, 500 mg tabs, 3 × 1 tab/d, 5 d *Gardnerella vaginalis vaginosis* *Amsel criteria* • Adherent bacteria (clue cells), anaerobes • Milky discharge • Stench (fish smell) • Elevated pH • Leukocytes are not elevated *Predisposing and risk factors* • Excessive vaginal hygiene • Inappropriate vaginal douche • Smoking • Recurrent STDs • Spermicides • Prolonged systemic antibiotics use • Steroids

Musculoskeletal

Contents

11.1 **History: Questions to Ask** 150

11.2 **Physical Examination** 151

11.3 **Clinical Features That Differentiate Inflammatory from Mechanical Pain** ... 151

11.4 **Cardinal Paramedical Musculoskeletal Examinations** 151

11.5 **Musculoskeletal Red Flags** 151

The study of musculoskeletal diseases, also termed rheumatology, entails disease entities such as rheumatism, arthritis, and other disorders of the joints, muscles, and ligaments (Fig. 11.1 and Table 11.2).

Patients with rheumatic diseases may experience both localized pains directly resulting from those conditions and chronic widespread pain, as in fibromyalgia. This generalized, widely spread pain may be felt by patients with osteoarthritis (OA), rheumatoid arthritis (RA), spondyloarthritis (SpA), psoriatic arthritis, and systemic lupus erythematosus (SLE). Generalized pain is also prominent in many musculoskeletal pain disorders including chronic trauma-induced low back pain and neck pain, such as following a motor vehicle accident; complex regional pain syndrome; joint hypermobility syndrome; carpal tunnel syndrome; and lateral epicondylitis.

Muscular and skeletal pathologies are common. Etiologic factors may include genetic defects, injuries incurred during the perinatal period, traumatic lesions, nutritional deficiency, or degenerative wear and tear of the osteoarticular structures.

Rheumatoid arthritis is encountered in young adults. In most cases, the family history will be positive.

Joint aches secondary to wear and tear commonly affect the large joints: knee, coxo-femoral, shoulder, and lower back. Advanced age, male gender, physically demanding professions, a history of trauma, and a lower social status are predicting factors.

Trauma is the sole etiology of a significant number of patients presenting with musculoskeletal afflictions. The cause of the trauma may be sports, professional accidents, road traffic, and auto- and hetero-aggressions. Cultural and religious factors may affect the quality of the history taking; for example, a battered woman is very unlikely to reveal inflicted aggression. A victim of a road traffic accident may not recount the incident accurately because of legal concerns (Table 11.1).

© The Author(s), under exclusive license to Springer Nature Switzerland AG 2021

M. Touray, A. Touray, *Clinical Work and General Management of a Standard Minimal-Resource Facility*, Sustainable Development Goals Series, https://doi.org/10.1007/978-3-030-71032-3_11

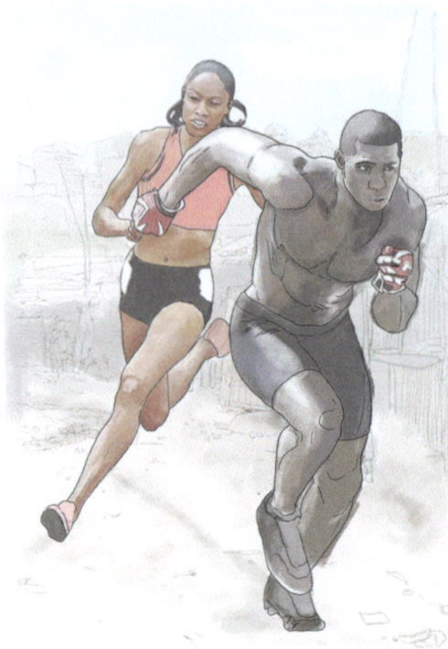

Musculoskeletal

List of musculoskeletal disorders that are described in the text.
For easy reference, the corresponding page on which the
disease condition is described is in brackets.

Acute septic arthritis (p151)
Ankylosing spondylitis (p151)
Bechet syndrome (p152)
Compartment syndrome (p152)
Coxo-cruralgia (p153)
Fibromyalgia (p153)
Lumbago (p154)
Osteoarthritis (p154)
Osteomyelitis (p154)
Osteoporosis (p155)
Rheumatoid arthritis (p155)
Sjogren syndrome (p156)
Spondylarthritis (p156)

Fig. 11.1 Musculoskeletal: A mnemonic illustration representing main anatomic musculoskeletal features of the human body and their corresponding pathologies

Table 11.1 How to distinguish Inflammatory from mechanical pain

Inflammatory pain	Mechanical pain
Pain at night	Pain during the day
Pain at rest	Pain during activity
Sleep impairment due to pain	Nocturnal pain only induced by movement
Morning stiffness	May feel difficulty initiating movement but no stiffness
Insidious onset	Prompt onset
Improvement with exercise	Worse with exercise
No improvement with rest	Improves with rest
For example, rheumatoid arthritis	For example, osteoarthritis

Vitamin D deficiency leading to deforming osteopathy may still be seen in the pediatric age group, for example, in bowed knees.

Oncologic entities are rare but should be considered. An otherwise healthy young adult presenting with recurrent localized bone pain may turn out to have osteomyosarcoma.

Infectious conditions include septic arthritis, osteomyelitis, and necrotizing myositis. Articular aspiration and microbiologic examinations of swabs are not readily available. Empiric antibiotherapy should be rapidly instituted when the clinical suspicion is high.

Significant clinical findings with respect to the joints include warmth, pain, and tumefaction, especially with associated systemic signs, including fever, poor general condition, and weight loss.

In this chapter, we address common musculoskeletal disorders that are encountered in a standard minimal resource facility (Table 11.2).

11.1 History: Questions to Ask

- Do you have muscle and joint pain?
- Any swollen joints? Any trauma, be it recent or past?
- Does any family member have severe joint pain?
- Characterize the extent of the trauma: quantity of energy received by the injured body part (i.e., fall from height, weight impacted), the intensity of the pain, deformations, loss of function, active bleeding.
- GALS (Gait, Arms, Legs, Spine) screening: Do you have any stiffness or pain in your back or in any muscles or joints? Can you dress yourself without any problem? Can you walk up and down stairs without a problem? (Table 11.1)

11.2 Physical Examination

- Observe the patient's gait.
- Inspect, palpate, and move the joints: tumefaction? hot? hematoma? pain? loss of function?
- Appreciate the passive and active range of movements of the concerned joints.

11.3 Clinical Features That Differentiate Inflammatory from Mechanical Pain

- The following table describes typical inflammatory and mechanical pain.
- Bear in mind that overlapping or atypical presentations exist.

11.4 Cardinal Paramedical Musculoskeletal Examinations

- Full blood count
- Erythrocyte sedimentation rate
- X-ray

11.5 Musculoskeletal Red Flags

- Spinal cord or cauda equina compression
- Metastatic cancer
- Spinal epidural abscess
- Vertebral osteomyelitis
- Compression fracture

Table 11.2 Osteoarticular system/rheumatic disease conditions and their treatment

Diagnosis and classification	Treatment and relevant clinical features: osteoarticular conditions
Acute septic arthritis Acute inflammation of joints, usually big joints; may be caused by bacteria, fungi, mycobacteria *Terminology* • Septic arthritis • Pyogenic arthritis • Suppurative arthritis • Purulent arthritis • Pyarthrosis	*Treatment* • Co-amoxicillin, tab, 1 g, 2 × 1 tab/d, 10 d *or* • Cloxacillin, tab, 500 mg, 4 × 1 tab/d, 10 d *and* • Paracetamol, tab, 500 mg, 3 × 2 tab/d, 5 d • Ibuprofen, tab, 400 mg, 3 × 1 tab/d, 5 d *Differential diagnosis* • Transient (or toxic) synovitis • Trauma • Slipped capital femoral epiphysis • Tumor (e.g., leukemia, osteosarcoma, osteoid osteoma) • Villonodular synovitis *Common bacteria involved* • Gonococcus • Staphylococcus • Streptococcus • Hemophilus • Influenza in infants • Salmonella in sickle cell disease
Ankylosing spondylitis A potentially disabling inflammatory arthritis of the spine, usually presenting as chronic back pain, typically before the age of 45 Also known as axial spondyloarthritis	*Treatment* • Physiotherapy, 2 sessions weekly • Paracetamol, tab, 500 mg, 3 × 2 tab/d, 5 d *and* • Naproxen, tab, 500 mg, 2 × 1 tab/d, 5 d

(continued)

Table 11.2 (continued)

Diagnosis and classification	Treatment and relevant clinical features: osteoarticular conditions
Nomenclature: Spondyloarthropathies entail • Ankylosing spondylitis • Undifferentiated SpA • Reactive arthritis • Psoriatic arthritis • Juvenile SpA • Arthritis and spondylitis associated with inflammatory bowel diseases (Crohn's disease and ulcerative colitis)	*Characteristic clinical features* • Inflammatory back pain • Heel pain (enthesitis) • Dactylitis • Uveitis • Positive family history for SpA • Inflammatory bowel disease • Alternating buttock pain • Psoriasis • Asymmetric arthritis • Positive response to NSAIDs • Elevated acute phase reactants (ESR or CRP) *Clinical features* • Chronic lower backache in a young adult, generally worse in the morning • Progressive limitation of back motion and/or chest expansion • Transient or persistent peripheral arthritis • Anterior uveitis • Diagnostic radiographic changes in the sacroiliac joints • HLA-B27 testing is most helpful when there is no intermediate probability of disease
Behçet syndrome Recurrent oral aphthae and any of several systemic manifestations, including genital aphthae, ocular disease, skin lesions, gastrointestinal involvement, neurologic disease, vascular disease, or arthritis	*Treatment* • Paracetamol, tab, 500 mg, 3 × 2 tab/d, 5 d *and* • Ibuprofen, tab, 400 mg, 2 × 1 tab/d, 5 d *and/or* • Prednisolone, 50 mg tab, 1 tab/d, 5 d • Omeprazole, tab, 20 mg, 1 tab/d 10 d *Diagnostic features* • Recurrent pain • Oral or genital aphthous ulcers • Erythema nodosum-like lesions, follicular rash • Anterior or posterior uveitis • Posterior uveitis may be asymptomatic until significant damage occurs to the posterior chamber • Neurologic lesions can mimic multiple sclerosis
Compartment syndrome A condition in which increased pressure within one of the body's anatomical compartments results in insufficient blood supply to tissue within that space *Pathophysiology* Compartment pressure increases, which threatens tissue vascularization Since compartment syndrome involves capillaries, pulse is usually conserved *Absolute emergency:* Ischemia and irreversible necrosis leading to loss of function	*Treatment* • Appropriate evaluation Analgesia: • Paracetamol, tab, 500 mg, 3 × 2 tab/d, 5 d *and* • Ibuprofen, tab, 400 mg, 2 × 1 tab/d, 5 d *and/or* • Proper documentation and referral to a tertiary center for emergency surgical decompression fasciotomy *Etiologies:* may be either intrinsic or extrinsic • Bleeding • Edema • Snakebite • Tight bandage • Complication of orthopedic surgery fasciotomy *Evaluation* • History • Physical examination • Directed neurologic examination • Measure compartment pressure where available: Pdiastolic—Pcompartment ≤30 mmHg

Table 11.2 (continued)

Diagnosis and classification	Treatment and relevant clinical features: osteoarticular conditions
	Signs and symptoms • Pain with passive stretch • Pallor • Palpable tense compartment • Paresis • Paresthesia, pulselessness sometimes
Coxo-cruralgia Pain felt in the hip and/or thigh mainly due to an impairment of the femoral nerve *Differential diagnosis* • Rheumatoid arthritis, spondyloarthritis (e.g., psoriatic arthritis or reactive arthritis) • Crystal arthropathies (e.g., gout or pseudogout) • Osteoarthritis • Aortoiliac arterial insufficiency • Septic arthritis • Osteonecrosis • Primary or secondary bone tumors	*Treatment* • Determine etiology • Paracetamol, tab, 500 mg, 3 × 2 tab/d, 5 d *and* • Ibuprofen, tab, 400 mg, 3 × 1 tab/d, 5 d *or* • Gabapentin, tab, 100 mg, 2 × 1 tab/d, can be increased up to 3 × 300 mg as needed *and* • Physiotherapy where available and as needed *Clinical signs and symptoms* • Burning or electric like pain felt in the buttocks, proximal and distal thigh down the leg • The anterior and inner part of the thigh and down the leg in case of infringement of the nerve at the third lumbar spine • It may be at the middle part of the buttock, the outer part of the upper thigh, extending along the front of the leg in case of damage of the fourth lumbar vertebra • In case of damage to the root of the nerve, the pain goes down the lower back: this is called lumbo-cruralgie *Clinical evaluation* *History*: thorough pain history consisting of OPQRS ST • *O*nset (e.g., sudden, gradual, traumatic or nontraumatic) • *P*rovocative and palliating factors (e.g., increased pain with weight-bearing) • *Q*uality • *R*adiation (e.g., to or from the low back) • *S*ite (e.g., lateral, anterior, or posterior hip) • *S*ymptoms associated with pain (e.g., paresthesia, mechanical symptoms such as catching, systemic symptoms such as fever) • *T*ime course (overall duration, length of episodes) *Physical examination* • Gait assessment by observing the patient walking • Walk on their heels and then on the toes to assess for distal limb weakness indicating lumbar radiculopathy • A "waddling" or Trendelenburg gait may be indicative of hip joint pathology causing restricted joint motion (e.g., osteoarthritis, osteonecrosis) • Inability to bear weight may indicate a hip fracture or weakness from lumbar radiculopathy • *Note*: Intraabdominal conditions may refer pain to the hip
Fibromyalgia Significant musculoskeletal pain accompanied by fatigue, sleep, memory, and mood issues *Nomenclature* Fibromyalgia shares many features with chronic fatigue syndrome, namely, increased frequency among women over 50 years, absence of objective findings, and absence of diagnostic laboratory test results	*Treatment* • Multidisciplinary approach is indicated • Paracetamol, tab, 500 mg, 3 × 2 tab/d, 5 d • Psychological support *Diagnostic features* • Most frequent in women age 20–50 • Chronic widespread musculoskeletal pain syndrome with multiple tender points • Fatigue, headaches, numbness • Objective signs of inflammation absent • Laboratory studies normal • Sleep disorders

(continued)

Table 11.2 (continued)

Diagnosis and classification	Treatment and relevant clinical features: osteoarticular conditions
Lumbago Pain felt in the lower back mainly comprising of the lumbar spine region and may irradiate to buttock, thigh, calf down to the ankle and foot *Terminology* • *Spondylolysis:* A fracture in the *pars interarticularis* where the vertebral body and the posterior elements protecting the nerves are joined • *Spinal stenosis:* Local, segmental, or generalized narrowing of the vertebral canal by bone or soft tissue elements • *Radiculopathy:* Impairment of a nerve root, usually causing radiating pain, numbness, tingling, or muscle weakness that corresponds to a specific nerve root • *Sciatica:* Pain, numbness, tingling in the distribution of the sciatic nerve, radiating down the posterior or lateral aspect of the leg, usually to the foot or ankle • *Cauda equina syndrome:* Loss of bowel and bladder control and numbness in the groin and saddle area of the perineum, associated with weakness of the lower extremities	*Treatment* • Identify and treat etiology: • Promote mobilization • Ibuprofen, tab, 400 mg, 3 × 1 tab/d, 5 d *and* • Paracetamol, tab, 500 mg, 3 × 2 tab/d, 5 d • Physiotherapy • Refer to tertiary center for neurosurgical review and management *Etiology* • Nonspecific back pain • Trauma • Metastatic cancer • Spinal cord or cauda equina compression • Spinal epidural abscess • Vertebral osteomyelitis • Vertebral compression fracture • Radiculopathy • Spinal stenosis • Systemic disease *Static changes* • *Kyphotic curves:* Outward curve of the thoracic spine (at the level of the ribs) • *Lordotic curves:* Inward curve of the lumbar spine (just above the buttocks) • *Scoliotic curving:* A sideways curvature of the spine, always abnormal *Management tips* • Perform thorough physical examination • Order lumbar X-ray (lateral and anterior-posterior (AP) for men over 50 years) *Emergency* • Refrain from X-ray for under fifties • Cauda equina syndrome
Osteoarthritis Degenerative joint disease that damages the articular cartilage leading to reactive new bone formation. The newly formed reactive bone, termed osteophytes, have characteristic radiographic features and constitute the main diagnostic feature of osteoarthritis	*Treatment* • Paracetamol, tab, 500 mg, 3 × 2 tab/d, 5 d *and/or* • Naproxen, tab, 500 mg, 2 × 1 tab/d, 5 d *or* • Indomethacin, tab, 25 mg, 2 × 1 tab/d, 5 d • Physiotherapy • Dietary advice, weight loss, and lifestyle modification • Counseling *Management tips* • Patient education • Results from wear and tear • Avoid unnecessary imaging • Encourage physical activity • Prescribe physiotherapy with the goal of muscle tonification
Osteomyelitis Infection involving bone *Classification* based on the mechanism of infection: • Hematogenous *or* • Nonhematogenous *Classification* based on duration of illness: • Acute versus • Chronic	*Treatment* • Treat predisposing factors: malnutrition, furuncles, cutaneous ulcers • When tuberculous osteomyelitis is clinically suspected, address to tertiary center • If sequestrum detected, refer to tertiary center for surgical consultation for subsequent debridement

Table 11.2 (continued)

Diagnosis and classification	Treatment and relevant clinical features: osteoarticular conditions
	Antimicrobial therapy • Co-amoxicillin, tab, 1 g, 2 × 1 tab/d, for 14 d *or* • Cloxacillin, tab, 500 mg, 4 × 1 tab/d, for 4 weeks *or* • Cephalexin, tab, 500 mg, 3 × 1 tab/d, 21 d *or* • Chloramphenicol, tab, 500 mg, 4 × 1 tab/d, 21 d., especially if sickle cell disease present *or* • Erythromycin, tab, 500 mg, 4 × 1 tab/d, at least 21 d • Limb immobilization • Drainage and removal *Microbiology* May be polymicrobial or monomicrobial *Staphylococcus aureus* (including methicillin-resistant *S. aureus*), coagulase-negative *Staphylococci, Enterococci* Salmonella species in sickle cell patient *Management tips* • Patient education • Rest • Educate to ensure antibiotherapy adherence • Surgical drainage of any abscess
Osteoporosis Low bone mass, microarchitectural disruption, and skeletal fragility, resulting in decreased bone strength and an increased risk of fracture	*Treatment* • Maintain good calcium intake and physical activity • Refrain from smoking • Adequate vitamin D supplementation • Hormone therapy where indicated *Diagnostic criteria* Fragility fracture, particularly at the spine, hip, wrist, humerus, rib, and pelvis *Clinical manifestations* • Vertebral fracture • Hip fractures • Distal radius fractures (Colles fractures)
Rheumatoid arthritis Chronic systemic inflammatory disease Characterized by symmetrical inflammation of the synovial tissue of joints resulting in destruction of the joints and periarticular tissues More common in young- and middle-aged women	*Treatment* • Paracetamol, tab, 500 mg, 3 × 2 tab/d, 5 d *and/or* • Naproxen, tab, 500 mg, 2 × 1 tab/d, 5 d *or* • Indomethacin, tab, 25 mg, 2 × 1 tab/d, 5 d • Dexamethasone, 2 mg tab, 1 tab/morning, 3 d • In severe cases, methotrexate, tab, 5 mg, 1 tab/week • Rest of affected joints • Physiotherapy *Management tips* • The choice and dose of an NSAID should be personalized, with each NSAID tried for at least 1 week • Long-term use of high-dose corticosteroids is avoided, because of severe associated adverse effects • Avoid NSAIDs in renal failure in favor of paracetamol

(continued)

Table 11.2   (continued)

Diagnosis and classification	Treatment and relevant clinical features: osteoarticular conditions
Sjögren syndrome A chronic autoimmune inflammatory disorder characterized by diminished lachrymal and salivary gland function, with resultant dryness of eyes and mouth	*Treatment* • Address specific symptoms • Physiotherapy • Corticoid therapy where needed • Refer to appropriate center for tertiary care *Diagnostic features* • 90% of patients are women, average age 50 years • Dryness of eyes and mouth • Rheumatoid factor and antinuclear antibodies are common • Increased incidence of lymphoma *Clinical signs* • Keratoconjunctivitis and order ocular symptoms • Dryness of mouth, i.e., xerostomia • Dysphagia • Small vessel vasculitis • Eye disease • Obstructive airway disease and interstitial lung disease • Neuropsychiatric dysfunction • Renal dysfunction (tubular acidosis)
Spondyloarthritis Inflammatory disease of the vertebral spine and joints. Rheumatoid factor is characteristically negative and rheumatoid nodes are absent *Classification* • Ankylosing spondylitis • Reactive arthritis (Reiter syndrome) • Psoriatic arthritis • Juvenile chronic arthritis	*Treatment* • High index of suspicion and early diagnosis • Regular spinal and chest exercises • Paracetamol, tab, 500 mg, 3 × 2 tab/d, 5 d *and/or* • Indomethacin, tab, 25 mg, 2 × 1 tab/d, 5 d *or* • Diclofenac, tab, 25 mg, 2 × 1 tab/d, 5 d • Encourage regular physical activity *Clinical features* • Pain at night or morning stiffness • Alternating buttock pain • Arthritis • Dactylitis • Enthesitis (heel) • Inflammatory bowel disease • Psoriasis • Diarrhea <1 month before onset of arthritis • Positive family history for SpA • HLA-B27 positive • Elevated CRP • Sacroiliitis radiographic abnormalities consistent with sacroiliitis • Limitation in mobility of lumbar spine • Limitation in chest expansion *Nomenclature:* variants of the disease are described using localizing adjectives or acronyms • Axial spondyloarthritis • Ankylosing spondylitis • Spondyloarthritiden • Spondyloarthropathy • Enteropathic spondyloarthritis • Seronegative spondyloarthropathy • Seronegative spondyloarthritis • Spondyloarthritis ankylosans • Morbus Bechterew

Dermatology

12

Contents

12.1 **History Taking in Dermatology: Questions to Ask** 157

12.2 **Physical Examination in Dermatology** 158

Dermatology is a medical specialty which focuses on conditions and disorders that affect the skin, nails, and hair (Fig. 12.1). Cosmetic reasons may be the main motivation for some dermatologic consultations. In this chapter, we address common dermatologic disorders that are encountered in a standard minimal resource facility (Table 12.1).

The presence of skin eruptions is the chief complaint of a significant number of patients presenting at our facility. Efforts should be made by the clinician to characterize and describe the lesions as precisely as possible (Table 12.1).

Allergic-contact dermatitis is a common dermatological condition. The pathophysiologic basis may be allergic, toxic, and/or irritative. Associated fungal and/or bacterial infection may be present. These afflictions may present in all classic forms of dermatosis: macules, pustules, desquamation, erythema, etc. A good history may reveal the underlying etiology.

Therapies should be directed against etiologic factors where possible. Patients should be reminded of good skin care practices, and measures for eviction of the causative agent should be discussed and proposed.

Conditions due to viral and bacterial infections should not be missed.

Leprosy and tuberculous skin eruptions are rarely diagnosed. When suspected, they should promptly be referred to a major health facility along with a well-written accompanying document.

Suspected cancerous skin lesions present mainly as nevus, raised squamous lesions, dysmorphic nails, and chronic ulcers. These lesions should be carefully characterized and documented. Important clinical characteristics include their form, color, size, the irregularity of the borders, indolence, and their progressive nature. Oncologic diagnostic entities may include melanoma and basaliomas.

12.1 History Taking in Dermatology: Questions to Ask

- When did you first notice this skin problem?
- Did it appear suddenly? Is it increasing or decreasing?
- Does it itch?
- Does it bleed?

M. Touray, A. Touray, *Clinical Work and General Management of a Standard Minimal-Resource Facility*, Sustainable Development Goals Series, https://doi.org/10.1007/978-3-030-71032-3_12

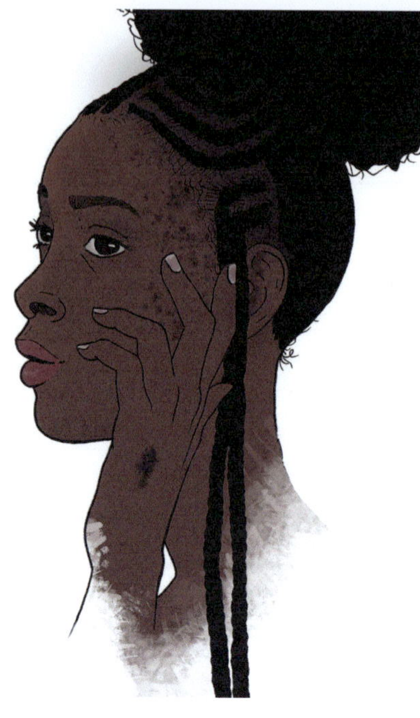

Fig. 12.1 Dermatology: A mnemonic illustration representing main anatomic dermatology structures and their corresponding pathologies

- Has any family member had skin cancer? Or any other cancer?

12.2   Physical Examination in Dermatology

- Location of the lesions: localized or generalized
- Analyze lesions and their evolution: identify the elementary lesion
- Primary skin lesions: vesicle, bulla, macula, nodule, papule, plaque, pustula, urticaria
- Secondary skin lesions: atrophy, crust, erosion, excoriation, fissure, lichenification, rhagade, scar, ulceration
- Basic characteristics of lesions: size, shape, border
- ABCDE mnemonic for describing a skin lesion: Asymmetrical, Borderless, Color change, Diameter, Evolving

Table 12.1 Dermatology conditions and their treatment

Diagnosis and classification	Treatment and relevant clinical features: dermatology conditions
Acne A skin disorder characterized by chronic or recurrent appearance of papules, pustules, or nodules on the face, neck, trunk, or proximal upper extremities *Classification* • Comedonal acne (closed or open) • Post-adolescent acne • Papulopustular • Nodular acne • Acne conglobata • Excoriated acne • Infantile acne • Acne fulminans • Drug-induced acne • Acne cosmetica • Acne mechanica • Occupational acne • Chloracne *Clinical features and complication* • Disfiguring • Scarring • Post-inflammatory hyperpigmentation • Gram-negative folliculitis • Psychological effect: low self-esteem, depression, and anxiety • Negative psychosocial effects	Treatments include non-pharmacological, topical, oral, and procedural therapies *Non-pharmacological* Good lifestyle adoption (sleep, diet, physical exercise), good skin hygiene *Topical medication* • Benzoyl peroxide; apply 2× daily • Salicylic acid (0.5–2.0%) • Sulfur • Topical retinoids: tretinoin, adapalene, tazarotene, trifarotene *Oral medication* • Doxycycline 100 mg tabs, 1 tab/day, 10 days or • Tetracycline 100 mg, tabs, 1 tab/day, 10 days • Isotretoin, tabs 10 mg and tabs 20 mg: 0.5 mg/kg/day in 2 divided doses for 1 month, then increase to 1 mg/kg/day in 2 divided doses as tolerated *Pathogenesis* Inflammatory disorder of the pilosebaceous unit, which includes the hair follicle and sebaceous gland. A complex interplay of host factors, such as androgen-mediated stimulation of sebaceous glands, dysbiosis within the microbiome of the pilosebaceous follicle, and innate and cellular immune responses. Genetics and diet may be influencing factors. As a result, there may be increased sebum production by sebaceous glands and hyperproliferation of bacteria *Contributory factors* • Skin trauma • Diet (milk, high glycemic load diets) • Stress • Insulin resistance • Body mass index *Clinical assessment* • History: puberty, menarche, skin conditions, diet, physical activity, sleeping habits, screen time, cosmetic use, soaps-detergents used • Physical examination: whole body skin review • Acne lesion types: comedones and/or inflammatory papules, pustules, or nodules • Acne severity: distribution and degree of skin involvement • Presence of complications: post-inflammatory hyperpigmentation, post-inflammatory erythema, scarring, psychological distress • Potential contributing factors: comedogenic skin care products, acne-inducing medications, signs or symptoms of endocrine disorders associated with acne vulgaris

(continued)

Table 12.1 (continued)

Diagnosis and classification	Treatment and relevant clinical features: dermatology conditions
Alopecia Hair loss *Classification* • Androgenic alopecia • Telogen effluvium • Effluvium • Alopecia areata • Alopecia universalis • Scar alopecia *Pediatric alopecia* • Hypotrichosis • Congenital dysplasia • Infection	*Treatment* • Good hair hygiene • Antifungal shampooing: Ketoconazole shampooing, 5%, 3×/w, 3 months • Exclude deficiency conditions • Ferrous sulfate, tab, 100 mg, 1 tab/d where needed *Physiology* Throughout life, hair follicles undergo cycling characterized by: • *Anagen:* periods of growth • *Catagen:* periods of involution and rest • *Telogen:* period of rest At any given time, 90% of hair follicles on the scalp are in anagen *Differential diagnosis* • Acne keloidalis nuchae • Androgenetic alopecia in men • Androgenetic alopecia in women • Central centrifugal cicatricial alopecia • Alopecia related to systemic cancer therapy • Alopecia areata • Dissecting cellulitis of the scalp • Folliculitis decalvans • Lichen planopilaris • Tinea capitis • Traction alopecia • Frontal fibrosing alopecia • Erosive pustular dermatosis *Etiology* • Polycystic ovarian syndrome • Iron deficiency • Vitamin B12 deficiency • Malnutrition • Significant weight loss • Exoparasitic infestation • Compromised personal hygiene • Tenia capitis • Dysthyroidy • Major psychological stress • Poisoning from arsenic, mercury, or thallium *Description of hair loss* • Duration and rate of progression of hair loss • Location and pattern of hair loss • Extent of hair loss • Associated symptoms: pain, tenderness, pruritus, or burning sensation

Table 12.1 (continued)

Diagnosis and classification	Treatment and relevant clinical features: dermatology conditions
Angioedema Localized subcutaneous (or submucosal) swelling, which results from extravasation of fluid into interstitial tissues. Often self-limiting *Classification* • Clinical type of "deep urticaria" • 50%: associated with urticaria • 10%: isolated *Clinical features* • Anaphylaxis: an acute, potentially life-threatening, multisystem syndrome caused by the sudden release of mast cell mediators into the systemic circulation • Angioedema • Bronchospasm • Urticaria (hives) • Hypotension • Hypersensitivity reaction	*Treatment* • Eviction where possible • Cetirizine, tab, 10 mg, 2 × 1 tab/d, 5 d *and/or* • Prednisone, tab, 20 mg, 1 × 2 tabs/d, 3 d (to be taken in the morning) • Evaluate need for permanent prescription of EpiPen • EpiPen: 0.3 mg Adrenaline in a ready-to-use vial, IM administration in the anterolateral aspect of the middle third of the thigh is preferred in the setting of anaphylaxis *Signs and symptoms* • More painful than itchy • Localized firm tumefaction • Distribution: on extremities, tongue, lips, eyelids, external genitalia • Dysphonia • Respiratory distress (pharynx, larynx) *Pathophysiology* • Angioedema • Results from a loss of vascular integrity that allows fluid to move into tissues • Exposure of the vasculature to inflammatory mediators causes dilation and increased permeability of capillaries and venules • Fluid collects asymmetrically in the areas in which the vasculature has been altered, and these areas, for example, face, larynx, and bowel wall • Cause is divided into mast cell-mediated etiologies, bradykinin-mediated etiologies, and etiologies of unknown mechanism • May be triggered by foods, drugs, latex, exercise, insect stings, and other uncommon allergens
Bacterial skin infections Inflammation of the surroundings, including hair follicles. This condition may be complicated by an abscess *Classifications* • Impetigo • Furunculosis • Folliculitis • Carbuncles	*Treatment* • Amoxicillin, tab, 500 mg, 3 × 1 tab/d, 5 d *or* • Cloxacillin, tab, 500 mg, 3 × 1 tab/d, 5 d *or* • Erythromycin, tab, 500 mg, 4 × 1 tab/d, 5 d *or* • Doxycyclin, tab, 100 mg, 2 × 1 tab, 5 d *Indications for antibiotherapy* Antibiotics should only be initiated if there are signs of regional or systemic spread, or the skin lesions are on the hand, feet, or face A single abscess may be treated locally without any system antibiotic
Burns Tissue injury caused by extremes of temperature, chemical, electrical, or radiation energy *Classification* • *First degree:* Epidermis, sunburn, erythema, and pain • *Second degree (superficial):* Superficial derma, blisters, erythema, pain • *Second degree (deep):* Deep derma, torn blisters, little pain, hair falls out easily • *Third degree:* Hypoderm, "leather skin," no pain, hair loss	*Treatment* • Pour water on the affected area (especially in the first hour after the burn). This may reduce the depth of injury if started immediately • Clean with water and soap • Apply Silver Sulfadiazine (Flamazine) cream generously • Cover with clean dressing • Do not puncture the blisters • Paracetamol, tab, 500 mg, 3 × 2 tab/d as needed • If signs of infection, Amoxicillin, tab, 500 mg, 3 × 1 tab/d, 5 d *Management tips* • Encourage good fluid intake (>3 L/d) • Good skin hygiene with daily dressing • Avoid malnutrition

(continued)

Table 12.1 (continued)

Diagnosis and classification	Treatment and relevant clinical features: dermatology conditions
Cellulitis, erysipelas Areas of skin erythema, edema, and warmth; develop as a result of bacterial entry via breaches in the skin barrier *Classification* • *Cellulitis* involves the deeper dermis and subcutaneous fat and • may present with or without purulence *S. aureus*, Group A β-hemolytic streptococcus, *H. Influenzae, Pneumococcus* • *Erysipelas* is nonpurulent and involves the superficial dermis Group A β-hemolytic streptococcus	*Treatment* • Amoxicillin, tab, 500 mg, 3 × 1 tab/d, 10 d *or* • Co-amoxicillin, tab, 1 g, 2 × 1 g/d, 10 d • Erythromycin, tab, 500 mg, 4 × 1 tab/d, 7 d Severe or advanced cellulitis: • Penicillin G, ampoule for injection, 1.2 million unit, 3 × 1 amp/d. *or* • Ceftriaxone, ampoule for injection 2 g, 1 amp/d, 2 d *then* • Amoxicillin, tab, 500 mg, 3 × 1 tab/d, 7 d *or* • Cloxacillin, tab, 500 mg, 4 × 1 tab/d, 7 d *and* • Paracetamol, tab, 500 mg, 3 × 2 tab/d, 5 d *Note:* Complications when localized on the face include sinus cavernous thrombosis with neurological deficit *Management tips* • Advise limb elevation • Maintain good skin hygiene and care • Patients with cellulitis tend to have a more indolent course with development of localized symptoms over a few days
Eczema (dermatitis) Itchy and recurrent erythema with crusting, scaling, and thickening *Classification* Can be classified according to mechanism, appearance as well as chronicity • Allergic • Atopic • Dyshidrotic • Irritative • Nummular • Seborrheic	*Treatment* • Patient education • Avoid irritants, for example, aggressive soaps *Mild cases* • Hydrocortisone 1% cream/ointment, apply on skin 2×/d *Severe cases* • Betamethasone, cream 0.1%, apply 1×/d, 7 d • Claritin, tab, 10 mg, 1 tab/bedtime *or* • Loratadine, tab, 10 mg, 1, tab, at bedtime, 5 d *or* • Chlorphenamine (Piriton), tab, 25 mg, 2 × 1 tab/d, 5 d • In bacterial superinfection, oral broad-spectrum antibiotic (Amoxicillin, tab, 500 mg, 3 × 1 tab/d, 5 d) • Avoid using steroids on the face • Steroids should be applied intermittently when used for a long time *Signs and symptoms* • Acute oozing • Subacute + redness + swelling but dry • Subacute oozing • Subacute crusted with pus, subacute dry, chronic dry crusted
Reactive mucocutaneous disorders Severe mucocutaneous reactions, most commonly triggered by medications, characterized by extensive necrosis and detachment of the epidermis Mucous membranes are affected in over 90% of patients, usually at two or more distinct sites (ocular, oral, and genital)	*Treatment* • Identify the cause • Prompt eviction of causative agent • High fluid intake • Institute antibiotherapy where need • Hydrocortisone ampoule for injection, 100 mg, 3 amps in 500 ml of 0.9% NaCl, 1× d, 3 d

Table 12.1 (continued)

Diagnosis and classification	Treatment and relevant clinical features: dermatology conditions
Disease entities: • Erythema multiforme • Stevens-Johnson syndrome • Toxic epidermal necrolysis *Complications* Infections Pulmonary complications Gastrointestinal complications	*Etiology* • Drugs, for example, sulfonamides, allopurinol • Typical exposure period before reaction onset is 4 d to 4 weeks of first continuous exposure • Mycoplasma pneumoniae infection • Bone marrow transplantation • Others: vaccinations, systemic diseases, contrast medium, external chemical exposure, herbal medicines, and foods • Idiopathic *Diagnostic features* • Medication-induced • Mucocutaneous lesion, target ring-form • Predilection of trunk and mucous membranes • May progress to cover most of the body surface • Can be life-threatening • Herpes simplex maybe involved *Differential diagnosis* • Erythema multiforme • Erythroderma and erythematous drug eruptions • Acute generalized exanthematous pustulosis • Generalized bullous fixed drug eruption • Phototoxic eruptions • Staphylococcal scalded skin syndrome • Paraneoplastic pemphigus • Chikungunya fever
Erythema nodosum A delayed-type hypersensitivity reaction that most often presents as erythematous, tender nodules in the subcutaneous tissue on the pretibial regions (shins) *Nomenclature* • Panniculitis: inflammation of the subcutaneous fat	*Treatment* • Identify and treat underlying cause • Alleviate discomfort by leg elevation rest and compression application where tolerated • Ibuprofen, tab, 400 mg, 3 × 1 tab/d 5 d *or* • Indomethacin, tab, 25 mg, 2 × 1 tab/d, 5 d *or* • Prednisone, tab, 20 mg tabs, 1 tab/d, 5 d *and* • Omeprazole, tab, 20 mg, 1 tab/d *Etiology* • A *hypersensitivity reaction* of unknown etiology in most cases • In some cases, it is associated with an identified infection, drug, inflammatory condition, or malignancy • *Infections:* Throat infections, streptococcal disease, primary tuberculosis, Yersinia infection; chlamydia, fungal (histoplasmosis), amoebiasis, giardiasis, herpes simplex, viral hepatitis, HIV infection, *Campylobacter* infection, and *Salmonella* infection • *Inflammatory conditions:* Sarcoidosis or gastrointestinal diseases; however, many cases are idiopathic • *Drugs:* Oral contraceptives, penicillin, sulfonamides • *Inflammatory bowel disease:* Crohn's disease, ulcerative colitis • *Malignancies:* Lymphoma, leukemia, internal carcinomas • Other associated conditions: Sarcoidosis, pregnancy, Behçet disease

(continued)

Table 12.1 (continued)

Diagnosis and classification	Treatment and relevant clinical features: dermatology conditions
	Clinical signs and symptoms • Manifests as erythematous, usually tender, nonulcerated, immobile nodules on the bilateral shins • Nodules are slightly preeminent • May present in other body areas: on other areas such as the ankles, thighs, arms, buttocks, calves, or face • Prodrome of fatigue, fever, malaise, arthralgias, or upper respiratory infection symptoms and joint swelling, erythema, or pain • Nodules may remit spontaneously *Differential diagnosis* • Nodular vasculitis (erythema induratum) • Subcutaneous bacterial, fungal, or mycobacterial infections • Cutaneous polyarteritis *nodosa* • Malignant subcutaneous infiltrates • Pancreatic panniculitis • Alpha-1 antitrypsin deficiency
Fungal skin infection Fungal infection of the skin, hair, and nails *Nomenclature* Dermatophytes Mycosis Onychomycosis Candidiasis Aspergillosis *Diagnostic entities* • Taenia corporis • Tinea pedis • Tinea capitis • Tinea unguium • Tinea cruris • Tinea manum • Intertrigo • Diaper rash • Intertrigo	*Treatment* Topical treatment • Clotrimazole cream, apply on affected skin 2×/d *or* • Miconazole cream, apply on affected skin 2×/d Systemic treatment • Fluconazole, tab, 50 mg, 1 tab/d, 10 d *or* • Griseofulvin, tab, 500 mg, 2 × 1 tab/d, 14 d *or* • Terbinafine (Lamisil), tab, 250 mg, 1 tab/d, 3–6 weeks (monitor liver function test before and during therapy) • Good perineal hygiene: no nylon underwear, avoid prolonged groin sweating. Change cotton underwear daily *Management tips* • Continue applying even after lesions have disappeared • High risk of recurrence • Educate to avoid "wet feet" for prolonged periods • Advise to dry feet after ablution or showering
Herpes simplex Type 1 and 2 (HSV-1 and 2), also known as herpes labialis, is the etiologic agent of vesicular lesions of the oral mucosa and genitalia respectively *Clinical note* • *HSV-1* mainly causes infections in the mouth and facial area ("fever vesicles"). Said to be "above the belt" • *HSV-2* infections mainly found genital, herpes genitalis. Said to be "below the belt"	*Treatment* • Acyclovir, 400 mg tabs, 4 × 1 tab/d, 5 d • Apply acyclovir cream every 4 h/d • Inspect for secondary bacterial infection and treat accordingly *Signs and symptoms* • Asymptomatic • Oral infections of mucosal surfaces, epidermis and dermis • Localized, itchy, slightly painful vesicles • More severe in seropositive HIV patients • Cutaneous manifestations: infection of the finger (herpetic whitlow), skin infection on the face, neck, and arms of wrestlers (herpes gladiatorum), erythema multiforme, eczema herpeticum, • Ocular manifestations: vision loss and blindness, keratitis, acute retinal necrosis, conjunctivitis and blepharitis, chorioretinitis • Neurologic syndromes: encephalitis, Bell's palsy (facial nerve palsy), aseptic meningitis • Other manifestations: Hepatitis, respiratory tract infections, HSV esophagitis

Table 12.1 (continued)

Diagnosis and classification	Treatment and relevant clinical features: dermatology conditions
Classification May done according to organ system infected • Genitalia • Liver • Lung • Eye • Central nervous system	*Transmission of HSV* • Occurs when someone with no prior infection with HSV-1 comes in contact with herpetic lesions, mucosal secretions, or skin that contain HSV-1 • Transmission typically occurs via oral-oral, oral-genital, or genital-genital contact, as well as contamination of skin abrasions with infected oral secretions *Population at risk* • Sexually active adolescents • Athletes involved in contact sports • Neonates • Health care workers
Herpes zoster (shingles) Varicella zoster virus (VZV) infection causes two clinically distinct diseases *Primary infection* with VZV results in varicella (chickenpox), which is characterized by vesicular lesions on an erythematous base in different stages of development; lesions are most concentrated on the face and trunk *Herpes zoster, or shingles*, results from reactivation of latent VZV that gained access to sensory ganglia during varicella. Herpes zoster is characterized by a painful, unilateral vesicular eruption, which usually occurs in a restricted dermatomal distribution	*Treatment* • Clean the lesions or wash them gently with soap and water *and* • Paint the lesions twice daily with gentian violet or calamine lotion *and* • Paracetamol, tab, 500 mg tabs, 3 × 2 tab/d *and* • Acyclovir, tab, 800 mg, 4 × 1 tab/d, 5 d • Apply acyclovir cream every 4 h/d *Risk factors* • Age • Immunocompromised patients • Transplant patients • Autoimmune disease *Complications* • Postherpetic neuralgia • Herpes zoster ophtalmicus • Acute retinal necrosis • Herpes zoster oticus (Ramsay Hunt syndrome) • Aseptic meningitis • Encephalitis • Peripheral motor neuropathy • Myelitis • Guillain-Barré syndrome • Stroke syndromes • Bacterial infections *Note:* A common presentation in HIV positive patients
Hirsutism Excessive terminal hair growth, affects between 5% and 10% of women of reproductive age *Clinical note:* Presence of excess terminal hair growth (dark, coarse hairs) in androgen-dependent areas (e.g., upper lip, chin, midsternal, upper and lower abdomen, upper and lower back, and buttocks) where women typically have little or no hair	*Treatment* • Identify and treat underlying cause • A gynecologist or endocrinologist may be involved in the overall management • Refer to tertiary for endocrinologic care *Physiopathology* • Humans are born with five million hair follicles distributed in the scalp and other body parts • Vellus (fine, soft, and not pigmented) or • Terminal (long, coarse, and pigmented) • Hirsutism is a result of the effect of high circulating serum androgens on hair follicle • The secreted active androgens are: testosterone, dehydroepiandrosterone sulfate and androstenedione

(continued)

Table 12.1 (continued)

Diagnosis and classification	Treatment and relevant clinical features: dermatology conditions
	Etiology • Idiopathic hirsutism • Congenital adrenal hyperplasia • Severe virilizing hyperandrogenemia • Post-menopausal • PCOS • Spironolactone induces
Hyperkeratosis Palmoplantar keratoderma is a heterogeneous group of inherited or acquired disorders characterized by excessive epidermal thickening of the palms and soles	*Treatment* • Salicylic acid in Vaseline, 50%, to be applied at night in occlusion, using socks or nylon fittings; wash off in the morning • Avoid exhaustive scrubbing *Advice to patient:* reactive hyperkeratosis of areas of the body that are recurrently exposed to pressure and frequent fiction (palms of a physical worker, soles) is physiologic. Attempts to remove such by excessive scrubbing may not be effective
Insect bite or sting The bites of insects and other arthropods may be a minor nuisance or may lead to serious medical problems, including transmission of insect-borne illnesses and severe allergic reactions	*Treatment* If allergic reaction: • Hydrocortisone, ampoule for injection, 100 mg, 2 amps in 500 ml of 0.9% NaCl, iv infusion in 2 h single dose, *then* • Oral antibiotic if skin integrity is compromised: Doxycycline, tab, 100 mg, 2 × 1 tab/d, 10 d
Classification • Bite • Sting	*Management note* Anaphylaxis is a possible complication of insect bite/sting. Treat as per protocol
Lichen planus Noncontagious inflammatory dermatosis, involves skin and/or mucosa (mouth, external genitalia)	*Treatment* • Topical corticoids (occlusion): Hydrocortisone cream, 1% • Systemic corticoids: Prednisolone tab, 20 mg, 1ta/d, 5 d • PUVA (320–400 mm), UVB, UVA *Clinical notes* • Associated with chronic hepatic disease • Cicatricial alopecia • Nail destruction • Pruriginous • Purplish color • Wickham striae
Lower limb ulcer Disruption of the normal structure and function of the skin and soft tissue structure and may be due to a variety of mechanisms and etiologies	*Treatment* • Identify and treat underlying cause • Provide good diet with appropriate nutrients, protein, and calories • Empiric and/or etiologic antibiotherapy. Commonly used regimen: • Co-amoxicillin, tab, 1 g, 2 × 1 tab/d, 7 d *or* • Cloxacillin tab, 500 mg, 4 × 1 tab/d, 7 d • Metronidazole, tab, 500 mg, 3 × 1 tab/d, 7 d

Table 12.1 (continued)

Diagnosis and classification	Treatment and relevant clinical features: dermatology conditions
Classifications • Acute versus chronic • Arterial versus venous • Diabetic ulcer • Infected ulcer • Trauma or surgery • Tissue loss	*Etiology* • *Venous ulcers:* may be caused by multiple factors including chronic venous insufficiency, deep vein thrombosis, and venous valvular incompetence • *Pressure-induced skin injury:* where structures are compressed between osseous prominences and/or hard external surfaces • *Diabetic foot ulcers:* multifactorial, due to a combination of diabetic neuropathy, autonomic dysfunction, and vascular insufficiency. Location at areas of repeated trauma, such as the plantar metatarsal heads or dorsal interphalangeal joints • *Ischemic ulcers:* result of hypoperfusion due to arterial obstruction as a result of atherosclerosis (i.e., peripheral artery disease, patients with diabetes, thromboangiitis obliterans, vasculitis, scleroderma) • *Ulcers associated with malignancy:* squamous cell or basal cell carcinoma • *Hypertensive ulcers:* typical located in the supra-malleolar region of the anterolateral leg or Achilles tendon, and bilateral ulcers are common *Clinical evaluation* • *History:* Query onset and perceived etiologic factors, change in size, painful? Differentiating the most common chronic ulcers. Pain, wound history, medico-surgical and social history • *Ulcer assessment:* location and number of wounds. Wound location, length, width, depth, and the presence and position of undermining, dried necrotic wound surface. Presence of cellulitis, and drainage (amount, type, color, odor) should also be documented. Determine whether vital structures such as bone, tendons, nerves, and vessels have been exposed • *Vascular assessment:* Signs of arterial obstruction include lack of peripheral pulses with poor capillary refill, thin atrophic skin, lack of hair on the feet and lower leg, and hypertrophic deformed nails • *Laboratory workup:* Hematology—Complete blood count and differential. Chemistries—Metabolic panel, liver function tests, albumin, hemoglobin A1c. Microbiology—Cultures/pathology (wound, urine, blood) *Local signs of ulcer infection* • Induration of the margins of the ulcer • Cellulitis extending >2 cm beyond the margin of the wound • Augmented local warmth • Pain on palpation • Drainage from the site *System signs of serious ulcer infection* • Increasing erythema/cellulitis of the surrounding skin >2 cm • Lymphangitis • Increase in the size of the ulcer • Large amount of drainage • Fever • Wound odor

(continued)

Table 12.1 (continued)

Diagnosis and classification	Treatment and relevant clinical features: dermatology conditions
Lupus erythematous Chronic inflammatory autoimmune disorder, genetic susceptibility Involves skin and other organs Young adults (20–40 years old) F:M = 6:1 *Classification* • Discoid • Subacute • Cutaneous • Systemic	*Treatment* Chronic and subacute • Topical or intralesional corticosteroids • Photoprotection: antimalarials (hydroxychloroquine or chloroquine) • Systemic therapy • Anti-malarials: Chloroquine (Plaquenil), tab, 200 mg, 3 × 1 tab/d • Corticosteroid therapy, immuno-suppressants (e.g., azathioprine/cyclophosphamide)
Orbital cellulitis Infection involving the contents of the orbit (fat and ocular muscles)	*Treatment* • Co-amoxicillin tabs, 1 g, 2 × 1 tab/d, 7 d *Etiology* • Bacterial rhinosinusitis • Ophthalmic surgery: strabismus surgery, blepharoplasty, radial keratotomy, retinal surgery • Peribulbar anesthesia • Orbital trauma with fracture or foreign body • Dacryocystitis • Infection of the teeth, middle ear, or face • An infected mucocele that erodes into the orbit • Fungal rhinosinusitis *Clinical features* • Ocular pain • Restricted eye movement • Swelling and redness of the affected eyelid • Intravenous antibiotherapy
Purpura Nonblanchable, hemorrhagic skin lesions that result from the leakage of red blood cells into the cutaneous tissue *Nomenclature* • Retiform purpura • Purpura fulminans *Differential diagnostic* • Livedo reticularis • Livedo racemose • Vasculitis	*Treatment* Identify and treat underlying cause *Pathogenesis* Thrombosis, intravascular deposition of abnormal proteins, and embolic phenomena may result in the development of retiform purpura *Associated disorders* • Disseminated intravascular coagulation (DIC): Occur in the setting of sepsis, organ failure, trauma • Malignancy, malaria, and meningococcemia are common causes of DIC • Hypercoagulable states: Antiphospholipid syndrome • Warfarin-induced skin necrosis • Heparin-induced thrombocytopenia • Paroxysmal nocturnal hemoglobinuria • Embolic disorders: Cholesterol and septic emboli, atrial myxoma • Vessel wall pathology: Vasculitis *Clinical evaluation* • History and physical examination: Pay special attention to the presence of red flags, for example, DIC • Laboratory: FBC and punch biopsy

Table 12.1 (continued)

Diagnosis and classification	Treatment and relevant clinical features: dermatology conditions
Pruritus A localized stimulus or urge to scratch the area of concern. Occurs in a wide variety of clinical settings, such as dermatologic disorders, neuropathic disorders, and systemic or psychiatric disease	*Treatment* • Identify and treat cause: Dry skin, diabetes, renal failure, hepatic disease, scabies, etc. • Cetirizine, tab, 10 mg, 1 tab/d, 5 d *or* • Chlorpheniramine, tab, 25 mg, 3 × 1 tab/d, 5 d If superimposed infection • Amoxicillin, tab, 500 mg, 3 × 1 tab/d, 5 d • *Xeroderma* (dry skin) is the most common cause. Advise about the use of mild soap. Use a dry, clean cotton towel to dry after showering. Hydrate body with good lotion • Do not shower using soap more than 1×/d *Etiology* • Cutaneous disorders: inflammatory (dermatitis, urticaria, psoriasis, pityriasis rosea, pityriasis rubra pilaris, acne, dermatitis herpetiformis, bullous pemphigoid), neurodermatitis (prurigo nodularis, lichen simplex chronicus), burns and scars • Renal disease: end-stage chronic renal failure • Liver disease: cholestatic jaundice, cholestasis of pregnancy • Hematopoietic disease: iron deficiency anemia, polycythemia vera, mastocytosis, multiple myeloma • Endocrine and metabolic disorders: hyperthyroidism, hypothyroidism, diabetes, carcinoid syndrome • Infectious and parasitic disorders: superficial fungal infections, Scabies, HIV infection, varicella • Autoimmune disorders: dermatomyositis, scleroderma, Sjögren syndrome • Neurologic disorders: brachioradial pruritus, postherpetic neuralgia, multiple sclerosis, cerebrovascular accident • Psychogenic disorders: depression, psychogenic excoriation, delusional infestation, anorexia nervosa
Psoriasis A chronic, noncontagious, incurable autoimmune disease Twenty percent of patients who suffer from a severe form of psoriasis will develop arthritis *Note:* • Type I occurs <40 years old • Type II occurs >40 years old	*Treatment* • Diprosalic, cream, apply on skin 2×/d • Corticosteroid cream: Hydrocortisone 1%, apply on skin 2× /d • Emollients *Management tips* Good skin care: mild soap usage, rehydration with neutral cream or Vaseline *Classification* based of body areas, disease extension, and appearance • Erythroderma • Guttate • Inversa • Pustulosa • Ungual • Vulgaris • Scalp • Intertriginous psoriasis
Scabies Skin infestation with the ectoparasite *Sarcoptes scabiei*	*Treatment* • Benzyl benzoate, cream, 25%; apply to whole body from the neck down. Ensure all parts of the skin are covered and allow the medication to dry and remain on the skin for at least 10 h *or* • Ivermectin, tab, 3 mg, 0.25 mg/kg, single dose, to be repeated 10 d after. For example, for a 70-kg patient, give 6 tabs on day one as a single dose, then repeat 10 d after • Cetirizine, tab, 10 mg, 2 × 1 tab/d, 5 d

Table 12.1 (continued)

Diagnosis and classification	Treatment and relevant clinical features: dermatology conditions
	Eradication procedure • Rigorous eradicative hygiene: • Wash bedding (can live up to 2 d in clothes) at 20–55 °C • Treat the whole family and any other close contacts *Signs and symptoms* • Pruritus • Generalized eczematiform dermatitis • Intraepidermal burrows (pathognomonic), nodular scabies
Snakebite	*Treatment* First aid • Apply firm pressure bandage over bite • Immobilize limb • Identify snake type • Give 0.5 ml of Tetanus toxoid injection IM When envenomation is suspected • Early use of antivenom (slow intravenous infusion) • Have epinephrine (adrenaline) at standby for any allergic reactions to antivenom • General supportive measures: iv fluids for hypotension, diazepam for anxiety • Institute treatment for acute respiratory, cardiac, and renal failure as necessary *Management tips* • Avoid use of arterial tourniquets • In 50% of cases, no venom has been injected in the bite • Refer after first aid or initial resuscitation to appropriate facility for possible antivenom injection *Note: compartment syndrome*
Urticaria Skin eruption of papulas or wheals with intense itching	*Treatment* • Cetirizine, tab, 10 mg, 2 × 1 tab/d, 5 d • Chlorpheniramine, tab, 4 mg, 2 × 1 tab/d as needed *Clinical notes* • Acute or chronic (>6 weeks) • 70% of chronic urticaria are idiopathic • 10–15% are associated with Hashimoto thyroiditis • Spontaneous or reactional • Take good directed history to identify causative allergen • Advise on eviction
Varicella (chicken pox) Vesicular pustules (croups) on face, hands, or trunk, with extreme itching, which may lead to widespread infection and disfigurement *Differential diagnosis* • Shingles • Herpes • Impetigo	*Treatment* • Calamine lotion, 2%, apply to affected skin areas 3×/d • Paracetamol, tab, 500 mg, 3 × 2 tab/d as needed *or* • Ibuprofen, tab, 400 mg, 2 × 1 tab/d, as required • Treat superinfection: Amoxicillin, tabs, 500 mg, 3 × 1 tab/d • Antiviral if patient presents in acute phase: Acyclovir, tabs, 200 mg, 4 × 1 tab/d, 5 d • If ophthalmic sphere is involved, urgent ophthalmic referral is required • Propose retroviral serology

Hematology 13

Contents

13.1 History: Questions to Ask 171

13.2 Physical Examination 171

13.3 Cardinal Paramedical Hematology Examinations 172

13.4 Hematology Red Flags 172

Hematology is the medical specialty composed of the diagnosis, treatment, and prevention of diseases of the blood and bone marrow as well as of the immunologic, hemostatic blood clotting, and vascular systems (Fig. 13.1). Because of the dynamic and multisystemic nature of blood, the science of hematology profoundly affects the understanding of many diseases (Table 13.1).

Parasitic infection of the hematological system remains the most significant cause of mortality and morbidity. The *Plasmodium* family of protozoa comprise the most lethal infectious diseases. Species include *P. falciparum*, *P. vivax*, and *P. malariae*. As malaria is a multisystemic and rapidly fatal disease, it should always be on the mind of the clinician during history taking and during the physical examination.

Anemias resulting from occult or frank hemorrhages, iron and/or folic acid deficiency, and genetic defects are common.

BMC encounters oncologic conditions of the hematological and lymphatic system. Specific diagnostic entities may be leukemia, lymphomas, and Vasquez syndrome. Unfortunately, therapeutic options are presently limited.

In this chapter, we address common hematologic disorders that are encountered in a standard minimal resource facility (Table 13.1).

13.1 History: Questions to Ask

- Do you have a fever?
- Are you unusually tired?
- Do you have a headache?
- Do you have nausea?
- Did you vomit?
- Are you dizzy?

13.2 Physical Examination

- Observe general clinical status
- Do a systemic directed review

© The Author(s), under exclusive license to Springer Nature Switzerland AG 2021

M. Touray, A. Touray, *Clinical Work and General Management of a Standard Minimal-Resource Facility*, Sustainable Development Goals Series, https://doi.org/10.1007/978-3-030-71032-3_13

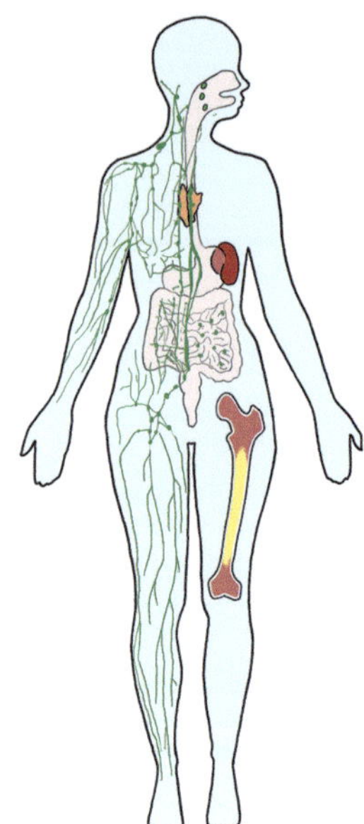

Fig. 13.1 Hematology: A mnemonic illustration representing main anatomic hematology structures and their corresponding pathologies

13.3   Cardinal Paramedical Hematology Examinations

- Full blood count
- Erythrocyte sedimentation rate

13.4   Hematology Red Flags

- Documentation of high parasitemia on thick blood film (>5) parasites/high field 40×
- Presence of B symptoms: nocturnal transudation, fever >38 °C, significant loss of weight, that is, >10%
- Adenopathy
- Hepatomegaly and/or splenomegaly
- Petechia and ecchymosis
- Jaundice
- Persistence of anemia despite proper substitutive treatment (iron, vitamin B12, and folic acid)
- Associated digestive symptoms

Table 13.1 Hematology conditions and their treatment

Diagnosis and classification	Treatment and relevant clinical features: hematology conditions
Anemia Hemoglobin less than 10 g/dl. Make allowance for gender and age *or* Reduced absolute number of circulating red blood cells (i.e., a reduced red blood cell mass) *or* Serum ferritin less than 12 ng/mL or less than 27 pmol/L *Classification of anemia by means of blood cell volume* *Microcytic anemia* • Iron deficiency • Thalassemia • Anemia of chronic disease • Lead toxicity • Zinc deficiency *Macrocytic anemia* • Vitamin B12 deficiency • Folate deficiency • DNA synthesis inhibitors *Aplastic anemia* • Myelodysplasia • Liver disease • Hypothyroidism • Bone marrow failure *Normocytic anemia* • Kidney disease • On-thyroid endocrine gland failure	*Treatment* • Treat underlying cause • Iron supplementation: Ferrous sulfate, tab, 100 mg, 1 × 1 tab/d, 3–6 months, to be taken in the morning with citrus juice *and* • Acid folic, tab, 5 mg, 1 tab/d, 3–6 months • Advice on iron rich diet: green vegetables, for example, spinach and beans *If digestive suspicion:* • Mebendazole 200 mg stat in suspected helminthiasis • Triple therapy (Omeprazole + Doxycycline + Flagyl) for *H. pylori* infection • Ferrous sulfate, tab, 100 mg, 1 tab/d, 90 d *and* • Folic acid, tab, 5 mg, 1 tab/d, 90 d *Etiology of microcytic anemia* • Iron deficiency • Inflammatory (cancer, infection, inflammatory disease, etc.), hemoglobinopathy (thalassemia and sickle cell disease) • Chronic bleeding, uterine myofibroma, gastroduodenal ulcers *Etiology of normocytic anemia* • Acute hemorrhage, beginning of iron deficiency, inflammation, leukemia *Etiology of macrocytic anemia* • Vitamin B12 deficiency • Alcohol abuse *Etiology of anemia* • Gastrointestinal parasites (e.g., hookworm, whipworm) • Traumatic hemorrhage • Hematemesis or melena • Hemoptysis • Menorrhagia • Pregnancy and delivery • Hematuria • Occult bleeding, typically gastrointestinal (e.g., gastritis, malignancy, telangiectasia) *Management tips* • Review Hb at least 30 d after commencement of therapy • Avoid long-term proton-pump inhibitor use (e.g., Omeprazole) • Provide iron supplements • Provide dietary advice *Signs and symptoms* Chronic anemia is characterized by • Fatigue • Pallor • Small for age • Impaired cognition Acute anemia is clinically distinguished by dyspnea *Causes of iron deficiency* • Deficient diet intake • Decreased absorption, for example, *H. pylori* gastritis • Increased requirements, for example, pregnancy and lactation • Blood loss, for example, gastrointestinal, menstrual, blood donation, hemoglobinopathics • Iron sequestration • Idiopathic

(continued)

Table 13.1 (continued)

Diagnosis and classification	Treatment and relevant clinical features: hematology conditions
Eosinophilia Peripheral blood eosinophilia, absolute eosinophil count of ≥500/microL *Calculation of absolute eosinophil count* WBC count/microL X percentage of eosinophils = eosinophils/micro L *Eosinophilia—AEC ≥500 eosinophils/ micro L* *Hyper eosinophilia—≥1500 eosinophils/ micro L* *Hyper eosinophilic syndromes ≥1500/micro L* (on two occasions ≥1 month apart) *plus* organ dysfunction attributable to eosinophilia	*Treatment* Identify and treat underlying etiology *Etiology* Can be a result of numerous disorders • *Infectious diseases:* Helminths (e.g., strongyloidiasis, trichinellosis, filariasis, toxocariasis, schistosomiasis, hookworm), ectoparasites (e.g., scabies, myiasis), protozoans, fungi, and viruses, for example, HIV • *Allergic disorders:* Asthma, allergic rhinitis, atopic dermatitis, drug hypersensitivity • *Neoplastic disorders:* Acute or chronic eosinophilic leukemia and other myeloid neoplasms (e.g., chronic myeloid leukemia, systemic mastocytosis) • *Immunologic disorders:* immune deficiencies, autoimmune and idiopathic disorders *Clinical evaluation* • *History:* query symptoms that may reflect organ involvement by eosinophils, including a complete review of systems, family history, medication, and occupation 　　*Constitutional:* Fever, night sweats, unintentional weight loss, fatigue 　　*Cutaneous:* Eczema, pruritus, urticaria, angioedema, rash, ulcers 　　*Cardiac:* Dyspnea, chest pain, palpitations, symptoms of heart failure 　　*Respiratory:* Nasal/sinus symptoms, wheezing, cough, chest congestion 　　*Gastrointestinal:* Weight loss, abdominal pain, dysphagia, nausea, vomiting, diarrhea, food intolerance, changes in stools 　　*Nervous system:* Transient ischemic attack, cerebrovascular accident, behavioral changes, confusion, balance problems, memory loss, change in vision, numbness, weakness, pain • *Physical examination:* sought for evidence of organ involvement and/or possible causes of eosinophilia
Hematopoietic cancer Malignancies of the hematopoietic and lymphoid tissues, including lymphomas, leukemias, myeloproliferative neoplasms, mast cell neoplasms, plasma cell neoplasms, histio-leucomia cystic tumors, and dendritic cell neoplasms *Classification* • Myeloid • Acute myeloid • Myeloproliferative neoplasms • Mastocytosis • Myelodysplastic syndrome *Lymphoid* • Hodgkin's lymphoma • Precursor lymphoid neoplasm	*Treatment* • Hematopoietic cancers are usually suspected based on history, physical examination, and a simple blood count • Refer suspected case to a specialist for adequate treatment *Diagnostic features* • B symptoms: fever, night sweats, and weight loss • Hemorrhagic events • Thromboembolic events • Hepatosplenomegaly • Leukocytosis • Leucopenia • Anemia
Hemophilia Congenital disorders of coagulation *Classification* • *Hemophilia A* is a congenital deficiency of coagulation factor VIII • *Hemophilia B* is a congenital deficiency of coagulation factor IX	*Treatment* • Refer to a tertiary center for tertiary hematology care *Diagnostic features* • Recurring hemarthrosis and arthropathy • Risk of development of inhibitory antibodies to factor VIII and factor IX • Exposed to risks related to transfusion

Table 13.1 (continued)

Diagnosis and classification	Treatment and relevant clinical features: hematology conditions
Human immunodeficiency virus (HIV) Acute HIV infection presents with a constellation of nonspecific symptoms *Differential diagnosis* • Mucocutaneous ulceration is common in syphilis • Rash is uncommon in EBV/CMV mononucleosis and toxoplasmosis and tends to spare the palms and soles in rubella • Pharyngeal edema with little associated tonsillar exudate or hypertrophy • SLE can closely resemble acute HIV infection	*Treatment* Refer to tertiary health facility for specialized care for tri-therapy based on reverse transcriptase inhibitors and protease inhibitors Give empirical PCP prophylaxis: • Cotrimoxazole 800/160, tab, 2 × 1tab/14 d • Fluconazole, tabs, 50 mg, 1×/d, 5 d • Multivitamins, tabs, 3 × 1 tab/d, 3 months *Signs and symptoms* • Constitutional symptoms (fever, fatigue, myalgia) • Adenopathy • Oropharyngeal findings: sore throat • Mucocutaneous ulcers: shallow, sharply demarcated ulcers with white bases surrounded by a thin area of erythema on the oral mucosa, anus, penis, or esophagus • Rash • Gastrointestinal symptoms: nausea, diarrhea, anorexia, and weight loss • Neurologic findings: aseptic meningitis *General assessment* • CD4 to evaluate the progression of the disease • Chest X-ray • Evaluate nutritional status • Social network and support system • Address stigmatization issues • Reassurance • Opportunistic infections • Oral and esophageal candidiasis • CMV infection (proctitis, colitis, and hepatitis) • Pneumocystis jirovecii pneumonia • Prolonged, severe cryptosporidiosis *Management tips* • Patient education about national treatment and support programs • Gain patient confidence by ensuring confidentiality • Provide nutritional advice • Offer provider-initiative counseling and testing (PICT) • Assess presence and degree of risk to others
Infectious mononucleosis A systemic infectious disease characterized by a triad of fever, tonsillar pharyngitis, and lymphadenopathy *Nomenclature* • Glandular fever • Epstein-Barr virus mononucleosis • Kissing disease	*Treatment* Symptom control and supportive treatment *Etiology* • Epstein-Barr virus (EBV) is a widely disseminated herpes virus that is spread by intimate contact between susceptible persons and EBV shedders • Contact of EBV with oropharyngeal epithelial cells allows replication of the virus, the release of EBV into the oropharyngeal secretions, and infection of B cells in the lymphoid-rich areas of the oropharynx • Transmission: person-to-person, breastfeeding, sexual transmission *Clinical presentation* • *Symptoms*: Anorexia, nausea, headache cough, chills, myalgia, ocular muscle pain, chest pain, arthralgia, photophobia • *Signs*: Adenopathy, fever, pharyngitis, splenomegaly, bradycardia, periorbital edema, palatal enanthem, liver/spleen tenderness, hepatomegaly, skin rash, rhinitis, jaundice, pneumonia

(continued)

Table 13.1 (continued)

Diagnosis and classification	Treatment and relevant clinical features: hematology conditions
	Complications • Splenomegaly and splenic rupture • *Rash:* generalized maculopapular, urticarial, or petechial rash • *Neurologic syndromes:* include Guillain-Barré syndrome, facial and other cranial nerve palsies, meningoencephalitis, aseptic meningitis, transverse myelitis, peripheral neuritis, optic neuritis, and encephalomyelitis • *Other:* any organ system such as hepatitis or cholestasis, pneumonia, pleural effusions, myocarditis, pancreatitis and acalculous cholecystitis, mesenteric adenitis, myositis, acute renal failure, glomerulonephritis, gastric pseudo-lymphoma, and genital ulceration. Jaundice and hepatomegaly are less common, although ascites and fatal cases of hepatitis have been described
Jaundice and hyper bilirubinemia Yellowing of skin, sclera, and other mucosa due to deposition of overt production of bilirubin *Disorders associated with jaundice* • Overproduction of bilirubin • Extravascular hemolysis • Extravasation • Intravascular hemolysis • Dyserythropoiesis • Gallstones • Hepatitis	*Etiology* *Unconjugated hyperbilirubinemia may be caused by:* • Hemolysis • Extravasation of blood into tissue • Dyserythropoiesis • Stress situations (e.g., sepsis) leading to increased production of bilirubin • Impaired hepatic bilirubin uptake • Impaired bilirubin conjugation *Conjugated hyperbilirubinemia may be caused by:* • Biliary obstruction (e.g., gallstones, pancreatic or biliary malignancy, parasites) • Viral hepatitis • Alcoholic hepatitis • Nonalcoholic steatohepatitis • Primary biliary cholangitis • Drugs and toxins • Ischemic hepatopathy • Liver infiltration • Inherited disorders • Total parenteral nutrition • Postoperative jaundice • Intrahepatic cholestasis of pregnancy • End-stage liver disease • Organ transplantation (e.g., bone marrow, liver)
Malaria, uncomplicated Malaria is caused by *Plasmodium* parasites Transmission requires an intermediate mosquito (*Anopheles*) host, which is found worldwide	*Treatment* *Adults* • Coartem (artemether 20 mg and lumefantrine 120 mg), tab, 20/120, 2 × 4 tab/d, 3 d *or* • Artesunate-amodiaquine, tab, 1 × 2 tab/d, 3 d *or* • Quinine, tab, 300 mg, 2 × 1 tb/d, 5 d *and* • Doxycyclin, tab, 100 mg, 2 × 1 tab/d, 5 d *Children* • Artesunate-amodiaquine, tab, 1 × 1 tab/d, 3 d *or* • Coartem, 1–3, tab, 2×/d, 3 d *or* • Quinine, tab, 300 mg 2 × 1 tab/d, 5 d *and* • Fansidar (Sulfadoxine and Pyrimethamine), 2, tab, single dose *Human plasmodium species* • *Plasmodium falciparum* • *Plasmodium vivax* • *Plasmodium ovale* • *Plasmodium malariae*

Table 13.1 (continued)

Diagnosis and classification	Treatment and relevant clinical features: hematology conditions
	Pathogenesis of malaria • Following exposure (an infected mosquito bite) the incubation period varies between 1 and 4 weeks in most cases • Depending on the plasmodium species involved, much longer incubation periods are possible • Once the plasmodia multiply inside the red blood cells, fever and multi-organ disease may ensue, which can be life-threatening when *P. falciparum* is involved • Symptoms are much reduced if the patient is semi-immune by a repeated previous infection • Several drugs are available for both treatment and prophylaxis
Malaria, severe/complicated • More than two convulsions in 24 h • Persistent vomiting • Impaired consciousness, including unarousable coma • Generalized weakness • Respiratory distress • Radiological or clinical evidence of pulmonary edema • Abnormal bleeding • Clinical jaundice plus evidence of other vital organ dysfunction • Severe pallor • Hemodynamic instability or shock with systolic blood pressure < 50 mm hg • Hemoglobinuria (dark urine)	*Treatment* *Adults* • Quinine, ampoule for injection, 600 mg, 2 amps in 500 ml of 5% dextrose, iv infusion, single dose, *then* • Quinine, ampoule for injection 600 mg, 1 amp in 500 ml of 5% dextrose/12 hours for 48 h *Children* • Quinine 20 mg/kg iv in 10 mL/kg of 5% dextrose single dose, *then* • Quinine 10 mg/kg iv in 10 mL/kg of 5% dextrose every 12 h for 48 h *Management tips* • Patients who vomit constantly are treated as severe malaria patients, even in the absence of signs of severity such as seizures, shock, severe anemia, etc. • *Plasmodium falciparum* is the most dangerous form (more common in West Africa) • *Plasmodium vivax* (more common in East Africa) is known to cause recurrence of malaria without exposure to mosquito bites, due to dormant form in the liver *Note: Switch to oral formula as soon as emesis subsides* *Most admitted patients will return home with a 5-d course of:* • Quinine, tab, 300 mg 3 × 1 tab/d *and* • Doxycyclin, tab, 100 mg 2 × 1 tab/d
Malaria in pregnancy (MIP) Infection of the pregnant woman by malaria-inducing *Plasmodium* species *Complications* Abortion Intrauterine fetal death Premature labor Low birth weight Intrauterine growth retardation Stillbirth Anemia	*Treatment* *First trimester* • Uncomplicated malaria: Quinine, tab,300 mg, 3 × 2 tab/d, 7 d • Severe malaria: Quinine, ampoule for injection, 600 mg, 1 amp im, 2 × 1 amp/d then change to quinine, tab, 300 mg, 3 × 2 tab/d, (per oral, as soon as tolerated), 7 d *Second & third trimesters (16–34 weeks)* • Uncomplicated malaria: artemisinin-based combination therapy (ACT), tab • Severe malaria: ruinine injection, as above • Treat hypoglycemia and anemia accordingly: Glucose 5%, infusion bag, 2 bags in 4 h, monitor blood sugar level *Intermittent preventive treatment (IPT)* • Malaria prevention strategy that involves administration of four doses of sulfadoxine + pyrimethamine (SP). This has to be administered by direct observed treatment (DOT) • Antenatal visits up to 14 weeks (3 tabs) • 16–20 weeks (3 tabs) • 24–28 weeks (3 tabs) • 32 weeks (3 tabs) • 36 weeks up to delivery (3 tabs)

(continued)

Table 13.1 (continued)

Diagnosis and classification	Treatment and relevant clinical features: hematology conditions
	Clinical notes Malaria is frequently more severe in pregnancy Treat for malaria if: • Fever above 37.5 °C in the absence of other reasons • Headache, abdominal pain, vomiting • Hb drop over 1 g/dl in 2 d
Sickle cell disease *Evaluation* • Family and personal medical history • Rigorous systematic physical history • Full blood count • Electrophoresis • HbsAg	*Treatment* • Patient education • In severe cases requiring transfusion, refer to tertiary center • Treat *sickle-cell crisis* as appropriate • iv fluids: 500 cc, 0.9% NaCl • Paracetamol, tab, 500 mg, 3 × 2 tab/d • Naproxen, tab, 500 mg, 2 × 1 tab/d • Tramadol, tab, 50 mg, 2 × 1 tab/d • Prophylaxis: penicillin, tab, 500 mg, 1×/d • Polyvalent pneumococcal vaccine and Hemophilus influenza type B *Long-term treatment* • Folic acid, tab, 5 mg, 1 tab/d *Complications* • Recurrent multiple organ infarctions: brain, bone, heart • Failure to thrive • Small for age • Adverse effects of stigmatization • Absenteeism at school and workplace *Precipitating factors of sickle-cell crisis* • Infection • Dehydration • Exposure to extremes of temperatures
Splenomegaly Enlargement of the spleen, measured by size or weight *Pathophysiology* The spleen is a hematopoietic organ capable of supporting elements of the erythroid, myeloid, megakaryocytic, lymphoid, and monocyte macrophage (i.e., reticuloendothelial) systems *Terminology* • Hypersplenism • Hypersplenism and asplenia • Splenosis • Splenic infarction • Splenic infarction • Massively enlarged spleen	*Treatment* • Treat underlying cause • Address to tertiary center for specialized hematological management if persistent *Etiology* • Splenic engorgement due to sequestration of red blood cells • Extramedullary hematopoiesis in the spleen • Splenic trauma with intracapsular hematoma formation, sequestration crisis in sickle cell disease, and portal hypertension • Chronic inflammation or infection, as in systemic lupus erythematosus • Splenic hemangioma, hamartoma, or cysts *Associated clinical scenarios* • Chronic myeloid leukemia • Myelofibrosis, primary or secondary to polycythemia vera or essential thrombocytosis • Gaucher disease • Lymphoma, usually indolent, including hairy cell leukemia • Kala-azar (visceral leishmaniasis) • Hyperactive malarial splenomegaly syndrome, also called tropical splenomegaly syndrome • Beta thalassemia major or severe beta-thalassemia intermedia • AIDS with mycobacterium avium complex

Endocrinology

14

Contents

14.1 **History: Questions to Ask** 180

14.2 **Physical Examination** 180

14.3 **Cardinal Paramedical Endocrinology Examinations** 180

14.4 **Endocrinology Red Flags** 180

Endocrinology is the study of the medical aspects of hormones, including diseases and conditions associated with hormonal imbalance, damage to the glands that make hormones, or the use of synthetic or natural hormonal drugs (Fig. 14.1 and Table 14.1). This interesting subspeciality of internal medicine deals with the endocrine system, the organs that are associated with it, the diseases and conditions that may arise from any of the associated glands and organs, and the overall metabolic function of the body. Endocrinology also include any behavior or mental activity that can be associated with or develop because of changes in the endocrine system.

The major endocrine affliction seen at a standard minimal facility is diabetes, including both inaugural Type 1 and Type II. History taking is the leading diagnostic tool; ask about polyuria, polydipsia, and family history. An associated physical finding for Type II diabetes is obesity and hypertension.

Afflictions of the thyroid gland are also encountered, both hypo- and hyperthyroidism. Unfortunately, though crucial, laboratory sup-port for these afflictions is scarce in The Gambia. The clinician should exercise caution when interpreting obtained laboratory results from a thyroid panel, including TSH, T3 and T4, and thyroglobulin. It is important to interpret such results in the light of obtained historical and physical findings.

Dysfunctions of the pituitary axis should also not escape the vigilance of the clinician. This group of pathologies includes diabetes insipidus, sexual dysfunction, infertility, Cushingoid dimorphism, and visual field defects. History and physical findings may include galactorrhea, reduced libido, visual field obliterations, headache, and gynecomastia. Correlating laboratory findings may include inappropriate serum levels of TSH, FSH, prolactin, testosterone, estrogen, and progesterone. A gynecologist, endocrinologist, or urologist may be included in the care of affected patients.

Pathologies of the suprarenal gland malfunctions should also be addressed, including Addisonian crises, hirsutism, hypercortism (Cushing syndrome), and alopecia.

M. Touray, A. Touray, *Clinical Work and General Management of a Standard Minimal-Resource Facility*, Sustainable Development Goals Series, https://doi.org/10.1007/978-3-030-71032-3_14

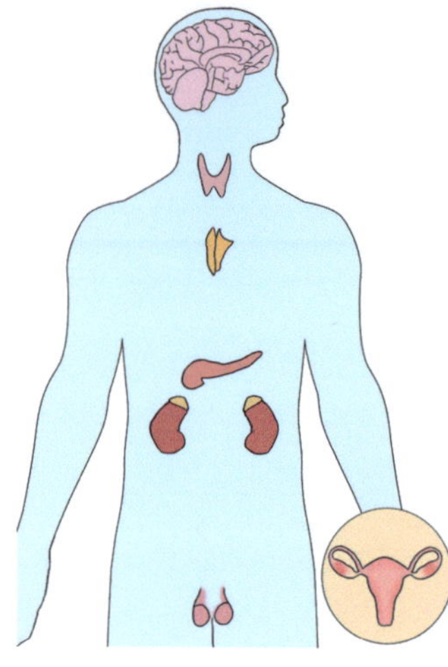

Fig. 14.1 Endocrinology: A mnemonic illustration representing main anatomic endocrinology structures and their corresponding pathologies

In this chapter, we address common endocrinologic disorders that are encountered in a standard minimal-resource facility (Table 14.1).

14.1   History: Questions to Ask

- Do you have diabetes, or does anyone in your family have it?
- How many times do you get up to urinate? Are you often thirsty, and are you drinking a lot more than usual?
- Are you unusually tired?
- Have close friends or family said your neck looks bigger? Or your eyeball?
- Do you feel that you are growing hair at unusual sites?

14.2   Physical Examination

- Appreciate the general appearance: Moon face? Abnormal hair growth? Scalp hair loss?
- General internal medical physical.

14.3   Cardinal Paramedical Endocrinology Examinations

- Full blood count
- Fasting blood sugar
- Thyroid panel
- Urine sticks, urine microalbumin
- Ultrasonographic imaging
- Chest X-ray

14.4   Endocrinology Red Flags

- Signs of imminent thyrotoxicosis: Hemodynamic instability: tachyarrhythmia, decompensated cardiac failure, myocardial ischemia
- Suggestive neuropsychological signs: confusion, manic decompensation
- Hypothyroidy: poorly tolerated bradycardia, decompensated cardiorespiratory status
- Laboratory findings of hypo- or hyperglycemia

Table 14.1 Endocrinology conditions and their treatment

Diagnosis and classification	Treatment and relevant clinical features: endocrinology conditions
Adrenal insufficiency Acute or chronic disease conditions characterized by dysfunction of the adrenal gland	*Treatment* • *Appropriate hormone supplementation* • *Involve endocrinology in caregiving where available* • *Long term corticosteroid supplementation: Hydrocortisone, tab, 10 mg, 1, tab, /d,* *Etiology* • Prolonged administration of pharmacologic doses of synthetic glucocorticoids • Addison disease • Adrenal gland infarction *Clinical manifestations* • Fatigue • Weight loss • Nausea, vomiting, abdominal pain • Muscle and joint pain • Skin hyperpigmentation • Postural hypotension • Salt craving • Dehydration, hypotension, or shock out of proportion to the severity of current illness • Unexplained hypoglycemia • Hyponatremia, hyperkalemia, azotemia, hypercalcemia, or eosinophilia
Cushing syndrome A complex clinical syndrome resulting from chronic exposure to excess glucocorticoid *Cushing disease* is pituitary ACTH-dependent Cushing syndrome	*Treatment* • Avoid systemic corticoids where possible *Etiology* • Chronic use of high dose glucocorticoids • Cushing disease • Adrenal adenoma • Adrenal carcinoma *Clinical manifestations* • Decreased libido • Obesity/weight gain • Plethora • Round face • Menstrual changes • Hirsutism • Hypertension • Ecchymoses • Lethargy • Depression • Dorsal fat pad • Abnormal glucose tolerance • ECG abnormalities or atherosclerosis striae • Edema • Proximal muscle weakness, osteopenia, or fracture • Headache • Backache • Recurrent infections • Abdominal pain • Acne • Female balding

(continued)

Table 14.1 (continued)

Diagnosis and classification	Treatment and relevant clinical features: endocrinology conditions
	Diagnostic features • Central obesity • Muscle wasting • Hirsutism • Hyperpigmented striae • Psychological changes • Osteoporosis • Hypertension • Poor wound healing • Hypoglycemia, leukocytosis, lymphocytopenia, hypokalemia • Elevated serum cortisol • Lack of normal suppression by dexamethasone
Diabetes insipid Is characterized by decreased release of antidiuretic hormone (ADH), resulting in polyuria. nocturia, polydipsia (initially) *Synonym* Central diabetes insipidus	*Treatment* • Identify the underlying cause • Desmopressin, ampoule for injection, 2 mcg, 05.5–1 ml, iv or subcutaneous/d or • Chlorpropamide, tab, 125 mg, 1 × 1 tab/d • Carbamazepine, tab, 200 mg, 1 × 1 tab/d *Etiology:* cause by reduced action of ADH. Lack of ADH can be caused by disorders that act at one or more of the sites involved in ADH secretion: • The hypothalamic osmoreceptors; • The supraoptic or paraventricular nuclei; • The superior portion of the supra optico-hypophyseal tract • Primary or secondary tumors or infiltrative diseases, for example, Langerhans cell histiocytosis, craniopharyngiomas, • Neurosurgery, and trauma • Idiopathic • Familial and congenital disease • Congenital hypopituitarism • Septo-optic dysplasia • Hypoxic encephalopathy • Anorexia nervosa • Post-supraventricular tachycardia *Clinical manifestations* • Polyuria, nocturia, polydipsia • Decreased bone mineral density at the lumbar spine and femoral neck
Diabetes mellitus (DM) High blood glucose levels: Fasting whole blood glucose level is 7 mmol/L or more and/or Random blood glucose, taken 2 h after a meal is 11.1 mmol/L or more *Classification* • *Type 1 diabetes:*insulin-dependent diabetes mellitus or juvenile diabetes • *Type 2 diabetes:*noninsulin-dependent diabetes mellitus or maturity onset diabetes	*Treatment* • Patient education • Dietary advice • Lifestyle modification: regular exercise, weight reduction, alcohol, and smoking cessation • Optimal blood pressure control *Pharmacotherapy* *Type 1 DM* • 0.3–0.5 units/kg of soluble insulin (rapid/short-acting) in three divided doses • Mixtard, 0.3–0.5 units/kg twice daily plus insulin glargine (long-acting at bedtime) • Soluble insulin, 0.3–0.5 units/kg twice daily plus insulin glargine daily (at bedtime) *Type 2 DM* • Educating the patient about signs and symptoms of diabetes is paramount • Metformin, tab, 500 mg, 2 × 1 tab/d, maximal dose 3 g/d, to be taken after food • Glibenclamide, tab, 5 mg, 2 × 1 tab/d, to be taken after food

Table 14.1 (continued)

Diagnosis and classification	Treatment and relevant clinical features: endocrinology conditions
• *Gestational diabetes:* diabetes that develops during pregnancy in previously nondiabetic individuals. (See section on Diabetes in Pregnancy)	*Acute complications* • Hypoglycemia • Diabetic ketoacidosis • Hyperosmolar nonketotic coma • Hyperglycemic hyperosmolar state (HHS) • Diabetic nephropathy *Chronic complications of diabetes* • Ocular complications: cataracts, retinopathy, glaucoma • Diabetic neuropathy: peripheral neuropathies, neuropathic cachexia, autonomic neuropathy • Cardiovascular complications: myocardial infarction • Skin on mucosa membrane complication • Bone and joint complications • Diabetic gastroplasty • Renal failure • Diabetic foot ulcers *Short-term complications* • Recurrent infections: UTI, upper respiratory tract infection (URTI) *Long-term complications* • Blindness • Amputation *Microvascular complications* • Peripheral neuropathy • Retinopathy • Nephropathy *Macrovascular complications* • Coronary • Cerebral • Peripheral vessels
Diabetic foot Foot wounds in a diabetic patient characterized by suppuration and necrosis	*Treatment* • Rigorous glycemic control • Proper footwear • Intravenous antibiotics: • Ceftriaxone, ampoule for injection, 1 g, 1 amp/3 d • Metronidazole (Flagyl), tab, 500 mg 3 × 1 tab/d, 7 d *and* • Co-amoxicillin, tab, 1 g, 2 × 1 tab/d, 7 d • Closely monitor glycemia and control • In very severe cases, refer to a tertiary center for surgical intervention *Etiology/risk factors* • Loss of protective sensation due to neuropathy • Secondary foot deformity leading to excess pressure, external trauma, and infection • Effects of chronic ischemia, typically due to peripheral artery disease *Management tips* • Ensure good footwear • Patient education • Assess degree of foot involvement • Do simple wound debridement under local anesthesia if tissue involvement is minimal • Clean and dress wound with normal saline, povidone-iodine, and hydrogen peroxide

(continued)

Table 14.1 (continued)

Diagnosis and classification	Treatment and relevant clinical features: endocrinology conditions
Diabetic ketoacidosis A serious acute complication of diabetes characterized by metabolic acidosis with high ketoacid accumulation Moderately high serum glucose concentration	*Treatment* • Aggressive intravenous fluid resuscitation • NaCl, 0.9%, 500 ml bags for iv infusion, 4 bags in first 6 h; monitor urine output • Insulin administration as required *Note: This is a medical emergency* If in a coma or in difficult circumstances, refer to tertiary for intensive care management *Differential diagnosis* Hyperosmolar hyperglycemic state • No ketoacid accumulation • Serum glucose concentration frequently exceeds 56 mmol/L • Plasma osmolality (Posm) may reach 380 mOsmol/kg • Neurologic abnormalities are frequently present (including coma in 25–50%)
Gynecomastia A benign proliferation of the glandular tissue of the male breast, caused by an increase in the ratio of estrogen to androgen activity *Clinical definition* Palpable enlargement of the male breast, often asymptomatic and unilateral *Classifications* based on tissue involved, distribution, and location • Glandular gynecomastia; normally tender • Fatty gynecomastia; typically, nontender • Unilateral • Bilateral • Areolar	Treatment • Focused assessment including Good history and physical examination, Paramedical: FBC, TSH, and prolactin Imaging: CT or MRI of the brain with pituitary axis where available • Refer to a tertiary center for tertiary endocrinology care *Etiology* • Hyperthyroidism • Liver disease • Drugs: estrogen, cannabis, diamorphine, or antiandrogens (spironolactone, cimetidine) • Tumors: HCG-producing (testis, lung); estrogen-producing tumors (testis, adrenal); carcinoma of breast and pituitary adenoma • Excessive chronic alcohol consumption • Past bodybuilding • Aging • Endocrine disorders • Systemic diseases • Drugs, for example, alcohol *Management tips* • Psychological support • Reassure if physiological: neonatal, pubertal, and old age, ex-body builder • Perform histopathology brain CT with pituitary axis
Hirsutism and virilization Excessive male-pattern hair growth, affects between 5% and 10% of women of reproductive age	*Treatment* • Etiologic assessment, refer to tertiary for gynecological or endocrinology tertiary care *Etiology* • Idiopathic • Familial • Polycystic ovary syndrome • Neoplastic disorders *Diagnostic features* • Hirsutism, acne, menstrual disorders • Virilization: muscularity, androgenic alopecia, deepening voice, clitoromegaly • Occasionally a palpable pelvic tumor • Serum testosterone is often elevated

Table 14.1 (continued)

Diagnosis and classification	Treatment and relevant clinical features: endocrinology conditions
Hot flushes Sensation of warmth accompanied by transient on the face, neck, ears, chest, epigastrium, and arms *Modes of presentation* • Episodic • Transient • Persistent • Menopausal	*Treatment* • Identify and characterize underlying condition/predisposing factors • Tailor treatment accordingly • Menopausal-related • Flushing related to nicotinic acid can be prevented by administration of aspirin prior to a dose of nicotinic acid and by use of longer-acting formulations of nicotinic acid • Alcohol-induced flushing can be prevented by avoiding alcohol consumption *Pathogenesis* • Increased cutaneous blood flow secondary to vasodilation and represents part of a synchronized physiologic response of cutaneous vascular smooth muscle to a variety of autonomic or vasodilator stimuli • Appearance varies depending on skin color, temperature, visibility of blood vessels beneath the skin, and capacitance of those vessels for erythrocytes *Etiology* • Autonomic mediated flushing • Hyperthermia • Menopause • Emotional blushing • Rosacea *Classification* • *Autonomic mediated flushing:* Fever, exercise, heat exposure: ambient or ingested hot beverage, menopause, emotional flushing, neurologic disorders (cranial tumors, epilepsy, cluster headache, spinal cord injuries, Parkinson disease, multiple sclerosis, orthostatic hypotension) • *Vasodilator mediated flushing*: rosacea, may be stimulated by emotion, heat or cold, exercise, spicy or hot foods, and alcohol. Often associated with burning sensation. Xerosis, edema, and plaque formation. Medication (Nifedipine), food injection, alcohol, carcinoid syndrome, mastocytosis, pheochromocytoma, medullary thyroid carcinoma, serotonin syndrome, anaphylaxis, pancreatic tumor, renal cell carcinoma, sarcoidosis *Clinical evaluation* *History*: presence of sweating associated with flushing suggests an autonomic mediated etiology of flushing and distinguishes this from a direct vasodilator etiology Physical examination
Hyperthyroidism Production of excessive amounts of thyroid hormones	*Treatment* • Patient education • Antithyroid drugs: • Carbimazole, tab, 5 mg, 3 × 2 tab/d, 14 d, *then* • Taper to 5 mg daily *and,* • Propranolol, tab, 40 mg, 1 tab/d (watch out for asthma) • High index of suspicion for carbimazole-induced agranulocytosis: presents with signs of infection

(continued)

Table 14.1 (continued)

Diagnosis and classification	Treatment and relevant clinical features: endocrinology conditions
	Diagnostic features • Weight loss in spite of a good or excessive appetite • Excessive sweating • Heat intolerance • Anxiety and emotional irritability • Accelerated bowel movements • Palpitation • Fatigue • Menstrual irregularities • Tachycardia • Warm, moist skin, stare • Graves' disease: majority • Palpable goiter • Suppressed TSH in primary hyperthyroidism *Management tips* • Surgery indicated in cases of large goiters with compressive symptoms (dyspnea, hoarseness, dysphagia) • Resistance to medical therapy • Monitor serum TSH regularly, every 3–6 months
Hypothyroidism and myxedema Underactive thyroid gland deficiency of thyroid hormones causing changes in metabolism, growth, and reproductive function *Classifications* • Iodine deficiency with endemic goiter • Primary (autoimmune) hypothyroidism or Hashimoto's disease • Congenital hypothyroidism (cretinism)	*Treatment* • Patient education • Levothyroxine, tab, 0.1 mg, start with half tab/d, increase biweekly by 50 μm as tolerated *Diagnostic features* • Fatigue, cold intolerance • Constipation • Depression • Menorrhagia • Hoarseness • Dry skin • Bradycardia • Delayed return of tendon reflexes • Anemia, hyponatremia, hyperlipidemia • TSH elevated in primary hypothyroidism *Management considerations* • Good skin care • Diets rich in fiber • Serial TSH measurements after at least 6 weeks of commencing therapy, to determine the optimal dose
Obesity An excess of adipose tissue *Classifications* Body mass index (BMI) is calculated by dividing body weight in kilograms by the height in meters squared • *Normal* BMI: 18.5–24.9 • *Overweight*: BMI 25.0–29.9 • *Class I* obesity: BMI 30.0–34.9 • *Class II* obesity: BMI 35.0–39.9 • *Class III* obesity: BMI >40	*Treatment* • Evaluate to exclude and treat secondary causes • Multidisciplinary care entailing diet advice, cognitive-behavioral counseling *Diagnostic features* • Excess adipose tissue, BMI >30 • Upper body obesity (abdomen and flank) is of greater health consequences than lower body obesity (buttocks and thighs) • Associated with consequences including diabetes mellitus, hypertension, and hyperlipidemia

Table 14.1 (continued)

Diagnosis and classification	Treatment and relevant clinical features: endocrinology conditions
Thyroid nodule Present as solid or fluid-filled lumps that form within the thyroid gland.	*Treatment* • Reassure • Cytologic studies of fine needle aspirate will determine the management course to adopt *Etiology* • Overgrowth of normal thyroid tissue • Thyroid cyst • Chronic inflammation of the thyroid • Multinodular goiter • Thyroid cancer • Iodine deficiency *Clinical evaluation* • History and physical examination • Measurement of serum thyroid-stimulating hormone • Ultrasound to confirm the presence of nodularity, assess sonographic features, and assess for the presence of additional nodules and lymphadenopathy *Clinical signs and symptoms of hormone producing nodule* • Weight loss • Increased sweating • Tremor • Nervousness • Tachyarrhythmia *Complication* • Odynodysphagia • Hyperthyroidism *Increased prevalence of associated cancer* • Children • Adults less than 30 years of age • Past history of head and neck irradiation • Positive family history of thyroid cancer
Thyroid storm A rare, life-threatening condition characterized by severe clinical manifestations of thyrotoxicosis	*Treatment* • Propranolol, tab, 40 mg, 3 × 1 tab/d as tolerated • Hydrocortisone, amp 100 mg, 1 amp in 500 cc slow iv drip *Note: This is a medical emergency* Appropriate supportive measures: iv fluids, antipyretics

Ophthalmology

15

Contents

15.1 **History: Questions to Ask** 190

15.2 **Physical Examination** 191

15.3 **Cardinal Paramedical Ophthalmology Examinations** 191

15.4 **Ophthalmology Red Flags** 191

Ophthalmology is the branch of medical science dealing with the structure, functions, and diseases of the eye (Fig. 15.1).

The main structures of the eye are:

- Upper and lower eyelids (palpebra) with the eyelashes
- Lachrymal glands
- Cornea
- Aqueous humor: the fluid beneath the cornea
- Iris and pupil
- Lens
- Vitreous humor: a transparent watery gel that supports the eye
- Retina and the optic nerve

Diseases of the eye are a common cause of ambulatory consultation.

Viral and bacterial eye infections such as conjunctivitis, scleritis, and blepharitis are easily diagnosed based on history and physical findings. In general, these entities do not affect the visual acuity nor the visual field.

Afflictions that impact visual acuity and the visual field include retinopathies of various etiologies (hypertensive, diabetic, degenerative, and oncologic), affliction of the refractory system (cataract), ophthalmic shingles, herpetic keratitis, and some spontaneous hemorrhagic conditions. These potentially debilitating ophthalmic conditions need prompt recognition and referral. The Gambia is blessed with an excellent International Eye Centre, which readily accepts patients.

The implications of a systemic disease should always be borne in mind when taking history and when performing an ophthalmic physical examination. Common internal medical diseases with ophthalmic complications include hypertension, diabetes, and hyperthyroidism.

Affliction of the eyelid and the lachrymal gland and its draining system should be queried. Specific diagnoses include blepharitis, dacryocystitis, stye, and chalazion.

The eye is often involved in facial trauma. Thorough eye examination should be aimed at detecting traumatic ocular lesions and addressing the patient appropriately.

M. Touray, A. Touray, *Clinical Work and General Management of a Standard Minimal-Resource Facility*, Sustainable Development Goals Series, https://doi.org/10.1007/978-3-030-71032-3_15

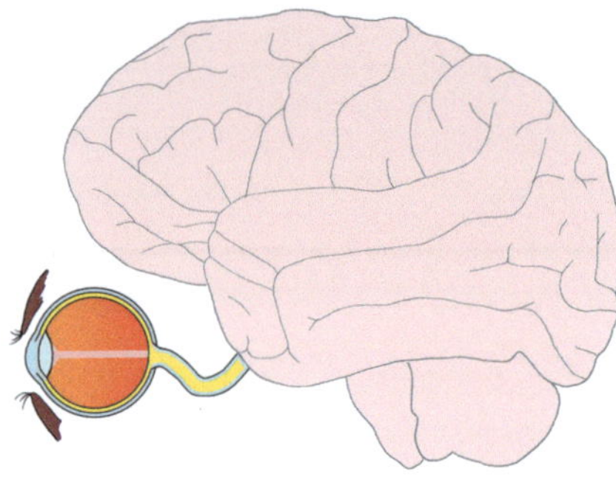

Fig. 15.1 Ophthalmology: A mnemonic illustration representing main anatomic ophthalmology structures and their corresponding pathologies

There are endemic pockets of protozoal eye infection by *Onchocerca cysticus*; onchocerciasis is commonly called river blindness. Successful sensitization of affected communities in conjunction with the effective use of ivermectin has led to a drastic decrease in the prevalence of onchocerciasis.

In this chapter, we address common ophthalmologic disorders that are encountered in a standard minimal resource facility (Table 15.1).

15.1 History: Questions to Ask

- Does your eye hurt? Both eyes or only one?
- When did it start? Any trauma, any possibility of a foreign object flying into your eye?
- If the eye pain is of sudden onset, what were you doing when it started: carpentry, welding, farming, etc.?

- Do you see well? Diplopia? Blurry vision? Any photophobia? Tearing?
- Contagiousness: Does anybody around you also have an eye affliction? Do you have white stuff in the corner of your eyes when you wake up in the morning?
- Where did you live before (river blindness)?

15.2 Physical Examination

- Inspect for any visible structural anomalies: symmetry, swelling, hematoma.
- Inspect the conjunctiva: both lid and bulbar for erythema, foreign objects, secretions.
- Palpate the globe and appreciate any mass, any tenderness, resistance against reasonable pressure.
- Test ocular motor skills; is it smooth and harmonious? Any nystagmus?
- Test visual acuity and visual field by confrontation.
- Fundus examination.

15.3 Cardinal Paramedical Ophthalmology Examinations

- Full blood count
- Erythrocyte sedimentation rate

15.4 Ophthalmology Red Flags

- Suspicion of glaucoma
- Ocular trauma with suspicion of corneal injury
- Fracture: blow-out, white-eyed, trap door
- Deteriorating visual acuity
- Amaurosis fugax: sudden loss of vision
- Long history of poorly controlled hypertension and/or diabetes
- Clinical suspicion of shingles affecting the ocular region
- Severe palpebral swelling and erythema

Table 15.1 Ophthalmology conditions and their treatment

Diagnosis and classification	Treatment and relevant clinical features: ophthalmology conditions
Amputation of visual field *Amaurosis fugax* A sudden and transient loss of vision in one or both eyes *Terminology* • Transient visual loss • Transient binocular visual loss • Transient monocular blindness	*Treatment* • Prompt ophthalmic referral *Etiology* • Carotid artery disease • Giant cell arteritis • Cardiogenic embolism • Hypotension • Coagulopathy • Retinal vein occlusion • Retinal vasospasm and retinal migraine • Optic neuropathy • Papilledema • Optic nerve compression • Ocular causes: angle-closure glaucoma, spontaneous hyphemia, vitreous floaters, congenital optic disc anomalies *Pathophysiology:* ischemic origin: • Large artery occlusive disease: atherothrombosis, embolus, dissection • Small artery occlusive disease (anterior ischemic optic neuropathy, vasculitis), venous disease, cardiac disease, hypercoagulable disorders, and systemic hypoperfusion, resulting in ischemia of the retina, the optic nerve, or both

(continued)

Table 15.1 (continued)

Diagnosis and classification	Treatment and relevant clinical features: ophthalmology conditions
	Clinical assessment *History* • Whether the visual loss affected one or both eyes, • The duration of the episode, and a • Specific description of the symptoms and precipitating factors *Examination*: • Test visual acuity and visual fields • Examine optic fundus *Signs and symptoms* • Eye redness • Pain and tearing associated with visual loss (intermittent angle-closure glaucoma) • More prolonged episodes • Relief of symptoms with blinking or rubbing the eye (dry eye) • Squinting (refractive error)
Anisocoria Asymmetric pupil size. The anisocoria is usually less than 0.4 mm difference between sides, and there is no dilation lag	*Treatment* • Identify and treat the underlying cause *Etiology* • Intracranial aneurysm • Meningitis • PCA or pituitary gland apoplexy • Stroke • Urgent Horner syndrome: • Carotid artery dissection • Pediatric: mediastinal neuroblastoma • Pharmacologic mydriasis, for example, atropine • Traumatic mydriasis • Physiologic anisocoria *Pathophysiology* *CN III paralysis:* neurological emergency, often associated with intracranial pathologies
Bacterial conjunctivitis Inflammation of the conjunctiva due to bacteria characterized by purulent or mucopurulent secretion *Classification*: base on etiology • Infectious • Bacterial • Viral • Noninfectious • Allergic • Nonallergic *Causative bacteria* • *Chlamydia trachomatis* • *Neisseria gonorrhea* • *Staphylococcus aureus* • *Streptococcus pneumoniae* • *Haemophilus influenzae* • *Moraxella catarrhalis*	*Treatment* • Cold compression Topical • Chloramphenicol eye drop, 3 × 5 drops in each eye, 5 d Severe cases • Amoxicillin, tab, 500 mg, 3 × 1 tab/d, 5 d *Advice* • Frequent hand washing • Limit sharing of towels and linens • Caregiver notes • Ensure proper hygiene • Often highly contagious *Signs and symptoms* • Redness • Irritation/foreign body sensation • Conjunctival discharge • Eyelid edema

Table 15.1 (continued)

Diagnosis and classification	Treatment and relevant clinical features: ophthalmology conditions
Blepharitis Inflammation of the eyelid margin associated with eye irritation *Classification* • Posterior blepharitis • Anterior blepharitis	*Treatment* • Chloramphenicol eye drops, 3 × 5 drops in each eye, 5 d In severe cases: • Amoxicillin, tab, 500 mg, 3 × 1 tab/d, 7 d *or* • Cephalexin, tab, 500 mg, 3 × 1 tab/d, 5 d *Differential diagnosis* • Xanthelasma • Molluscum contagiosum • Seborrheic keratosis • Actinic keratosis • Squamous papilloma • Benign nevi • Milia • Dermoid cyst • Demangioma • Basal cell carcinoma *Management tips* • Improved eyelid hygiene • Use mild rehydrating creams • Referral to ophthalmologist if treatment with steroids is indicated *Signs and symptoms* • Red, swollen, or itchy eyelids • Burning sensation • Excessive tearing • Crusting of eyelashes in the morning • Flaking or scaling of the eyelid skin • Photophobia • Blurred vision that improves with blinking
Cataract Opacification of the eye lens secondary to various medical	*Treatment* • Prevent onset or progression by controlling modifiable etiologies • Blood glucose control in diabetics • Discontinue use of drugs such as corticosteroids, phenothiazines, amiodarone, etc. • *Definitive treatment* of choice is cataract extraction (phakectomie) and insertion of an intraocular lens • Referral to tertiary center for specialized eye care *Etiology* • Atopic dermatitis • Diabetes • Inflammatory diseases • Pilocarpine • Senility • Steroids • Trauma *Note:* Free surgical treatment is periodically available at some regional eye centers, for example, check for dates with appropriate health authorities

(continued)

Table 15.1 (continued)

Diagnosis and classification	Treatment and relevant clinical features: ophthalmology conditions
Allergic conjunctivitis Conjunctivitis that develops upon episodic or seasonal exposure to an allergen *Classification* base on etiology, seasonality, and chronicity • Acute allergic conjunctivitis • Chronic • Perennial • Seasonal • Atopic	*Treatment* • Eviction of the etiologic allergen • Oral antihistamine: • Cetirizine, 10 mg tab, 2 × 1 tab/d, 5 d • Chlorpheniramine (Piriton), tab, 25 mg, 2 × 1 tab/d, 5 d • Paracetamol, tab, 500 mg, 3 × 2 tab/d, 5 d • Patient education *Symptoms* • Ocular pruritus • Eye burning • Redness • Eyelid edema • Mild nonpurulent crusting upon awakening • Mild photophobia *Differential diagnosis* • Infectious conjunctivitis • Blepharitis • Xeropthalmia (dry eye) • Vernal keratoconjunctivitis presents with intense ocular pruritus, stringy mucoid discharge, and cobblestoning • Giant papillary conjunctivitis is a form of hypersensitivity reaction to various insults; for example contact lenses, ocular sutures, or ocular implants • Atopic keratoconjunctivitis: chronic and severe disorder that can affect the eyelid, conjunctiva, and cornea • Viral infection • Toxic conjunctivitis • Keratitis • Angle-closure glaucoma • Episcleritis/scleritis *Note:* Eye pain is not characteristic of allergic conjunctivitis
Eye injuries Trauma to the eye *Classification:* based on mechanic, causative agent, and extent of organ damage • Ocular: trauma to the eye • Periocular: trauma to the orbit • Chemical: acid or caustic • Physical: object, burns, smoke	*Treatment* • Wash abundantly with running water where available • Control pain • Cover the globe and address to Eye Center *Trauma threatening vision* • Eye contact with acids or alkalis • Orbital compartment caustic syndrome: occurs after contusive traumas. It is a vision-threatening elevation of intra-orbital pressure which exceeds the vascular perfusion pressure of the ophthalmic artery. It can result in ischemia and irreversible vision loss if not corrected emergently
Keratoconjunctivitis Viral concomitant inflammation of the cornea and the conjunctiva *Nomenclature* *Keratoconjunctivitis sicca* is commonly known as dry eye syndrome. It results in redness and burning of the eye, accompanied by foreign body sensation, which are caused by a disturbance of the tear film	*Treatment* • Reassure patient of self-limiting nature • Strict hygiene • Cold compression • Artificial tears, 2 drops, 4×/d as needed *Signs and symptoms* • Upper respiratory tract infection • Burning ocular pain • Mild photophobia • Watery nonpurulent secretion

Table 15.1 (continued)

Diagnosis and classification	Treatment and relevant clinical features: ophthalmology conditions
Corneal abrasion Bruises on the corneal epithelium	*Treatment* • Tetracycline eye ointment 1%, apply 2×/d, *and* • Eye pad for 24 h (promote corneal endothelial healing) *then* • Gentamicin eye drop, 0.3%, 4×/d, 7 d • Evert upper eyelid in search of foreign body *Signs and symptoms* • Mild to severe pain • Photophobia • Redness • Tearing
Corneal ulcer A break in the continuity of the corneal epithelium, stroma, or endothelium usually detected by corneal staining with fluorescence	*Treatment* • Gentamicin eye drop, every 1 h, 48 h *or* • Tetracycline, eye ointment, 1%, at night *Clinical manifestation* • Severe pain • Redness • Discharge • Hypopyon (pus in the anterior chamber) • Reduced vision • Headache • Fever • Tearing
Diplopia Double vision either in one eye or in both eyes *Classification* • Monocular diplopia • Binocular diplopia • Vertical diplopia • Horizontal diplopia	*Treatment* • Identify underlying cause • Prompt referral to tertiary center for tertiary care where indicated *Etiology* • Third cranial nerve palsy • Fourth cranial nerve palsy • Sixth nerve palsy • Internuclear ophthalmoplegia • Myasthenia gravis • Thyroid ophthalmopathy • Ophthalmoplegic migraine • Wernicke syndrome • Orbital myositis • Acute inflammatory demyelinating polyneuropathy (Guillain-Barré syndrome) • Tick bite paralysis and botulism • Structural lesions (metastases, infections) • Giant cell arteritis *Physiopathology* Dysfunction of the extraocular muscles may be the result of an abnormality of the muscle itself or an abnormality of the motor nerve to the muscle. The major symptom associated with this dysfunction is binocular diplopia, which is present with both eyes open and absent when either eye is closed

(continued)

Table 15.1 (continued)

Diagnosis and classification	Treatment and relevant clinical features: ophthalmology conditions
Endophthalmitis Bacterial or fungal infection within the eye; usually implies infection of the vitreous and/or aqueous *Pan ophthalmitis* is the inflammation of all coats of the eye, including the intraocular structures	*Treatment* • Institute empiric antibiotherapy: Co-amoxicillin, tab, 1 g, 2 × 1 tab/d, 7 d • Refer to tertiary center for specialized care *Signs and symptoms* • Floaters and a subtle decrease in vision • Progressive loss of vision • Photophobia • Eye erythema • Palpebral edema (sometimes) • Eye pain may be minimal or absent • Patient may not have fever, chills, or leukocytosis • Hypopyon
Exophthalmia Protrusion of one or both eyes	*Treatment* • Artificial tears should be applied • Humidification of bedroom where applicable • Treat underlying etiology *Etiology* • Hyperthyroidism • Blow out fracture (pseudoproptosis: enophthalmos of fellow eye) • Rhabdomyosarcoma • Cavernous hemangioma • Orbital cellulitis *Management tips* • Protective eyeglasses are recommended • Rule out tumor/infection *Differential diagnosis* • Mass effect • Enophthalmos of the contralateral eye • Asymmetric eye position
Foreign body in eye Corneal ulcerations are common eye injuries that frequently result from eye trauma, foreign bodies, and improper contact lens use	*Treatment* • Evert upper eyelid and remove foreign body • Topical broad-spectrum antibiotic, chloramphenicol, eye drops, 4 × 5 drops in each eye/d, 5 d *Clinical evaluation* • Exclusion of an open globe and hyphemia • Measurement of visual acuity • Penlight and fluorescein examination • Lid eversion to assess for a conjunctival foreign body *Management tips* Advise carpenters, welders, and at-risk laborers and their employers to invest in goggles or spectacles
Glaucoma Is a group of eye diseases characterized by increased intraocular pressure. It is an optic neuropathy *Glaucoma: angle-closure* Angle-closure glaucoma is characterized by narrowing or closure of the anterior chamber angle	*Treatment* • Urgent referral to tertiary center for specialized eye care • Laser peripheral iridotomy where available *Predisposing (anatomic) factors* • Hyperopia • Narrow iridocorneal angle *Precipitating factors: anticholinergics* • Mydriasis • SSRIs

Table 15.1 (continued)

Diagnosis and classification	Treatment and relevant clinical features: ophthalmology conditions
	Signs and symptoms • Unilateral intense ocular, periocular, or orbital pain • High intraocular pressure (IOP) • Acute visual acuity decrease • Conjunctival hyperemia • Pupil mid-dilated and unresponsive • Corneal edema • Headache, nausea, emesis
Glaucoma: Open angle First cause of irreversible blindness worldwide	*Treatment* • Urgent referral to the tertiary center for specialized eye care • A possible regimen would be one drop each, 1 min apart, of: • 0.5% timolol maleate; 1 drop daily • 1% Apraclonidine; *and* • 2% pilocarpine • 500 mg of oral or intravenous acetazolamide *Signs and symptoms* • Usually asymptomatic in early stages: painless, peripheral loss of vision • High intraocular pressure • Cup/disc ratio >0.5 *Risk factors* • African origin • Age over 50 • Positive family history • High IOP • Myopia • Systemic steroid use
Hemorrhagic conjunctiva Contagious inflammation of the conjunctiva caused by *Hemophilus Aegyptus* *Note:* Conjunctival hemorrhages are mostly benign and resorb within a week • Gonococcal infections may include urethritis, cervicitis, epididymitis, and proctitis	*Treatment* Azithromycin ophthalmic drops: Instill 1 drop into affected eye(s) 2×/d for 5 d *or* Tetracycline eye ointment, 1%, apply in the conjunctival sac, 2×/d, 5 d Severe forms Doxycycline, tab, 100 mg, 2 × 1 tab/d, 5 d *or* Azithromycin, tab, 250 mg, 4 tab, single dose *Etiologic classification* *Acute hemorrhagic* conjunctivitis a highly contagious form due to • *Enteroviruses*: highly contagious infection with enteroviruses *Gonococcal conjunctivitis*; a severe form, marked by greatly swollen conjunctivae and eyelids with a profuse purulent discharge. In newborns it is bilateral, acquired from an infected maternal vaginal passage. In adults, it is usually unilateral and is acquired by autoinoculation into the eye of other gonococcal infections, such as urethritis, either in oneself or in another person • *Inclusion conjunctivitis* primarily affecting newborn infants, caused by Chlamydia trachomatis, beginning as an acute purulent form and leading to papillary hypertrophy of the palpebral conjunctiva. Neonatal conjunctivitis ophthalmia

(continued)

Table 15.1 (continued)

Diagnosis and classification	Treatment and relevant clinical features: ophthalmology conditions
Hyphemia Grossly visible blood in the anterior chamber of the eye *Classification* • Traumatic hyphemia • Spontaneous hyphemia	*Treatment* • Gentamicin eye drops 0.3%, 5 drops in each eye, 4x/d, 5 d • With good infection prevention, hyphemia is gradually resorbed without visual loss • Judicious etiologic assessment and prompt referral to Eye Clinic for ophthalmologic care where indicated *Predisposing factors* • Sickle cell disease or sickle cell trait • Patients with bleeding tendency or conditions that cause ischemia and neovascularization or vascular anomalies of the anterior chamber structures, such as: • Diabetes mellitus • Iris melanoma, retinoblastoma, and other eye tumors • Juvenile xanthogranuloma • Clotting disorders (e.g., thrombocytopenia, hemophilia, Von Willebrand disease) • Medications that inhibit platelet function, such as warfarin or aspirin *Complications of hyphemia* • Increased intraocular pressure • Optic atrophy • Secondary permanent vision loss *Physical findings of globe rupture* • Markedly decreased visual acuity • Eccentric pupil • Increased or decreased anterior chamber depth • Low intraocular pressure • Extrusion of vitreous • External prolapse of the uvea or other internal ocular structures • Tenting of the cornea or sclera at the site of globe puncture
Hordeola and chalazion Painless localized eyelid swelling caused by obstruction of Zeiss or meibomian glands. Hordeola sometimes transform into chalazia after the inflammation resolves	*Treatment* • No antibiotic needed • Warm black tea compress • Lid massage, lid washing • Topical antibiotic *Management tips* • Examination of inner eyelid reveals a nontender rubbery nodule • Chalazia and hordeola can have a similar appearance • Chalazia tend to be painless and are less erythematous
Horner syndrome A classic neurologic syndrome whose signs include • Miosis • Ptosis • Anhidrosis *Nomenclature* • Oculo sympathetic paresis	*Treatment* • Clinical evaluation to identify cause • Refer to tertiary center specialized eye care where needed *Etiology* • Birth-trauma related • Congenital infections • Neuroblastoma • Rhabdomyosarcoma • Brainstem vascular malformations (AVM) • Brainstem tumors (glioma) • Demyelination (brainstem) • Carotid artery thrombosis • Neck trauma • Iatrogenic • Idiopathic

Table 15.1 (continued)

Diagnosis and classification	Treatment and relevant clinical features: ophthalmology conditions
Onchocerciases (river blindness) Caused by the filarial nematode *Onchocerca volvulus*. It is also known as "river blindness" because the blackfly vector breeds near fast-flowing streams and rivers *Disease classes* • Blindness • Skin disease, and onchocerciasis-associated epilepsy • Secondary extreme poverty	*Treatment* • Ivermectin, tab, 3 mg, 150 µg/kg, orally, single dose on an empty stomach, with lots of water • To be repeated every 3 or 6 months until clinical symptoms subside • This may take up to 10 years • The recommended treatment is ivermectin, which will need to be given every 6 months for the life span of the adult worms (i.e., 10–15 years) or for as long as the infected person has evidence of skin or eye infection. Ivermectin kills the larvae and prevents them from causing damage but it does not kill the adults *Clinical manifestations* • Ocular changes • Pruritus • Subcutaneous nodules • Onchocercid skin disease in addition to some systemic features
Ophthalmia neonatorum Caused principally by *N. gonorrhoeae* and *C. trachomatis* infection of the newborn during childbirth	*Treatment* • *Gentamicin* eye drop, 0.3%, every 15 min for first 48 h, *then* every 6 h, 7–14 d • *Tetracycline* eye ointment 1%, at night to be applied in the lower conjunctival sac *Clinical features and complications* • Purulent conjunctivitis • Profuse exudate • Swelling of the eyelids • Inflammation of subconjunctival connective tissue and the cornea • Corneal ulceration, scarring, and visual impairment *Good to know* • Often caused by untreated STI in pregnancy that is transmitted to the child during birth • The infection usually becomes manifest 2–5 days after birth
Ophthalmic shingles *Herpes zoster ophthalmic (HZO)* Herpes zoster, potentially sight threatening, signifies involvement of the ophthalmic division of the fifth cranial nerve *Complications* • Acute retinal necrosis • Ramsay Hunt syndrome (herpes zoster oticus) • Aseptic meningitis • Encephalitis	*Treatment* • Prompt referral for ophthalmic care • Valaciclovir, tab, 500 mg, 2 × 1 tab/d, 7 d • Acyclovir, tab, 200 mg, 4 × 1 tab/d, 7 d *Pathogenesis and clinical course* • HZO begins with a prodrome of headache, malaise, and fever. Unilateral pain or hypesthesia in the affected eye, forehead, and top of the head may precede or follow the prodrome • With the onset of the rash, hyperemic conjunctivitis, uveitis, episcleritis, and keratitis may occur • Acute keratitis involves the epithelial, stromal, or endothelial layers of the cornea. Patients who develop epithelial or stromal keratitis are most at risk for vision loss • Vesicular lesions on the side or tip of the nose correlate highly with eye involvement • Lesions in this area of the face signify involvement of the nasociliary branch of the trigeminal nerve, which also innervates the globe *Signs and symptoms* • Usually unilateral • Recurrences • Photophobia • Cornea sensitivity is decreased

(continued)

Table 15.1 (continued)

Diagnosis and classification	Treatment and relevant clinical features: ophthalmology conditions
Pterygium Conjunctival growth over the cornea, mostly within the interpalpebral fissure	*Treatment* • Betamethasone eye drop, every 6 h 5 d, *then* • Taper down gradually as inflammation subsides, Advanced pterygium • Refer to tertiary center for specialized eye care • If not taken care of, can lead to loss of vision over time • Patient education *Pathogenesis* • Represents a fibrovascular reaction to light exposure and chronic dryness
Ptosis Drooping of the upper eyelid that usually results from a congenital or acquired abnormality of the muscles that elevate the eyelid *Nomenclature* • Blepharoptosis	*Treatment* • Treat underlying etiology *Etiology* • CN III palsy • Edema • Horner syndrome • Muscle disinsertion • Trauma *Clinical evaluation* • Test oculomotricity • Test pupils
Refractive errors Inability to see clearly near and/or distant objects without any apparent ocular injury or disease *Classifications* • Hyperopia or farsightedness • Myopia or nearsightedness • Astigmatism	*Treatment* • Most can be corrected with spectacles, contact lenses, and surgery *Clinical manifestation* • Poor reading vision • Poor distant vision • Headache • Monocular diplopia • Irritation • Drowsiness • Lack of interest in near work, especially reading
Retinopathy Pathologic changes in the retina caused by various systemic diseases with a high potential of visual loss *Classification* • Nonproliferative retinopathy • Proliferative retinopathy	*Treatment* • Diabetic: good glycemia control • Hypertension: control blood pressure adequately • Diabetic retinopathies may be classified into nonproliferative, proliferative, and macula edema *Etiology* • Diabetes • Hypertension • Idiopathic
Strabismus (squint) A disorder in which eyes do not line up in the same direction, so they do not look at the same object at the same time *Classification* • Congenital (note amblyopia) • Acquired • Horizontal • Vertical	*Treatment* • Ophthalmic consultation is indicated *Signs and symptoms* • Diplopia (double vision) • Reduced visual acuity • Reduced depth perception

Table 15.1 (continued)

Diagnosis and classification	Treatment and relevant clinical features: ophthalmology conditions
Sty, hordeolum, orgelet An abscess of the eyelid that presents as a localized, painful, erythematous swelling It can be external or internal	*Treatment* • Ibuprofen, tab, 400 mg, 2×/d, 3 d when needed • Warm compresses, lid massage, lid washing • Topical antibiotic: • Erythromycin ointment, apply 2×/d *or* • Doxycycline, tab, 100 mg, 1 tab/d, 5 d • Reassure patient *Pathophysiology* • External hordeola arise from glands in the eyelash follicle or lid margin (Zeis and Moll glands) • Internal hordeola are caused by inflammation of the meibomian gland, resulting in swelling just under the conjunctival side of the eyelid • No impact on visual field and acuity
Trachoma A chronic follicular keratoconjunctivitis affecting the superior and inferior tarsal conjunctiva and cornea	*Treatment* • Azithromycin, tab, 250 mg, 4 tab, as single dose *Signs and symptoms* • Watery discharge and foreign body sensation • Recurrent conjunctivitis • Reduced vision • Follicles in the upper tarsal plate • Scarring • In-turning of lids, rubbing of lashes on cornea • Corneal scars in older children and adults
Uveitis Inflammation of the uveal tissue, iris, ciliary body, and choroid *Classification* • Anterior (iritis) • Posterior (choroiditis) • Pan uveitis (vitritis)	*Treatment* • Prednisolone eye drop, every 6 h, 1 week • Tropicamide eye drop, 1%, every 8 h • Consider systemic corticoid therapy • Refer to tertiary center for specialized eye care *Etiology* • Infections: herpes virus, cytomegalovirus, toxoplasmosis, syphilis • Systemic immune-mediated disease: spondylarthritis, sarcoidosis, juvenile idiopathic arthritis, psoriatic arthritis and inflammatory bowel disease, Sjögren's syndrome, Systemic lupus erythematosus, systemic vasculitis • Syndromes confined primarily to the eye
Visual acuity disorders Clarity of vision	*Treatment* • Optometry and acquisition of personalized glasses • Avoid excessive use of screens: TV, smartphones, tablets, etc. Factors also affect visual acuities • Diffraction • Photoreceptor density inside the eye • Refractive error • Illumination • Contrast • Location of the retina being stimulated

(continued)

Table 15.1 (continued)

Diagnosis and classification	Treatment and relevant clinical features: ophthalmology conditions
	Classifications • *Myopia* ("nearsightedness"): refractive disorder in which the axial length of the eye is either too long or the refractive power of the eye's optical system is too great. The image is focused in front of the retina • *Hyperopia* ("farsightedness"): refractive disorder in which the axial length of the eye is too short or the power of the eye's optical system is insufficient to produce a focused image on the retina. The image is focused behind the retina • *Astigmatism* ("lack of a pinpoint"): refractive condition in which a warped corneal surface causes light rays entering the eye along different planes to be focused unevenly. The patient reports blurred vision at all viewing distances • *Presbyopia* ("aging sight"): nonrefractive error that also affects visual acuity. Presbyopia occurs when the lens loses its normal accommodating power and can no longer focus on objects viewed at arm's length or closer
Dry eye syndrome Is a multifactorial disease of the ocular surface with loss of homeostasis of the tear film and ocular symptoms *Pathophysiology* • Tear film instability and hyperosmolarity • Ocular surface inflammation and damage • Neurosensory abnormalities	*Treatment* • Improve diet • Vitamin A supplementation: Adults: vitamin A capsules, 200,000 iu day 1, day 2, and day 14 Children: 100,000 iu day 1, day 2, and day 14 *Note:* Common cause of blindness in children *Etiology* • Vitamin A deficiency • Malnutrition • Measles • Malabsorption • Tear film instability and hyperosmolarity • Ocular surface inflammation and damage • Neurosensory abnormalities play etiological roles

16

Contents

16.1 **History: Questions to Ask** 204

16.2 **Physical Examination** 204

16.3 **Cardinal Paramedical Psychiatry Examinations** 204

16.4 **Psychiatry Red Flags** 204

Bibliography 215

Psychiatry focuses on the diagnosis, treatment, and prevention of mental, emotional, and behavioral disorders (Fig. 16.1).

Mood disorders are the most commonly encountered psychiatric conditions, especially depression and anxiety disorders (Table 16.1). Good psychiatric history taking requires tactfulness and some experience, as most individuals will not readily talk about their mental health issues. The clinician should exercise caution not to appear intrusive. The family situation should be carefully questioned: living conditions, marital situation, finances, professional well-being, communal interactions, school, etc.

The burden of substance abuse is high. Implicated substances include marijuana, alcohol, tobacco, and "green tea/attaya," to name a few. Disease entities may include marijuana-induced psychosis, encephalopathies resulting from chronic alcohol use, addictive personality changes, and dementia.

Personality disorders are also common. A complementary history from reliable close family members may be helpful. Eating disorders (anorexia, bulimia, pica) should be considered in the differential diagnosis when suggestive historical elements are evident. Schizophrenia is a rare condition.

In this chapter, we address common psychiatric disorders that are encountered in a standard minimal resource facility (Table 16.1).

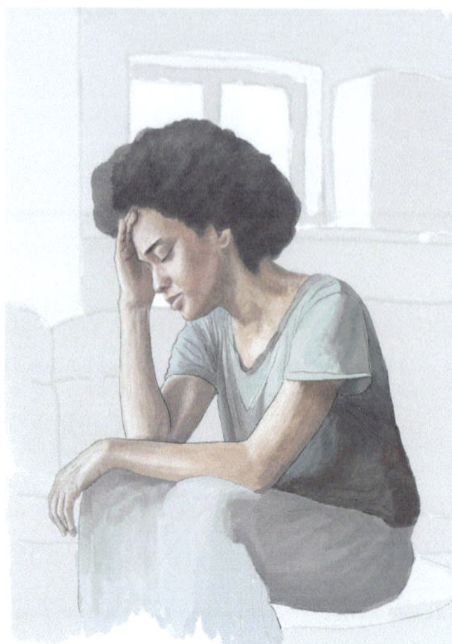

Psychiatry
List of psychiatry disorders that are described in the text.
For easy reference, the corresponding page on which
the disease condition is described is in brackets.

Addiction/substance use disorders (p 205)
Adjustment disorders (p 205)
Anxiety disorder (p 206)
Attention deficit hyperactivity disorder (p 206)
Autism spectrum disorder (p 206)
Child abuse (p 207)
Chronic pain disorder (p 207)
Delirium (p 207)
Mania (p 208)
Mood disorder (p 208)
Neuro-cognitive disorders (p 209)
Personality disorder (p 209)
Postnatal depression (p 211)
Psychosis of unspecified etiology (p 212)
Retarded mental development (p 212)
Schizophrenia spectrum disorder (p 213)
Sleep-wake disorders (p 213)
Suicide and suicide risk (p 214)

Fig. 16.1 Psychiatry: A mnemonic illustration representing characteristic psychiatric features and principles as well as their corresponding pathologies

16.1 History: Questions to Ask

- Do you feel sad? Guilty? Tired? Loss of energy? Insomnia? Hypersomnia? Inability to think or concentrate?
- Do you sometimes cry without having a specific reason to cry?
- Has your appetite and/or weight changed?
- Do you have little pleasure doing things you used to enjoy: seeing friends and family members, doing sports, going out, etc.?
- Do you hear or see things that others don't see?
- Any episodes of pica, especially geophagia?

16.2 Physical Examination

- Evaluate the facial expression: sad, anxious, confused, fugue, hypomimia.
- General appearance: hygiene, clothing, nutritional status.
- Language: content, volume, coherence.
- Memory: do Mini-Mental Status (needs cultural adapting).

16.3 Cardinal Paramedical Psychiatry Examinations

- Full blood count
- Liver function tests
- Serology: VDRL and HIV
- Chest X-ray
- Brain CT-scan
- Brain MRI
- Thyroid panel: TSH, T3, T4

16.4 Psychiatry Red Flags

- Known psychiatric comorbidity
- Unfavorable evolution
- Suicidal risks
- Psychotic symptoms: hallucination, delirious ideation
- Withdrawal syndrome
- Suspicion of auto- or hetero-aggression
- Complex family situation
- Severe depression

Table 16.1 Psychiatric/psychological conditions and their treatment

Diagnosis and classification	Treatment and relevant clinical features: psychiatric/psychological conditions
Addiction/substance use disorders A compulsive, chronic, physiological, or psychological need for a habit-forming substance, behavior, or activity having harmful physical, psychological, or social effects and typically causing well-defined symptoms (such as anxiety, irritability, tremors, or nausea) upon withdrawal or abstinence *Mental status examination includes:* • General appearance • Behavior and interaction • Speech and voice • Motor activity • Mood and affect • Perceptions • Thought process • Thought content (suicidal or homicidal ideation, hallucinations, delusions) • Insight • Judgment • Cognitive functioning *Comorbid conditions* Patients with addiction disorder are at higher risk of experiencing: • Depressive disorders • Bipolar disorder • Anxiety disorders • Posttraumatic stress disorder • Eating disorders • Schizophrenia • Attention deficit hyperactivity disorder	*Treatment* • Counseling and eventually behavioral therapy *Assessment using CAGE mnemonic:* • Have you ever felt you needed to *c*ut down on your drinking? • Have people *a*nnoyed you by criticizing your drinking? • Have you ever felt *g*uilty about drinking? • Have you ever felt you needed a drink first thing in the morning (*e*ye-opener) to steady your nerves or to get rid of a hangover? *Common substances* • Marijuana • Alcohol • Tobacco • Opioid dependency • Sedatives • Caffeine • Stimulants: amphetamines and cocaine • Gambling *Assessing withdrawal symptoms* • Nausea and vomiting • Tremor • Paroxysmal sweats • Anxiety • Tactile disturbances • Auditory disturbances • Visual disturbances • Headache, fullness of head *Alternative assessment tool* *WILD* mnemonic: • Interferes with obligations at *work*, school, or at home • Continued usage despite *interpersonal* or social consequences • *Legal* problems related to substance usage • Usage in *dangerous* situations
Adjustment disorders Emotional and behavioral distressing symptomatology in response to stress *Diagnostic features* • Anxiety or depression in reaction to identifiable stress, though out of proportion to the severity of the stress • Symptoms do not have the severity of a major depressive episode or the chronicity of generalized anxiety disorder	*Treatment* • Counsel accordingly • Define and include social network in the care • Exclude any somatic precipitating pathology • Refer to tertiary center for psychiatric care *Common individual reactions to stressors* • Become anxious or depressed • Develop physical symptoms • Running away • Drinking alcohol • Overeating • Staring from afar *Common subjective responses and emotions* • Anxiety • Sadness • Fear • Rage • Guilt • Shame

(continued)

Table 16.1 (continued)

Diagnosis and classification	Treatment and relevant clinical features: psychiatric/psychological conditions
Anxiety disorder Anxiety is the normal coping response that enables a person to take steps to deal with a threat. When anxiety is prolonged or interferes with normal functions of the individual, it constitutes the clinical condition of an anxiety disorder • Persistent excessive anxiety or chronic fear and associated behavioral disturbances • Somatic symptoms may involve the autonomic nervous system or a specific organ system, for example, dyspnea • Palpitation or paresthesia • Not a result of a physical disorder, psychiatric conditions, or drug abuse	*Treatment* • Empathy and psychological support • Patient education • Pharmacotherapy: • Lorazepam (Temesta), tab, 1 mg, 3 × 1 tab/d as needed • Diazepam, tab, 5 mg, 2 × 1 tab/d, 3 d • Propranolol, tab, 20 mg 2 × 1 tab/d, 5 d • Give half the dose to geriatric patients *Terminology* *Generalized anxiety disorder* • Excessive and persistent worrying that is hard to control, leading to debilitating distress or impairment; occurs on more days than not for at least 6 months • Concomitant psychological symptoms of anxiety may be apprehensiveness and irritability • Physical (or somatic) symptoms of anxiety may include increased fatigue and muscular tension *Classification and clinical features* • *Generalized anxiety:* Unrealistic, excessive worry about two or more life events • *Panic attacks:* Sudden onset of intense apprehension or terror; usually lasts a few minutes to 1 h • *Phobia:* Persistent fear of a known stimulus (object or situation), for example, animals, water, confined spaces • *Obsessive-compulsive disorder:* Repeated disturbing thoughts associated with time-consuming actions • *Post-traumatic stress disorder:* a person who experienced a major threatening life event, later in life begins to experience the same either in dreams or in clear consciousness
Attention deficit hyperactivity disorder A common neuropsychiatric disorder of childhood and adolescence; often persists in adults	*Treatment* • Methylphenidate (Ritalin) intermediate acting, tab, 10 mg, 2 × 1 tab/d • Refer to tertiary center for psychiatric care *Diagnostic features* • Persistent patterns of inability to sustain attention, excessive motor activity and impulsivity, or both • Symptoms interfere with daily functioning • Symptoms begun prior to age 12 in at least two settings, for example, school, work, home, with friends, or family
Autism spectrum disorder A biologically based neurodevelopmental disorder characterized by persistent deficits in social communication and social interaction as well as restricted, repetitive patterns of behavior, interests, and activities *Nomenclature* • Autism spectrum disorder • Pervasive developmental disorder	*Treatment* • Refer to tertiary center for geropsychiatric care *Diagnostic features* • Presentation in the first 2 years of life with deficits in social skills, language, or behavior • Intolerance to change • Plateau of social skills after typical early development • Persistent issues with social communication and interaction • Predictive behaviors, interests, or activities • Symptoms interfere with normal functioning • Accompanying language or intellectual impairment may be present

Table 16.1 (continued)

Diagnosis and classification	Treatment and relevant clinical features: psychiatric/psychological conditions
Child abuse Physical child abuse injury inflicted upon a child by a parent or caretaker. Varies widely among countries as well as among different ethnic and religious groups	*Treatment* • Determine nature of abuse: physical, sexual, psychological, etc. • Clearly document evidence of the above • Provide safety for the child from ongoing abuse • Conduct lab investigations to assess degree of exposure, such as HIV test, Hepatitis B (in cases of sexual abuse) • Liaise with officials from the social welfare services • Always report evidence of child abuse *Management tips* • Careful acquisition of witnessed evidence • Make use of entities such as UNICEF that may provide specialized support *Risk factors* • Certain child predisposing characteristics • Environmental factors • Certain caregiver features
Chronic pain disorder Pain that is enduring (>3 months) and multisystemic	*Treatment* • Develop a good caregiver–patient relationship • Determine which treatment category is best suited for the patient • Space out follow-up visits according to clinical condition *Treatment categories* • Physical medicine • Behavioral medicine • Neuromodulation • Interventional • Transcutaneous electrical neurostimulation • Surgical *Pharmacological agents* • Nonopioid analgesic • Tramadol • Opioids • Antidepressants (tricyclics and serotonin-norepinephrine reuptake inhibitors [SRIs]) • Antiepileptic drugs (gabapentin, pregabalin, and other anticonvulsants) • Muscle relaxants • Topical analgesic agents *Diagnostic features* • Complaints of pain • Symptoms frequently exceed signs • Minimal relief with standard treatment • History of having seen many clinicians • Frequent use of several nonspecific medications
Delirium Acute confusion state signifying impaired brain function resulting from diffuse physiological changes	*Treatment* • Identify causes and promptly address triggering factors • Provide appropriate psychological support • Be sensitive to religious, cultural, and traditional factors • Refer to tertiary center for psychiatric care

(continued)

Table 16.1   (continued)

Diagnosis and classification	Treatment and relevant clinical features: psychiatric/psychological conditions
Mania A disorder of mood control, usually in the excited form, with associated behavioral disorder in the form of elevated, expansive, or irritable moods	*Treatment* • Provide psychological support • Haloperidol, tab, 5 mg, initially 2 × 1 tab/d • Review and readjust dose *Clinical features* • Speech is increased with flight of ideas • Increased self-image, restlessness, and overactivity are common • Delusions of grandeur may occur • Increased libido • Increased appetite, but weight loss occurs due to overactivity • Auditory and visual hallucinations may be present
Mood disorder Low mood and loss of pleasure (anhedonia) *Classification* • Mild depression disorder • Severe or major depression disorder • Mania *Signs and symptoms* • Low mood and loss of interest or pleasure; apathy • Lack of energy, body weakness • Difficulty in concentrating • Sleep disorder • Poor appetite • Hyperphagia • Reduced libido • Diffuse pain syndrome • Suicidal thoughts occur in up to 65% of patients	*Treatment* • Provide ongoing psychological and emotional support appropriate to any of the mentioned triggers • Weekly visits in the acute phase, then space out visits accordingly • Screen for suicide risk *Severe depression* • Fluoxetine, tab, 20 mg, 1 tab/morning • Amitriptyline, tab, 25 mg, 1 tab/bedtime, 90 d *Clinical features* • Varies from mild sadness to intense despondency and feelings of guilt, weakness, and hopelessness • Difficulty in thinking, including inability to concentrate, ruminations, and lack of decisiveness • Loss of interest, with diminished involvement in work and recreation • Somatic complaints: disrupted and/or excessive sleep, loss of energy, change in appetite, decreased sexual drive, agitations • Delusions of somatic or persecutory nature • Withdrawal from activities • Physical symptoms of major depression: anorexia, insomnia, reduced sexual drive, weight loss, and various somatic complaints *Suicidal deviation: Possible triggers* • Job loss • Solitary home environment • Marital problems *Symptoms of mania* • Ranging from euphoria to irritability • Sleep disruption • Hyperactivity • Racing thoughts • Grandiosity or extreme overconfidence • Variable psychotic symptoms

Table 16.1 (continued)

Diagnosis and classification	Treatment and relevant clinical features: psychiatric/psychological conditions
Neurocognitive disorders Cognitive decline of sufficient magnitude to interfere with normal social and occupational functions or with usual daily activities *Nomenclature* • *Acute confusional state/Delirium*: a transient global disorder of attention, clouding of consciousness, usually a result of systemic problems, for example, medications, hypoxemia • *Dementia*: a chronic organic mental disorder characterized by failing memory, chronicity, and deterioration of selective mental functions	*Treatment* • Educate family members • Regular brain jogging if needed: reading simple text, solving puzzles • Haloperidol, tab, 1 mg, 1 tab/d • Adjust according to response, usual daily dose: 1.5–30 mg *Clinical features* • Fluctuating cognition with pronounced variations in attention and alertness • Recurrent visual hallucinations • One or more spontaneous cardinal features of parkinsonism (bradykinesia, rest tremor, rigidity) *Diagnostic features* • Transient or permanent brain dysfunction with alterations in awareness or attention • Cognitive impairment to varying degrees • Impaired recall and recent memory, inability to focus attention, and problems in perceptual processing, often with psychotic ideation • Random psychomotor activity such as stereotypy • Emotional disorders frequently present: depression, anxiety, irritability • Behavioral disturbances: Impulse control, sexual acting out, attention deficits, aggression, and exhibitionism *Management tips* In elderly people, think of normal pressure hydrocephalus when there is ataxia, incontinence, and dementia *Clinical findings* • Orientation problem • Short or fluctuating attention span • Loss of recent memory and recall • Impaired judgment • Emotional lability • Lack of initiative • Impaired impulse control • Inability to reason through problems • Depression • Confabulation • Constriction of intellectual functions • Visual and auditory hallucinations
Personality disorder Personality consists of enduring patterns of perceiving, relating to, and thinking about the environment and oneself that are exhibited across numerous social and personal contexts	*Treatment* • Social, behavioral, psychological, and pharmacological • Motivational intervention • Fluoxetine, tab, 25 mg, 1 tab/d *Approach to management* • Psychotherapy • Discussing the diagnosis • Foster the clinician–patient relationship • Referral to a mental health professional

(continued)

Table 16.1 (continued)

Diagnosis and classification	Treatment and relevant clinical features: psychiatric/psychological conditions
A personality disorder is diagnosed when personality traits are so inflexible and maladaptive across a wide range of situations that they cause significant distress and impairment of social, occupational, and role functioning. The thinking, displays of emotion, impulsivity, and interpersonal behavior of the individual must deviate markedly from the expectations of the individual's culture in order to qualify as a personality disorder	*Clinical manifestations* • *Paranoid:* distrust and suspicion of others such that their motives are interpreted as malevolent • *Schizoid:* detachment from social relationships and a restricted range of expression of emotions in interpersonal settings • *Schizotypal:* social and interpersonal deficits marked by acute discomfort with, and reduced capacity for, close relationships as well as by cognitive or perceptual distortions and eccentric behavior • *Antisocial:* disregard for and violating the rights of others, lying, stealing, defaulting on debts, neglect of children or other dependents • *Borderline:* instability of interpersonal relationships, self-image, affects, and control over impulses • *Histrionic:* excessively emotional and attention seeking • *Narcissistic:* Grandiosity (in fantasy or behavior), need for admiration, and lack of empathy • *Avoidant*: Social inhibition, feelings of inadequacy, and hypersensitivity to negative evaluation • *Dependent*: Feelings of inadequacy, inability to make own decisions, submissiveness, avoidance of confrontation for fear of losing source of support • *Obsessive-compulsive:* preoccupation with perfectionism, mental and interpersonal control, and orderliness at the expense of flexibility, openness, and efficiency *Suggestive behavior traits* • Frequent mood swings • Angry outbursts • Social anxiety sufficient to cause difficulty making friends • Need to be the center of attention • Feeling of being widely cheated or taken advantage of • Difficulty delaying gratification • Not feeling there is anything wrong with one's behavior (ego-syntonic symptoms) • Externalizing and blaming the world for one's behaviors and feelings *Diagnostic features* • Long history dating back to childhood • Recurrent maladaptive behavior • Difficulties with interpersonal relationships or society • Depression with anxiety when maladapting behavior fails

Table 16.1 (continued)

Diagnosis and classification	Treatment and relevant clinical features: psychiatric/psychological conditions
Postnatal depression Postpartum period is defined as the first 12 months after birth *Nomenclature* • Baby blues and postnatal depression share some symptoms but are two different entities, affecting 20% of new mothers • When it subsides within 1–2 weeks, it is called baby blues • When unresolved, may progress to postnatal psychosis	*Treatment* • Provide appropriate psychological support • Be sensitive to religious, cultural, and traditional factors *Risk factors* • Stressful life events (e.g., marital conflict or emigration) during pregnancy or after delivery • Poor social and financial support in the puerperium • Young age (<25 years) • Single marital status • Multiparity • Family history of postpartum depression or psychiatric illness • Intimate partner violence and lifetime history of physical and/or sexual abuse • Unintended/unwanted pregnancy • Negative attitudes toward pregnancy • Fear of childbirth • Poor perinatal physical health (e.g., obesity at the time of conception, pregestational or gestational diabetes, antenatal or postnatal hypertension, or infection following delivery) • Body image dissatisfaction (preconception, antenatal, and/or postpartum) • Personality traits, such as neuroticism (which is marked by an enduring tendency to worry and to feel anxious, angry, sad, and guilty) • History of premenstrual syndrome or premenstrual dysphoric disorder • Perinatal anxiety symptoms and disorders • Perinatal sleep disturbance • Season of birth • Adverse pregnancy and neonatal outcomes (e.g., including stillbirth, preterm birth, very low birth weight, and neonatal death) • Postpartum blues • Breastfeeding difficulty/shorter duration/cessation *Signs and symptoms* • Persistent low mood following delivery • Crying spells • Somatization • Palpitations • Dizziness • Gastrointestinal symptoms • Non-systemized gynecological complaints

(continued)

Table 16.1 (continued)

Diagnosis and classification	Treatment and relevant clinical features: psychiatric/psychological conditions
Psychosis of unspecified etiology a condition of the mind defined as a loss of contact with reality *Classification of psychosis* • Primary psychiatric disorders: schizophrenia and schizophrenia-related disorders • Medical disorders: physical trauma, temporal lobe epilepsy, dementia, neurologic and endocrine disease, metabolic abnormalities • Substance abuse disorders: amphetamines and hallucinogens	*Treatment* • Haloperidol, ampoule for injection, 5 mg, 1 amp/im unique dose, *then* • Haloperidol, 1 mg tab, half, tab, 3×/d, 5 d Consider: • Haloperidol decanoate, ampoule for injection, 25 mg, 1 amp im/4 weeks • Diazepam (Valium), ampoule for injection, 5 mg, 2 × 1 amp/d, 2 d as necessary • Ensure adequate fluid maintenance: NaCl 0.9%, 500 ml bag for iv infusion 2 × 1 bag/d and dextrose 5%, 500 ml bag for infusion, 1 bag/d *Clinical manifestations:* • *Delusions:* strongly held false beliefs that are not typical of the patient's cultural or religious background • *Hallucinations*: wakeful sensory experiences of content that is not actually present • *Thought disorganization*: may be derived from patients' patterns of speech during the interview • *Agitation/aggression*: an acute state of anxiety, heightened emotional arousal, and increased motor activity *Management tips* • Identify family member to provide added support by being as present as possible in the acute phase • Consider a convalescent stay on a convivial farm, for example, Kankanba farm
Retarded mental development (motor, intellectual) a neurodevelopmental disorder with multiple etiologies, characterized by deficits in intellectual and adaptive functioning of varying severity	*Treatment* • Family support • Frequently, the etiology may be perinatal anoxia *Terminology* • *Intellectual disability*—Intellectual disability (ID) is a neurodevelopmental disorder characterized by deficits in intellectual and adaptive skills, affecting at least one of three adaptive domains (conceptual, social, and practical) with varying severity • *Global developmental delay* describes intellectual and adaptive impairment in infants and children <5 years old who fail to meet expected developmental milestones in multiple areas of functioning

Table 16.1 (continued)

Diagnosis and classification	Treatment and relevant clinical features: psychiatric/psychological conditions
Schizophrenia spectrum disorder A psychiatric disorder involving chronic or recurrent psychosis. It is commonly associated with impairments in social and occupational functioning *Psychopathology* A chronic disorder with disturbance of form and content of thought, perception, sense of self, relationship to the external world, mood, and behavior	*Treatment* • Prompt referral to a tertiary care center *Clinical manifestations* • Positive symptoms include reality-distorting symptoms of hallucinations and delusions as well as disorganized thoughts and behavior • Negative symptoms include absence or diminution of normal processes, for example, decreased expressiveness, apathy, flat affect, and a lack of energy • Cognitive impairment • Mood and anxiety symptoms *Diagnostic features* • Social withdrawal, usually slowly progressive, with decreased emotional expression or motivation, or both • Deterioration in personal care, with disorganized behaviors or decreased reactivity to the environment, or both • Disorganized thinking, speech that switches topics oddly or is incoherent • Auditory hallucinations, often of a derogatory nature • Delusions, fixed false beliefs despite conflicting evidence, frequently of a persecutory nature
Sleep-wake disorders The intrinsic circadian timekeeping system influences consolidation of sleep and wake episodes and is critical for sleep health as well as optimal functioning of other organ systems. It modulates many physiological systems, including daily rhythms in core body temperature, cortisol, and appetite *Classification of sleep disorders* • Insomnia • Sleep-related breathing disorders • Central disorders of hypersomnolence • Circadian rhythm sleep-wake disorders • Parasomnias • Sleep-related movement disorders	*Treatment* • Provide personalized clinical assessment • Patient education • Weight reduction where needed • Encourage regular physical exercise *Sleep-related breathing disorders* • Sleep apnea syndromes (SAS) • Obstructive sleep apnea disorders • Sleep-related hypoventilation disorders • Sleep-related hypoxemia disorder *Sleep-related movement disorders include* • Restless leg syndrome • Periodic limb movement disorder • Sleep-related cramps • Sleep-related bruxism (teeth grinding) • Sleep-related rhythmic movement disorder

(continued)

Table 16.1 (continued)

Diagnosis and classification	Treatment and relevant clinical features: psychiatric/psychological conditions
Suicide and suicide risk The act or an instance of taking one's own life voluntarily and intentionally	*Treatment* • Counseling • Evaluate risk of passing from contemplation to action *Risk factors* • Mental disorders (e.g., major depression, substance use disorders, or psychotic disorders) • Previous suicide attempt • Sexual orientation: Gay, lesbian, or bisexual orientation, or transgender or gender non-conforming identity • History of physical or sexual abuse • Family history of suicidal behavior *Red flags* Use the mnemonic "is path warm?" to identify key warning signs for suicide: • *I*deation – Talking about or threatening to harm or kill oneself; looking for ways to kill oneself; talking or writing about death, dying, or suicide • *S*ubstance abuse – Increased substance use • *P*urposelessness • *A*nxiety – Worry, fear, agitation, or changes in sleep pattern • *T*rapped – Feeling like there is no way out of a bad situation • *H*opelessness • *W*ithdrawal from friends, family, and society • *A*nger • *R*ecklessness • *M*ood changes *Note:* Auto-hetero aggression should be quickly assessed and prompt medico-legal management be instituted where necessary

Bibliography

1. Papadakis MA, McPhee SJ, Rabow MW. Current medical diagnosis and treatment. New York: McGraw-Hill Education; 2019. https://accessmedicine.mhmedical.com/book.aspx?bookID=2449.
2. Preclinical and clinical lecture notes of the curriculum of medical studies, Faculty of Medicine, University of Lausanne, Course year 2015–2021.
3. Scientific-Units-Recommendations-Formulas (SURF), Guidelines, Médecine Interne General, Philippe Furger en collaboration avec Thierry Fumeaux et le SURF-team; 2020.
4. Pocket Book of Hospital Care for Children. Guidelines for the management of, common, childhood illnesses. 2nd ed. World Health Organisation; 2013.
5. Essential med notes, 2020 Comprehensive medical references and review for the United States Medical Licensing Exam (USMLE) step II and the Medical Council of Canada Qualifying Exam (MCCQE) Part 1, 36th ed, Sara Mirali and Ayesh Seneviratne.
6. WHO model list of essential medicines, 20th List. World Health Organization; March 2017, Amended August 2017. https://apps.who.int/iris/bitstream/handle/10665/273826/EML-20-eng.pdf?ua=1.
7. The Gambia Standard Drug Treatment Guidelines. Department of State for Health & Social Welfare, The Republic of the Gambia, 2nd ed. 2001. http://apps.who.int/medicinedocs/documents/s22418en/s22418en.pdf.
8. Cornuz J, Pasche O, Kermode-Noppel T. Compas: Stratégies de prise en charge clinique, Médecine interne générale ambulatoire. Lausanne: Institute of Social and Preventive Medicine; 2010.
9. Diseases and conditions: comprehensive guides on hundreds of conditions. Mayo Clinic. https://www.mayoclinic.org/diseases-conditions.
10. https://www.uptodate.com.
11. https://www.cdc.gov/ncbddd/actearly/milestones.
12. https://www.who.int/biologicals.

Pediatric Conditions and Their Treatment

17

Contents

17.1	**History Taking**	217
17.2	**Physical Examination**	219
17.3	**Laboratory Investigation**	219
17.4	**Initial Care After Birth**	219
17.5	**Pediatric Developmental Milestones**	220
17.5.1	Red Flags Signifying Developmental Retardation	220
17.5.2	Correlating Acquired Skills with Age	220
17.6	**Management of a Sick Child: Key Elements**	222
17.7	**General Pediatric Management Plan**	222
Bibliography		234

Pediatrics is a branch of medicine dealing with the development, care, and diseases of infants, children, and adolescents (Fig. 17.1).

Pediatric care is an important component in all medical facilities. A comprehensive pediatric approach encompasses assessing and attending to the physical, mental, and emotional needs of children at all developmental stages (Table 17.3). This approach applies to all children, whether sick or in good health. Thus, prevention is an important component of routine care.

Legally, the pediatric age is defined as the time period between birth and the child's eighteenth birthday. This birthday marks a significant change in the child's legal status as well as in medical procedures. It is assumed that responsibility will now be assumed by the child-become-adult, so the clini-

cian should be sensitive to such issues. However, individual developmental parameters, sociocultural attitudes, and religious affiliation should also be considered when dispensing healthcare to the child.

Here we outline general pediatric care and mention significant pediatric conditions we often encounter in our primary care setting (Table 17.3).

17.1 History Taking

The primary goal is to understand the present complaint and, subsequently, the present illness. This requires a flexible approach:

- Symptom-specific
- Vaccination

© The Author(s), under exclusive license to Springer Nature Switzerland AG 2021
M. Touray, A. Touray, *Clinical Work and General Management of a Standard Minimal-Resource Facility*, Sustainable Development Goals Series, https://doi.org/10.1007/978-3-030-71032-3_17

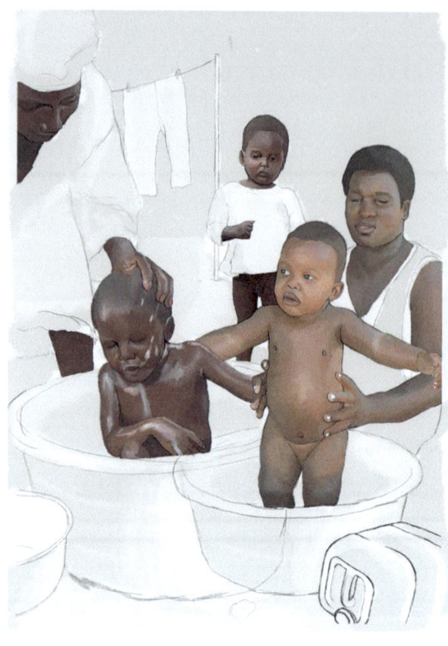

Paediatrics

List of paediatrics disorders that are described in the text.
For easy reference, the corresponding page on which the
disease condition is described is in brackets.

Acute otitis media (p230)
Acute sinusitis (p230)
Cardiac insufficiency (p226)
Choking child (p227)
Clubfoot (Talipes equinovarus) (p231)
Developmental dysplasia of the hip (p231)
Diarrhea (p223)
Epilepsy (p229)
Febrile seizure (p228)
Heart murmur (p226)
Hirschsprung disease (p224)
HIV infection (p234)
Jaundice in new born (p225)
Malnutrition (p102, p222)
Pediatric fractures (p232)
Perinatal sepsis (p232)
Pharyngitis (p230)
Pneumonia (severe) (p228)
Scoliosis (p231)
Sudden infant death syndrome (SIDS) (p228)
Urinary tract infections (p225)

Fig. 17.1 Key principles of pediatric healthcare: good hygiene, early socialization, protection, and loving care

- Personal, familial, social, and environmental history
- Young infants: history of pregnancy, birth, and feeding
- Older children: developmental milestones
- Adolescents: explore psychosocial aspects with HEEADSSS mnemonic while ensuring confidentiality
  - *Home:*
    - Where do you live?
    - Who lives with you?
    - How does each member get along?
    - Who could you go to if you needed help with a problem?
    - Parent(s) jobs? Recent moves? New people at home?
  - *Education:*
    - What do you like/not like about school/work?
    - What can you do well? What areas would you like to improve on?
    - How do you get along with teachers/other students?
    - Grades? Suspensions? Changes?
    - Many young people experience bullying at school—have you ever had to put up with this?
  - *Eating/Exercise:*
    - Sometimes when people are stressed, they can overeat/undereat. Have you ever experienced either of these?
    - In general, what is your diet like?
    - In screening more specifically for eating disorders, you may ask about body image, the use of laxatives, diuretics, vomiting, or excessive exercise, and rigid dietary restrictions to control weight.
  - *Activities and peer relationships:*
    - Relationships with peers? (What do you do for fun? Where? When?)
    - Relationships with family?
    - Sports—regular exercise?
    - Hobbies? Tell me about the parties you go to.
    - Gauge screen time: How much television would you watch a night? Smartphone usage? Favorite music?
    - Crimes? Arrests?

- *Drugs* (cigarettes/alcohols):
  - Many people at your age are starting to experiment with cigarettes/alcohol. Have any of your friends tried these, or maybe other drugs like marijuana, iv drugs?
  - How about you, have you tried any?
  - Then ask about the effects of drug taking/smoking or alcohol on them, and any regrets.
  - How much are they taking, how often, and has frequency increased recently?
- *Sexuality:*
  - Some people are getting involved in sexual relationships. Have you had a sexual experience with a guy or girl or both?
  - Degree and types of sexual experience?
  - Number of partners, masturbation, contraception?
  - Knowledge about STDs.
  - Has anyone ever touched you in a way that's made you feel uncomfortable or forced you into a sexual relationship? History of sexual or physical abuse?
  - How do you feel about relationships in general/about your own sexuality?
- *Suicide* (depression and mental mood screening):
  - How do you feel about yourself at the moment on a scale of 1–10?
  - What sort of things do you do if you are feeling sad/angry/hurt?
  - Is there anyone you can talk to?
  - Do you feel this way often?
  - Some people who feel really down often feel like hurting themselves or even killing themselves. Have you ever felt this way?
  - Have you ever tried to hurt yourself or take your own life? What have you tried?
  - What prevented you from doing so? Do you feel the same way now? Have you a plan… etc.
- *Safety:* immunization, bullying, carrying weapons
- *Spirituality:* Beliefs, religion, music, what helps them relax, etc.

17.2 Physical Examination

Children should be examined fully, as opposed to the systemic approach used for adults, to avoid missing a sign.

- Observe and record signs before touching the child.
- Perform invasive examination last.

17.3 Laboratory Investigation

Target the investigation based on the history taken and the examination conducted. A basic investigation includes:

- Hb or packed cell volume, full blood count
- Blood smear
- Sickle cell test
- Blood glucose
- Urine analysis
- Blood grouping
- HIV testing
- Blood bilirubin for sick newborns
- For further investigation:
- Pulse oximetry
- Chest X-ray
- Stool microscopy
- Blood cultures

17.4 Initial Care After Birth

The Apgar Score (Table 17.1):

- A method to quickly summarize the health of newborn children.
- Is determined by evaluating the newborn baby on five simple criteria on a scale from zero to two, then summing up the five values.
- The Apgar score should be assessed at 1 min, 5 min, and 10 min post-delivery (Table 17.1).
- First meal should be given as soon as possible and no later than 2 h after birth.
- Early feeding = offer of additional preventive liquid.

Table 17.1 Apgar score criteria for newborn assessment

	0	1	2
Skin color	Trunk blue or pale	Trunk pink but extremities blue	Completely pink
Respiratory effort[a]	Absent	Superficial	Good crying
Muscle tone	Flaccid	Some flexion of extremities	Well flexed extremities
Reactivity[b]	No response	Slow	Vigorous
Heart rate	0	<100/min	>100/min

[a]Assess respiratory effort in ventilated infants with a dash (−)
[b]Reactivity: spontaneous motor activity, crying, sneezing, coughing

- Indications:
  - Premature (34–37 weeks postmenstrual).
  - Intrauterine growth restriction/retardation (IUGR) (birth weight < P3), or < 2500 g.
  - Infants born to women with gestational diabetes mellitus (GDM) or birth weight >97 or birth weight >4500.
- Dietary supplement after each breastfeeding at 2–3 o'clock for the first 2 or 3 days.
- Supplement of 5–10 ml of dextrin-maltose (1×) and then formula or adapted milk.
- Blood glucose control before each meal, up to 3× greater than 2.6 mmol/L.

17.5 Pediatric Developmental Milestones

Developmental milestones are skills that most children can do by a certain age. It is important to monitor the achievement of these milestones, as gross deviation or inability of a child to accomplish certain skills at a given age should raise the suspicion of the caregiver for the presence of developmental impairment. Prompt identification and diagnosis will impact significantly on the clinical outcome. Key development characteristics include:

- Reflexes: present at birth and should disappear after 4–6 months
  - Moro
  - Galant
  - Grasping
  - Rooting
  - Suction
  - Tonic neck
  - Stepping
- Movement/physical development (e.g., weight)
- Social and emotional
- Language/communication
- Cognitive (learning, thinking, problem-solving)

17.5.1 Red Flags Signifying Developmental Retardation

- Gross motor: not walking >18 months
- Fine: hand preference <2 years
- Speech: <10 words at 18 months
- Social: not smiling at 3 months, not pointing at 18 months

17.5.2 Correlating Acquired Skills with Age

Children under 5 years should be periodically examined and acquisition of key developmental miles stones (gross motor, fine motor, speech, language, and adaptative and social skills) should be meticulously noted. Failure of the child to acquire such cardinal developmental milestones should prompt adequate timely actions.

2-month-old baby:

- Begins to smile at people
- Tries to look at parent
- Makes gurgling sounds
- Pays attention to faces
- Can hold head up and begins to push up when lying on tummy

4-month-old baby:

- Smiles spontaneously, especially at people
- Copies some movements and facial expressions, like smiling or frowning
- Begins to babble
- Cries in different ways to show hunger, pain, or being tired

- Lets you know if he/she is happy or sad
- Holds head steady, unsupported
- Brings hands to mouth
- May be able to roll over from tummy to back

6-month-old baby:

- Responds to other people's emotions and often seems happy
- Likes to look at self in a mirror
- Knows familiar faces and begins to know if someone is a stranger
- Responds to sounds by making sounds
- Babbling ("ah," "eh," "oh") and likes taking turns with parent while making sounds
- Responds to own name
- Looks around at things nearby
- Brings things to mouth
- Rolls over in both directions (front to back, back to front)
- Begins to sit without support

9-month-old baby:

- May be afraid of strangers
- May be clingy with familiar adults
- Understands "no"
- Makes a lot of different sounds like "mama-mama" and "babababababa"
- Moves things smoothly from one hand to the other
- Stands, holding onto a support
- Can get into sitting position
- Sits without support
- Pulls to stand

12-month-old baby:

- Is shy or nervous with strangers
- Cries when mom or dad leaves
- Responds to simple spoken requests
- Uses simple gestures, like shaking head "no" or waving "bye-bye"
- Explores things in different ways, like shaking, banging, throwing
- Follows simple directions like "pick up the toy"
- May take a few steps without holding on
- May stand alone

18-month-old baby:

- Shows affection to familiar people
- Says several single words
- Shows interest in a doll or stuffed animal by pretending to feed
- Walks alone
- May walk up steps and run

2-year-old child:

- Copies others, especially adults and older children
- Gets excited when with other children
- Shows defiant behavior (doing what he/she has been told not to)
- Says sentences with 2–4 words, vocabulary of at least 50 words
- Follows simple instructions
- Begins to sort shapes and colors
- Stands on tiptoe
- Kicks a ball
- Begins to run

3-year-old child:

- Copies adults and friends
- Shows concern for crying friend
- Understands the idea of "mine" and "his" or "hers"
- Follows instructions with 2 or 3 steps
- Can name most familiar things
- Understands what "two" means
- Copies a circle with pencil or crayon
- Climbs well
- Runs easily

4-year-old child:

- Enjoys doing new things
- Plays "mom" and "dad"
- Tells stories
- Can say first and last name
- Names some colors and some numbers
- Starts to understand time
- Hops and stands on 1 foot for up to 2 seconds
- Catches a bounced ball most of the time

5-year-old child:

- Wants to please friends
- Wants to be like friends
- Is aware of gender
- Speaks very clearly
- Tells a simple story using full sentences
- Counts 10 or more things
- Can draw a person with at least six body parts
- Stands on 1 foot for 10 seconds or longer
- Hops; may be able to skip, rides bicycles
- Can do a somersault
- Swings and climbs
- Injury prevention: injuries are the leading cause of death in children older than 1 year

17.6 Management of a Sick Child: Key Elements

The key components of providing medical care to the pediatric patient are similar to that of adult patient with special emphasis on developmental milestones, genetic or congenital etiologies, and environmental impact, socio-cultural, and other health determinants. The medical work-up varies significantly ranging from emergency hospital-based situations (Table 17.2) to outpatient and preventive type healthcare (Fig. 17.1 and Table 17.3).

17.7 General Pediatric Management Plan

- Physical examination
- Laboratory investigation if needed
- Diagnosis and differential diagnosis
- Treatment and/or referral
- Supportive care and monitoring
- Planning discharge
- Follow-up
- Emergency triage (Australian triage scale)
- Assess for emergency signs
- Check for priority signs
- Emergency treatment if needed

Table 17.2 Pediatric emergency/priority signs

Emergency signs: A-B-C-D	Priority signs: 3TPR MOB
• *Airway* and *Breathing* obstructed, absent breathing, central cyanosis, or severe respiratory distress • *Circulation*: Cold skin with capillary refill longer than 3 s; weak and fast pulse • *Coma/Convulsing* • Severe dehydration: *D*iarrhea plus lethargy and/or sunken eyes and/or very slow skin pinch and/or unable to drink or drinking poorly	• *T* for *T*iny infant <2 months, *T*emperature, *T*rauma • *P* for *P*allor, *P*oisoning, *P*ain • *R* for *R*espiratory distress, *R*estless (irritable or lethargic) • *M* for *M*alnutrition • *O* for (*O*)edema of foot or face • *B*urns

Table 17.3 Pediatric conditions and their treatment

Diagnoses and classification	Treatment and relevant clinical features: pediatric conditions
Gastroenterology	
Nutrition Very diverse methods and formulas *Factors influencing child feeding patterns* • Socioeconomic level • Tradition • Culture • Formal educational level • Religious background	*Birth to 6 months* *Weight loss (≤10% of birth weight) in first 7 d is normal* • During the first postpartum week while breastfeeding is being established, mothers should nurse whenever the infant shows signs of hunger or when 4 h have elapsed since the last feeding. This will usually result in 8–12 feedings in 24 h • Breastfeeding: Encourage exclusive breastmilk for 6 months and continuing as long as possible. The typical duration of breastfeeding in The Gambia is 12–18 months *7–18 months* Introduction to solid food

Table 17.3   (continued)

Diagnoses and classification	Treatment and relevant clinical features: pediatric conditions
	Above 18 months *Weaning*: Very sensitive developmental period. Child is prone to many infectious conditions because of lower immunity, due to lack of protective maternal antibodies in mother's milk *Clinical notes* • <6 months, avoid water or other fluid intake unless medically required • Avoid honey under 1 year old, as it may cause botulism • Vit K supplement: 2 mg at 4 h, 4 d, and at 28 d old • Vit D supplement: 400 UI/d first year • Each age has its specificities *Red flags* • Stunted growth (<P3 weight and height or fall across two major percentile curves) • Overweight (weight > P97) • Stunted development • Exclusive breastfeeding has benefits for both mother and child

Diarrhea
Passage of loose or watery stools at least three times in a 24-h period
Three pillars in the management of children with diarrhea are rehydration therapy, zinc supplementation, and counselling for continued feeding and prevention
	Treatment
	Fluid and electrolyte management consists of two phases:
	1/Rehydration:
	• No dehydration: Give fluid and food to treat diarrhoea, advise when to return to hospital, follow up if no improvement in 3-5 days
	• Moderate dehydration: treat with oral rehydration salts in the hospital over 4 hours 50 ml/kg, small and frequent sips, and gradually increat quantity if tolerates it (no vomiting), continues breastfeeding
	• Severe dehydration: in hospital treatment with iv resuscitation (NaCl 0.9% or ringer lactate) at 20 ml/kg over 1 h then give 50 ml/kg in 4-6h. If intravenous fluid is not available immediately, start with a nasagastric tube, 20 ml/kg of ORS in 1 h then 50 ml/kg in 4–6h
	
	2/*Maintenance rehydration:*
	  – 1–10 kg 100 ml/kg/d
	  – 11–20 kg: 1000 ml +50 ml for every kg above 10 kg
	  – >20 kg: 1500 ml + 20 ml for every kg above 20
	• Zinc supplementation 10–14 d:
	  – ≤ 6 months 10 mg/j
	  – ≥6 months 20 mg
	• Feeding and prevention
	• Antibiotics if bloody diarrhea (dd shigella)
	
	Prevention of diarrhea in infants
	• Exclusive breastfeeding until age 6 months
	• Consumption of safe food and water
	• Caregiver handwashing after defecating, disposing of a child's stool, and before preparing meals
	• The use of latrines; these should be located more than 10 m away and downhill from drinking water sources
	• Immunizations: Rotavirus vaccines
	
	Etiology/classification diarrhea in infants
	• *Infectious gastroenteritis*: *Rotavirus, Cryptosporidium, Shigella,* and enterotoxigenic *E. coli* (ETEC)
	• *Acute watery diarrhea:* In infants and young children, acute watery diarrhea is most often due to rotavirus; in older children, it is most often due to *E. coli*
	• *Invasive (bloody) diarrhea:* Shigellosis is the most common etiology of invasive or bloody diarrhea among children in resource-limited countries. It is a major cause of mortality and is associated with a high incidence of bacteremia, seizures, and several other life-threatening complications
	• *Persistent diarrhea:* Loose, watery, or bloody stools of ≥14 d
	• Assess dehydration status

Table 17.3 (continued)

Diagnoses and classification	Treatment and relevant clinical features: pediatric conditions
	Clinical assessment of a child with diarrhea A precise anamnesis (frequency, number of ill days, bloody stool, recent antibiotic use) physical examination and basic laboratory workup is performed Diarrhea in an infant is divided into four clinical entities to guide clinical management strategies: 1. Classification of type of diarrheal illness 2. Assessment of hydration status

Signs	*Classify as*
Two of the following signs: • *Lethargic or unconscious* • *Sunken eyes* • *Not able to drink or drinking poorly* • *Skin pinch goes back very slowly*	*Severe dehydration*
Two of the following signs: • *Restless, irritable* • *Sunken eyes* • *Drinks eagerly, thirsty* • *Skin pinch goes back slowly*	*Mild dehydration*
Not enough signs to classify as mild/some or severe dehydration	*No dehydration*

	3. Assessment of nutritional status
	4. Assessment of comorbid conditions
	  • *Fever* is common with diarrheal illness
	  • *Tachypnea* can be a sign of pneumonia with coughing or difficulty breathing
	  • *Abdominal pain* out of proportion to typical gastroenteritis raises the possibility of a surgical emergency
	  • *Central nervous system*: Moderate dehydration can lead to irritability; severe dehydration can lead to lethargy and coma. Encephalopathy and/or seizures can occur in the setting of severe disease, due to *Shigella*, and less commonly in systemic *Salmonella* infection
	
	Note: Diarrheal illness is the second leading cause of child mortality among children younger than 5 years worldwide
	V. cholerae is an important bacterial cause of childhood diarrhea in endemic areas, often occurring in large epidemics

Hirschsprung disease Congenital defect of the colon Described extensively above (see Table 8.1, "gastroenterology conditions and their treatment")	*Treatment* • Dietary advice to avoid constipation • Surgical treatment *Differential diagnosis of Hirschsprung disease* • Anorectal atresia/stenosis • Chronic intestinal pseudo-obstruction • Meconium ileus
Vomiting	*Red flag*: Bilious or bloody, projectile, abdominal distension, fever, signs of dehydration *Treatment* • Rehydration (see diarrhea) • Treat underlining cause Differential diagnosis (age dependent): Pyloric stenosis, GERD, sepsis, intestinal obstruction, Hirschsprung disease, gastroenteritis (with diarrhea), appendicitis, intussusception, increased intracranial pressure, toxic ingestion, pregnancy

Table 17.3 (continued)

Diagnoses and classification	Treatment and relevant clinical features: pediatric conditions
Jaundice in a newborn Yellow coloration of the sclera and skin	*Treatment* • Phototherapy • Intravenous phototherapy • Exchange transfusion, rarely practiced *Clinical notes* • May be normal or abnormal *Abnormal:* • Starts on day one of life • Lasts over 14 d in terms and >21 in preterms • Deep jaundice: Palms and soles • Causes: Bacterial infection, hemolytic disease due to blood group incompatibility, G6PD deficiency, congenital syphilis, liver disease, hypothyroid • *Laboratory workup*: Hb, Hematocrit, full blood count, blood type of mother and child, Coombs test *Nomenclature* • Hyperbilirubinemia in infants • Severe neonatal hyperbilirubinemia • Acute bilirubin encephalopathy • Kernicterus *Risk factors* • Prematurity • Feto-maternal incompatibility • Breastfeeding *Red flags* • If jaundice occurs <24 h after delivery • Prolonged jaundice >10 d • Sepsis signs • Hemolytic signs (splenomegaly) • Cholestatic signs (dark urine, discolored stool)
Urinary tract infections Bacterial and fungal growth in urethra, bladder, ureter, and kidney causing local and systemic symptoms *Nomenclature:* • Urethritis • Cystitis • Pyelonephritis	*Treatment* • <2 months, iv treatment: Amoxicillin 100–150 mg/kg/d in 3 doses and aminoglycoside (gentamicin/amikacin/tobramycin) 10–14 d • Triméthoprime sulfamethoxazole 2–3 mg/kg/d p.o. in 1 or 2 doses • Amoxicillin 10–20 mg/kg/d p.o. in 1 or 2 doses • Cefpodoxime 2–3 mg/kg/jour p.o. in 1 or 2 doses *Risk factors* • Age • Lack of circumcision • *Female infants*: Female infants have a two- to fourfold higher prevalence of UTI than male infants • *Genetic factors, race/ethnicity:* White children have a two- to fourfold higher prevalence of UTI than do black children • *Urinary obstruction:* Obstructive urologic abnormalities are at increased risk of developing UTI • Bladder and bowel dysfunction • Vesicoureteral reflux • *Sexual activity:* Strong association between sexual intercourse and UTI in females • *Bladder catheterization:* The risk of UTI increases with increasing duration of bladder catheterization

(continued)

Table 17.3 (continued)

Diagnoses and classification	Treatment and relevant clinical features: pediatric conditions
Microbiology: • Most common causative pathogen is *E. coli* • *Gram negatives: Klebsiella, Proteus, Enterobacter*, and *Citrobacter* • Gram positive: *Staphylococcus saprophyticus, Enterococcus*, and, rarely, *Staphylococcus aureus*	*Diagnostic features* • Infants: Fever and or strong-smelling urine • School-aged children: Dysuria, frequency, or urgency • Urinalysis is suggestive of infection with the presence of pyuria (leukocyte esterase or ≥5 WBCs per high-powered field), bacteriuria, or nitrites • Nitrites are not a sensitive measure for UTI in children and cannot be used to rule out UTIs
Cardiology	
Cardiac murmur Sounds during heartbeat made by turbulent blood in or out of the cardiac valves during diastolic and systolic phase of the heartbeat. A supplementary sound other than these two is referred to cardiac murmur Many healthy children have heart murmurs, most children do not have heart diseases	*Treatment/management* • Examine to distinguish innocent from pathologies murmur • Address to a tertiary center for pediatric evaluation *General approach* • Is it a newborn <72 h old? • Positive family history? • Abnormal physical findings? • Abnormal auscultation? • No fever? No anemia, age? • If yes to any of these questions, refer to cardiologist • Abnormal auscultation? • No fever? No anemia, age? • If yes to any of these questions, refer to cardiologist *Clinical classification of heart murmurs* • Functional/innocent heart murmur • Pathologic due to atrial and ventricular septal defects, pulmonary or aortic outflow tract abnormalities, and patent ductus arteriosus *Characteristics of pathologic murmurs* • Sound level of grade 3 or louder • Systolic murmur or an increase in intensity when the patient is standing
Cardiac insufficiency A clinical syndrome caused by low cardiac output. This morbid clinical syndrome is characterized by typical symptoms and signs associated with specific circulatory, neurohormonal, and molecular abnormalities	*Treatment* • Decompensated heart failure with fluid retention • iv diuretic: Furosemide • iv amines: Dopamine, NA • iv vasodilator • Compensated • PO diuretics • ACE-inhibitor • B-blocker *Etiology cardiac insufficiency* Causes depend on age of onset (differential diagnosis) • *Congenital heart diseases*: Ventricular septal defects, Complete atrioventricular canal defects, patent ductus arteriosus, aorto–pulmonary windows, mitral regurgitation, aortic regurgitation • *Cardiomyopathies* (inherited or acquired): Dilated cardiomyopathy, hypertrophic cardiomyopathy • *Arrhythmias*: Tachycardia induced cardiomyopathy • *Infection*: Sepsis-induced myocardial dysfunction • *High output state*: Severe anemia, thyrotoxicosis, systemic arteriovenous fistula
Pneumology	
Child presenting with wheeze Wheezing is continuous musical sound heard during chest auscultation that lasts longer than 250 ms	*Treatment* Similar principles as treatment of asthma that is facilitating air entry through the tracheobronchial tree • Short-acting beta agonist (SABA):

Table 17.3 (continued)

Diagnoses and classification	Treatment and relevant clinical features: pediatric conditions
Wheezing may occur during expiration or during inspiration and it is often associated with difficulty breathing *Differential diagnosis:* • Bronchiolitis • Asthma *Classification of wheezing* • Acute: Hours to days • Classification of wheezing • Acute: Hours to days • Chronic: Weeks to months	*Albuterol (salbutamol)*, two inhalations for symptom relief, then 2 puffs every 4–6 h as needed Albuterol solution for nebulization, nebulizer solutions: 0.021% (0.63 mg/3 mL), 2 i 4–6 h, as needed • Long-acting beta agonist (LABA) Beclomethasone (200 mcg twice daily) Combination of salmeterol (50 mcg twice daily) plus beclomethasone (200 mcg twice daily) • Long-acting beta agonist (LABA) *Beclomethasone* (200 mcg twice daily) Combination of salmeterol (50 mcg twice daily) plus beclomethasone (200 mcg twice daily) *Etiology* • Asthma • Bronchiolitis • Viral infections: Viral lower respiratory tract infection typically in younger infants. Occurs seasonally • Atypical infection (*Mycoplasma* pneumonia) • Bacterial tracheitis • Foreign body aspiration • Esophageal foreign body • Anomalies of the tracheobronchial tree • Mediastinal masses • Cardiovascular disease *Clinical signs* • Wheezing: Fine crackles and wheeze on auscultation • Lower chest in-drawing • Difficulty in feeding
Presenting with stridor *Diagnostic entities* • Viral croup • Diphtheria • Epiglottis • Anaphylaxis	*Treatment:* Dexamethasone 0.6 mg/kg or equivalent dose of another steroid, e.g., prednisone *Etiology* • Bacterial infection by *H. influenza* • Viral infection of the air ways *Clinical classification of stridor* • Mild stridor: Fever, hoarse voice, barking cough, stridor when the child is agitated • Severe stridor: Stridor when child is at rest, tachypnoea and lower chest indrawing, cyanosis or $SpO_2 < 90$
Choking child Tracheobronchial foreign body aspiration	*Treatment* • Infant: 5× back blows; if persistent, 5 chest thrusts. Repeat sequence if needed • Child older than 1 year: 5 back blows; if persistent, perform Heimlich maneuver 5× • Rigid bronchoscopy where available *Anatomic locations of aspired foreign bodies* • Larynx • Trachea/carina • Right lung: 60% • Left lung: 23% • Bilateral *Clinical signs and symptoms* • Severe respiratory distress, cyanosis, and altered mental status • Partial airway obstruction: Classic triad of wheeze, cough, and diminished breath sounds

(continued)

Table 17.3 (continued)

Diagnoses and classification	Treatment and relevant clinical features: pediatric conditions
Pneumonia (severe) Signs and symptoms of an acute infection of the pulmonary parenchyma in an individual who acquired the infection in the community (community acquired) from hospital (nosocomial) pneumonia	*Treatment* • Admit to hospital • Administer O_2 if $SaO_2 < 90\%$ • Treat fever, pain, and dehydration • Amoxicillin 50 mg/kg or iv every 6 h, 7 d or • Ceftriaxone 80 mg/kg IM or iv Oral empiric antibiotics with activity against *S. pneumoniae* • Amoxicillin 90 mg/kg/d in 2 or 3 divided doses (maximum dosage 4 g/d), *or* • Amoxicillin-clavulanate 90 mg/kg per day of the amoxicillin component in 2 or 3 divided doses (MAX 4 g/d amoxicillin component) *or* • Sulfamethoxazole/trimethoprim (Septrin, cotrimoxazole, TMP and SMZ, bactrim): Standard dosage is 30 mg sulfamethoxazole and 6 mg trimethoprim/kg given in two equally divided doses • Case example: Septrin 200 mg/40 mg per 5 ml, pediatric suspension, give 2 × 5 ml/d to a 12-kg child *When allergic to penicillin* • Erythromycin 40–50 mg/kg per day in 4 divided doses (MAX 2 g/d as base, 3.2 g/d as ethyl succinate), *or* • Azithromycin 10 mg/kg on day 1 followed by 5 mg/kg daily for 4 more days (maximum 500 mg on day 1 and 250 mg thereafter) *Clinical presentation* • Combination of fever and cough • Tachypnea • Labored breathing • Pleuritic chest pain • Fever and leukocytosis • Malaise/lethargy • Emesis • Hypoxemia • Decreased breath sounds • Crackles • Retractions • Grunting • Abdominal pain • Chest pain
Sudden infant death syndrome (SIDS) Unexplained death, mostly occurring during sleep of a seemingly healthy baby	*Preventive measures* • Smoke-free environment • Baby sleeps on his or her back • Breastfeeding *Risk factors* • Sex: Boys are more likely • <2 years • Positive family history of SIDS • Second-hand smoking • Prematurity
Neurology	
Febrile seizure A febrile seizure is a convulsion in a child, correlated with body temperature >38 °C	*Treatment* • Lateral position of security • Diazepam rectal or midazolam (oral, nasal) • Paracetamol *and/or* • Ibuprofen

Table 17.3 (continued)

Diagnoses and classification	Treatment and relevant clinical features: pediatric conditions
Classification of febrile seizure • *Simple:* Most common type. Lasts a few seconds to 15 min. Does not reoccur within 24 h. General seizure and loss of consciousness • *Complex:* Lasts >15 min or >2 episodes in 24 h *or* post-ictal deficit *or* focal seizure	*Criteria for hospitalization* • Age <18 months • Prolonged postictal phase • Abnormal clinical status • Complex febrile seizure *Large differential diagnosis* • Infection • Craniocerebral trauma • Intoxication • Metabolic disorders • Electrolytic disorders • Epilepsy
Epilepsy A seizure represents the clinical expression of abnormal, excessive, synchronous discharges of neurons residing primarily in the cerebral cortex. This abnormal neural activity is intermittent and usually self-limited, lasting seconds to a few minutes *Differential diagnoses* • Cardiogenic syncope • Breath-holding spells • Reflex anoxic seizure	*Treatment:* Valproate, carbamazepine, and phenytoin have nonlinear kinetics. Care is exercised during daily dose increment to attain optimum target serum levels and corresponding clinical results. It may be prudent to do this increase every other day *Phenytoin:* Maintenance therapy: iv, Oral: Initial: 5 mg/kg/d in divided doses; usual range: 4–8 mg/kg/d; maximum daily dose: 300 mg/d *Proposed usual oral dosing range:* 6 months to 3 years: 8–10 mg/kg/d 4–6 years: 7.5–9 mg/kg/d 7–9 years: 7–8 mg/kg/d 10–16 years: 6–7 mg/kg/d Phenobarbital *Seizures, maintenance therapy:* Maintenance dose usually starts 12 h after loading dose: Dosage should be individualized based upon clinical response and serum concentration; once-daily doses usually administered at bedtime in children and adolescents Infants, children, and adolescents: Oral: 3–6 mg/kg/d Initial: Oral Infants and children ≤5 years: 3–5 mg/kg/d in 1–2 divided doses Children >5 years and adolescents: 2–3 mg/kg/d in 1–2 divided doses *Valproate:* *Children ≥5 years and adolescents ≤16 years* Oral: Initial 10–15 mg/kg/d in 2 divided doses; maximum initial dose: 250 mg/dose. Titrate as needed over 4–6 weeks to 40–45 mg/kg/d in 2 divided doses; maximum daily dose: 1000 mg/*d* Adolescents ≥17 years: Oral: 250 mg twice daily; adjust dose based on patient response; maximum daily dose: 1000 mg/*d* *Pathognomic features* • Tongue biting • Fecal incontinence • Urinary incontinence *Classification* • Clinical (full clinical expression) • Subtle (minimal clinical expression) • Subclinical (no clinical or outward manifestation of the electrical seizure activity) • Generalized onset seizures • Focal onset seizures

(continued)

Table 17.3 (continued)

Diagnoses and classification	Treatment and relevant clinical features: pediatric conditions
Ear, nose, and throat	
Acute otitis media Definitive bulging of tympanic membrane or new onset otorrhea	*Treatment* • Amoxicillin 25 mg/kg 2×/d, 5 d *or* • Co-amoxicillin 25 mg/kg *Common etiology* • Respiratory viruses • *S. pneumoniae* • Moraxella catarrhalis • Common in children <5 years *Complications* • Mastoiditis • Cerebral abscess • Meningitis *Clinical presentation* • Temperature <38 °C • Otorrhea • Local inflammation signs • Otalgia (holding, tugging, rubbing of the ear in a nonverbal child) or intense erythema of the tympanic membrane
Pharyngitis Sore throat	*Treatment* • Amoxicillin and penicillin V remain first-line therapy • If penicillin allergy is suspected, then cephalexin, cefadroxil, clindamycin, clarithromycin, or azithromycin are recommended *Clinical features* • Absence of cough • Presence of tonsillar exudates or swelling • History of fever • Swollen and tender anterior cervical lymph nodes • Age <15 years • Pharyngitis and rheumatic fever is uncommon
Acute sinusitis Infection of the sinuses by viruses or bacteria	*Treatment* • Nasal rinsing • Watchful waiting for up to 3 d • Amoxicillin or amoxicillin/clavulanate *Diagnostic features* • Halitosis • Fatigue • Headache • Decreased appetite *Clinical signs and symptoms of bacterial infection* • Persistent symptoms without improvement: Nasal discharge or daytime cough >10 d • Worsening symptoms: Worsening or new onset fever, daytime cough, or nasal discharge after initial improvement of a viral URTI • Severe symptoms: Fever ≥39 °C, purulent nasal discharge for at least 3 consecutive days • Imaging tests are no longer recommended for uncomplicated cases

Table 17.3 (continued)

Diagnoses and classification	Treatment and relevant clinical features: pediatric conditions
Orthopedic disorders in children	
Clubfoot (Talipes equinovarus) It is a complex condition that involves both the foot and lower extremity. It is characterized by the foot being excessively plantar flexed, with the forefoot swung medially and the sole facing inward *Classifications:* • Positional clubfoot • Congenital clubfoot • Syndromic clubfoot	*Treatment* • Mostly nonsurgical • Physiotherapy to stretch the contracted muscles • Casting 6–8 weeks *Nomenclature* • Plantar flexion of the foot at the ankle joint (equinus) • Inversion deformity of the heel (varus) • Medial deviation of the forefoot (adductus)
Developmental dysplasia of the hip Spectrum of conditions related to the development of the hip in infants and young children, which includes abnormal development of the acetabulum and proximal femur and mechanical instability of the hip joint	*Treatment* • Early identification • Carrying the child on the back (tradition African positioning) • Special physiotherapy *Diagnostic features* • Positive Ortolani test or limited/asymmetric abduction • Positive Barlow maneuver *Terminology of hip dysplasia* • *Dislocation:* Complete loss of contact between the femoral head and the acetabulum • *Subluxation*: Femoral head is partially outside the acetabulum but remains in contact • *Dislocable*: Femoral head is reduced (i.e., within the acetabulum) at rest but can dislocate in other positions or with examination maneuvers, that is, *instability* • *Subluxable*: Femoral head is reduced at rest but can be partially dislocated or subluxated with examination maneuvers: *mild instability or laxity* • *Reducible*: Hip is dislocated at rest, but the femoral head can be positioned into the acetabulum with manipulation (generally flexion and abduction) • *Dysplasia*: Abnormality of the shape of the hip joint (usually shallowness of the acetabulum, involving the superior and anterior margins) *Clinical presentation of hip dysplasia* • Limited abduction • Weakness of the hip abductors on the affected side may be indicated by a positive Trendelenburg pelvic • Hip instability
Scoliosis Lateral curvature of the spine associated with rotation of the involved vertebrae *Classification based upon patient's age at presentation:* • Infantile: 0–3 years • Juvenile: 4–9 years • Adolescent: ≥10 years	*Treatment* • Adequate vitamin D3 supplementation • Prompt institution of physiotherapy • Education on postural hygiene • Regular physical activity *Clinical presentation* • Truncal asymmetry noted by the patient or parents • Restrictive pulmonary disease • May have obstructive lung disease • Differences in height of the shoulders or scapulae • Asymmetries of the waistline

(continued)

Table 17.3 (continued)

Diagnoses and classification	Treatment and relevant clinical features: pediatric conditions
Pediatric fractures Frank disruption of the cortex on one side of the bone but no discernible cleavage plane on the opposite side *Fracture patterns* • Transverse • Oblique • Spiral	*Treatment* • Plaster of Paris (POP) cast • Radiographic control 7–10 d to confirm reduction is maintained in cast *Common fracture types* • *Buckle fractures* follow compression injury, often at the junction between the porous metaphysis and the denser diaphysis • *Plastic deformity (or bowing fracture)* occurs when a longitudinal force directed along the shaft of the bone exceeds the bone's ability to recoil to its normal position, leading to accentuation of the curvature of the bone, which indicates microscopic fractures within the periosteum of the bone • *Greenstick fracture:* a bone that is bent, with a fracture line that does not extend completely through the width of the bone • *Physeal (growth plate):* Growth plates are susceptible to fracture and represent a weak point in pediatric bone • *Stress fractures:* Represent overuse injuries that arise from accumulated microtrauma after repetitive strain • *Child abuse fractures:* Long bone fractures in non-ambulatory children, metaphyseal corner (or bucket handle) fractures, rib fractures, fractures of the sternum, scapula, or spinous processes, bilateral acute long-bone fractures • *Pathologic fracture* in a bone that is weakened by an underlying abnormality *Clinical features when describing a fracture* • Age and gender • Mechanism of injury • Anatomic location • Soft tissue involvement (e.g., open or closed) • Key physical examination findings, especially neurovascular status *Note:* The further the fracture is from the growing bone, the longer it takes to heal
Other infectious diseases in children	
Perinatal infections Bacterial or viral infection that a mother passes to her baby during pregnancy, during delivery, or immediately after the delivery *TORCH infections congenital infections:* • *Toxoplasma gondii, Treponema pallidum, Listeria, Varicella,* and parvovirus B19 • *R*ubella virus • *C*ytomegalovirus • *H*erpes simplex virus	*Treatment of perinatal infections* • Amoxicillin gentamicin • *Chlamydia:* Oral erythromycin, while neonatal infection can be treated at birth with erythromycin suspension • Cytomegalovirus: Ganciclovir • *Genital herpes:* Antenatally, the mother can be prescribed antiviral drugs like acyclovir or famciclovir • *Hepatitis B:* Hepatitis B vaccine at birth as part of the routine immunization schedule • *Hepatitis C (HCV) infection:* Pegylated interferon gamma (tertiary centers) • *Human immunodeficiency infection:* Retroviral drugs during pregnancy, and mothers should be counseled against breastfeeding their infants to avoid vertical transmission of the infection • *Human papillomavirus:* Maternal genital warts can be treated antenatally with cryotherapy, laser, electrocautery, or surgical excision and caesarean section • *Rubella:* Women with no previous history of exposure to rubella should receive the rubella vaccine immediately after their first pregnancy. No treatment for the disease • *Streptococcus (GBS):* Maternal GBS bacteriuria of any significance or a positive rectovaginal swab at 35–37 weeks is an indication for chemoprophylaxis • *Syphilis:* Penicillin in the antenatal period if the mother is suspected to have syphilis. If given in the first trimester, vertical transmission of the infection to the fetus can be prevented

Table 17.3 (continued)

Diagnoses and classification	Treatment and relevant clinical features: pediatric conditions
	Etiology • Vertical transmission, resulting in initial neonatal colonization that evolves into later infection • Horizontal transmission from contact with care providers or environmental sources • Etiologic agents: *Listeria monocytogenes*, *Staphylococcus aureus*, *Enterococcus* • Other gram-negative bacteria: *Klebsiella*, *Enterobacter*, *Citrobacter* spp., and *Pseudomonas aeruginosa* *Risk factors* • Chorioamnionitis defined as: $T > 38°C$ and at least 2 signs: Tachycardia maternal >100/min, fetal tachycardia >160/min, uterine pain, liquid amniotic purulent/malodor, maternal leukocytosis >15,000 • Colonization by SGB • Prematurity • Birth weight <2.5 kg • Membrane rupture ≥18 h *Terminology of neonatal infections* • *Neonatal sepsis* is a clinical syndrome in an infant 28 d or younger, manifested by systemic signs of infection and isolation of a bacterial pathogen from the bloodstream • *Term infants* are those born at a gestational age of 37 weeks or greater • *Late preterm infants* (also called *near-term infants*) are born from 34 through 36 completed weeks of gestation • *Preterm infants* are those born at less than 34 weeks of gestation *Clinical manifestations* • Temperature instability, primarily fever • Respiratory and cardiocirculatory symptoms: Grunting, hypoxia • Tachycardia, poor perfusion, hypotension, respiratory symptoms (e.g., tachypnea) • Neurological symptoms: Lethargy, poor tone, poor feeding, irritability, and seizures • Fetal and delivery room distress: Intrapartum fetal tachycardia, which may be due to intra-amniotic infection, meconium-stained amniotic fluid, Apgar score ≤6 • Others: Jaundice, hepatomegaly, poor feeding, vomiting, abdominal distension, diarrhea • Toxoplasmosis, other (syphilis), rubella, cytomegalovirus, herpes simplex virus (TORCH)

(continued)

Table 17.3 (continued)

Diagnoses and classification	Treatment and relevant clinical features: pediatric conditions
HIV infection	Treatment • Early and lifelong antiretroviral therapy (ART) • Inactivated vaccinations are recommended • Psychosocial support and mental health are critical, more so during adolescence *Clinical manifestations* • Failure to thrive. Poor weight gain and bone growth • Swollen abdomen due to hepatosplenomegaly • Swollen lymph nodes • Intermittent diarrhea • Recurrent pneumonia • Oral thrush. Fungal infection of the oral mucosa characterized by white patches on the cheeks and tongue. Painful to the infant Modes of HIV transmission • Vertical transmission. Babies born to, or breastfed by, mothers infected with the virus • Sexual contact. In adolescents, HIV is spread most commonly by sexual contact with an infected partner • Blood contamination. Contact with infected blood. Screening of donated blood for evidence of HIV infection is mandatory • Needles. By sharing needles, syringes, or drug use equipment with someone who is infected with the virus

Bibliography

1. Pocket Book of Hospital Care for Children. Guidelines for the management of common illnesses with limited resources, Maternal, newborn, child and adolescent health. World Health Organization; 2020.
2. Papadakis MA, McPhee SJ, Rabow MW. Current medical diagnosis and treatment. New York, NY: McGraw-Hill Education; 2019. https://accessmedicine.mhmedical.com/book.aspx?bookID=2449.
3. Preclinical and clinical lecture notes of the curriculum of medical studies, Faculty of Medicine, University of Lausanne, Course year 2015–2021.
4. Scientific-Units-Recommandations-Formulas (SURF), Guidelines 2020, Médecine Interne General, Philippe Furger en collaboration avec Thierry Fumeaux et le SURF-team.
5. Pocket Book of Hospital Care for Children. Guidelines for the management of, common, childhood illnesses. 2nd ed. World Health Organisation; 2013.
6. Essential med notes, 2020 Comprehensive medical references and review for the United States Medical Licensing Exam (USMLE) step II and the Medical Council of Canada Qualifying Exam (MCCQE) Part 1, 36th ed., Sara Mirali and Ayesh Seneviratne.
7. WHO model list of essential medicines, 20th List. World Health Organization; March 2017, Amended August 2017. https://apps.who.int/iris/bitstream/handle/10665/273826/EML-20-eng.pdf?ua=1.
8. The Gambia standard drug treatment guidelines, 2nd ed. Department of State for Health and Social Welfare, The Republic of the Gambia; 2001. http://apps.who.int/medicinedocs/documents/s22418en/s22418en.pdf.
9. Cornuz J, Pasche O, Kermode-Noppel T. Compas: Stratégies de prise en charge clinique, Médecine interne générale ambulatoire. Lausanne: Institute of Social and Preventive Medicine; 2010.
10. Diseases and Conditions: Comprehensive Guides on Hundreds of Conditions. Mayo Clinic. https://www.mayoclinic.org/diseases-conditions.
11. https://www.uptodate.com.
12. https://www.cdc.gov/ncbddd/actearly/milestones.
13. https://www.who.int/biologicals.

Palliative Care

18

Contents

18.1 **Key Elements of Palliative Care** 235

18.2 **Healthcare for the Terminal Patient** 237

18.3 **Suggestions for Delivery of Difficult News** 238

Bibliography 238

The World Health Organization defines palliative medical care as follows: "Palliative care is an approach that improves the quality of life of patients and their families facing the problem associated with life-threatening illness, through the prevention and relief of suffering by means of early identification and impeccable assessment and treatment of pain and other problems, physical, psychosocial and spiritual." These concepts are depicted in Fig. 18.1.

In this chapter, we address basic care to ensure the comfort and dignity of the palliative patient in a standard minimal resource facility (Table 18.1).

18.1 Key Elements of Palliative Care

- Provides relief from pain and other distressing symptoms (Fig. 18.2).

- Affirms life and regards dying as a normal, natural process (Fig. 18.1).
- Intends neither to hasten nor postpone death.
- Integrates the psychological and spiritual aspects of patient care.
- Offers a support system to help patients live as actively as possible until death.
- Offers a support system to help the family cope during the patient's illness and in their own bereavement.
- Uses a team approach to address the needs of patients and their families, including bereavement counselling, if indicated.
- Will enhance quality of life, and may also positively influence the course of illness.
- If applicable early in the course of illness, in conjunction with other therapies that are intended to prolong life, such as chemotherapy or radiation therapy, and includes those investigations needed to better understand and manage distressing clinical complications.

© The Author(s), under exclusive license to Springer Nature Switzerland AG 2021
M. Touray, A. Touray, *Clinical Work and General Management of a Standard Minimal-Resource Facility*, Sustainable Development Goals Series, https://doi.org/10.1007/978-3-030-71032-3_18

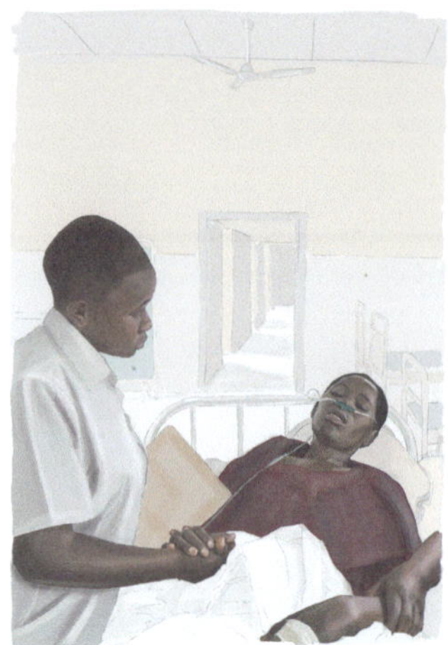

Fig. 18.1 Palliative care. A primary goal of palliative care is to enable the patient to understand that death is a natural process. Supportive care is provided to alleviate pain, anxiety, dyspnea, and to assert dignity

Table 18.1 Palliative care conditions and their treatment

Diagnosis and classification	Treatment and relevant clinical features: palliative care conditions
Palliative care Focus on improving quality of life for people living with serious illness	*Caring for patients at the end of life* • Prognosis of end of life • Expectation about the end of life • Communication of care of the patient • Caring for patient's family *Assessing nonpain symptoms* • Dyspnea • Nausea and vomiting • Constipation • Fatigue • Delirium and agitation.
Anxiety	*Treatment* • Diazepam (Valium), ampoule for injection, 10 mg, dilute in 500 ml of 0.9% NaCl, drip slowly over 2 h *Note: Cardiopulmonary arrest due to diazepam overdose*
Dyspnea	*Treatment* • Oxygen and oxygen concentrator • Hydrocortisone, ampoule for injection, 100 mg, 1 amp in 500 ml 0.9% NaCl, drip slowly over 4 h • Repeat as needed • Pulse oximetry
Nausea and vomiting	*Treatment* • Metoclopramide, ampoule for injection 10 mg, 3 × 1 amp iv/d *or* • Promethazine, ampoule for injection, 10 mg, 3 × 1 amp, iv/d as needed • Omeprazole, tab, 20 mg, 2 × 1 tab/d • Ensure adequate fluid intake but avoid fluid overload • Place urinary catheter • Watch out for extrapyramidal syndrome

Table 18.1 (continued)

Diagnosis and classification	Treatment and relevant clinical features: palliative care conditions
Pain and its management Definition: Sensory and emotional experience associated with actual or potential tissue damage. Pain may be acute or chronic	*Treatment* Adopt the WHO pain ladder as illustrated below (Fig. 18.2) • Step 1. Paracetamol, tab, 500 mg, 3 × 2 tab/d • Step 2. Naproxen, tab, 500 mg, 3 × 1 tab/d • Step 3. Tramadol, amp 100 mg in 500 ml 0.9% NaCl, drip for 4 h • Step 4. Morphine, tab, 10 mg, half, tab, every 4 h *or* • Fentanyl, tab, 0.2 mg, 1 tab/d Pain management strategies • *Acute pain* resolves within the expected period of healing time and is self-limited, for example, dental pain • *Chronic non-cancer* pain may begin as acute pain that then fails to resolve and extend beyond the expected period of healing. Chronic pain may be due to several conditions: Either cancer or non-cancer medical conditions • We use a WHO pain assessment scale to estimate the intensity of pain felt by the patient. Graded 1 (no pain) to 10 (maximum pain imaginable) *Management tips* Monitor and ensure adequate pain relief by clinical assessment Alternatively: • Oxycontin, tab, 5 mg, 2 × 1 tab/d *or* • Oxynorm, 10 mg/ml solution, 5 mg/6 h

18.2 Healthcare for the Terminal Patient

Most palliative conditions result from cerebrovascular accidents, commonly called stroke, as well as decompensated cardiovascular conditions (heart failure, myocardial infections, pericarditis), oncologic conditions (hepatocarcinoma, gastrointestinal carcinoma), and metastatic oncologic conditions (prostate, lung carcinoma, breast cancer, and lymphomas).

Conditions such as fulminant bronchopneumonia, cerebral malaria, severe asthmatic crises, acute fulminant renal failure, or exacerbation of a chronic renal failure commonly require palliation in our facility.

The primary objective of palliative care in a standard minimal-resource facility is to relieve pain, address anxiety, and maintain the dignity of the patient.

Available resources include intravenous pain and anxiety control, oxygen, and empathic, tender loving care.

Family members and friends should be comforted, and spiritual concerns may rise to the forefront during this time. According to the wishes of the patient and his or her family and based on the religious affiliation of the concerned patient, it is a common practice to call an imam or a priest to attend the patient and his or her family.

Extreme discretion is exercised in pronouncing prognoses. Sometimes close family members in distant countries must be notified of the condition of the palliative patient.

A pertinent clinical examination to diagnose, announce, and certify the death should be performed. Announcing the death formally to the family is done in a quiet and congenial room. All phones should be OFF. Time should be taken to explain the underlying disease that resulted in death. The family members should be given time and the opportunity to ask questions. Very clear answers using nonmedical jargon should be given to answer all questions asked by family members.

Prompt and discrete disposal of the remains of a patient is a significant part of palliative care. A standard minimal-resource facility should be sensitive to the psychological, religious, traditional, regulatory, and hygienic issues around disposal of patients' remains.

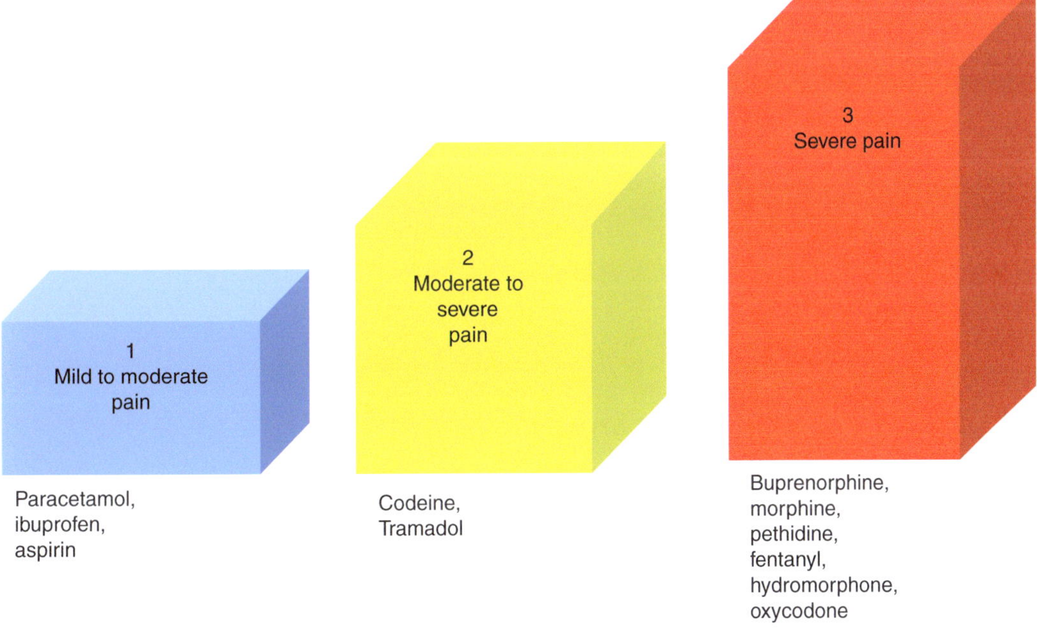

Fig. 18.2 The pain ladder (adapted from WHO pain scale)

18.3 Suggestions for Delivery of Difficult News

- Address basic and information needs.
- Be direct and avoid jargon and euphemisms.
- Assess and validate the patient's reaction.
- Listen actively and express empathy.
- Achieve a common perception of the problem.
- Reassure that pain relief is available.
- Ensure follow-ups and make specific plans for the future.

Bibliography

1. Papadakis MA, SJ MP, Rabow MW. Current medical diagnosis and treatment. New York, NY: McGraw-Hill Education; 2019. https://accessmedicine.mhmedical.com/book.aspx?bookID=2449.
2. Preclinical and clinical lecture notes of the curriculum of medical studies, Faculty of Medicine, University of Lausanne, Course year 2015–2021.
3. Scientific-Units-Recommandations-Formulas (SURF), Guidelines, Médecine Interne General, Philippe Furger en collaboration avec Thierry Fumeaux et le SURF-team. 2020.
4. Pocket Book of Hospital Care for Children. Guidelines for the management of, common, childhood illnesses. 2nd ed. World Health Organisation; 2013.
5. Essential med notes, 2020 Comprehensive medical references and review for the United States Medical Licensing Exam (USMLE) step II and the Medical Council of Canada Qualifying Exam (MCCQE) Part 1, 36th ed., Sara Mirali and Ayesh Seneviratne.
6. WHO model list of essential medicines, 20th List. World Health Organization; March 2017, Amended August 2017. https://apps.who.int/iris/bitstream/handle/10665/273826/EML-20-eng.pdf?ua=1.
7. The Gambia Standard Drug Treatment Guidelines, 2nd ed. Department of State for Health and Social Welfare, The Republic of the Gambia; 2001. http://apps.who.int/medicinedocs/documents/s22418en/s22418en.pdf.
8. Cornuz J, Pasche O, Kermode-Noppel T. Compas: Stratégies de prise en charge clinique, Médecine interne générale ambulatoire. Lausanne: Institute of Social and Preventive Medicine; 2010.
9. Diseases and conditions: comprehensive guides on hundreds of conditions. Mayo Clinic. https://www.mayoclinic.org/diseases-conditions.
10. https://www.uptodate.com.
11. https://www.cdc.gov/ncbddd/actearly/milestones.
12. https://www.who.int/biologicals.

Organization of Regular Standard Health Care

19

Contents

19.1   **Outpatient Triage and Patient Flow Within the Facility** 241
19.1.1 Standard Nursing Shifts 242
19.1.2 Nursing Duties During a Shift and How the Outgoing Shift Hands Over
to the Incoming Shift 242
19.1.3 The Pharmacy: How to Dispense Prescribed Drugs to Outpatients 242

19.2   **Patient Admission to the Hospital Wards and Inpatient Care** 244
19.2.1 Patient Admission to the Hospital Wards 244
19.2.2 Administration of Medication to Inpatients 245
19.2.3 Inpatient Monitoring and Vital Signs Measurement 246

19.3   **Discharging an Inpatient from the Wards to His/Her Home** 246

19.4   **Medical Follow-Ups After Initial Ambulatory or Inpatient Patient
Management** 247

19.5   **Physiotherapy Services** 247
19.5.1 Basic Requirements to Establish a Physiotherapy Unit 250
19.5.2 Scheduling Physiotherapy Sessions 251

References 251

The organization of daily healthcare delivery in a standard minimal-resource health care facility has the goal of optimally using the available human, logistic, and material resources to obtain the best possible clinical outcome for the ill. This needs pragmatic coordination of resources. The welfare of the human resources, the maintenance of the logistic facilities, and assurance of continuous availability of consumables are challenges that must be adequately addressed. In this section, we outline how best clinical practice may be successfully conducted in a minimal-resource setting.

19.1 Outpatient Triage and Patient Flow Within the Facility

As soon as the patient enters the gates of the hospital, it is the joint responsibility of all Bijilo Medical Center (BMC) team members to provide

M. Touray, A. Touray, *Clinical Work and General Management of a Standard Minimal-Resource Facility*, Sustainable Development Goals Series, https://doi.org/10.1007/978-3-030-71032-3_19

the best individual care possible. An efficient progression of the patient through the various stations of the hospital in a highly concerted spirit of teamwork is achieved through the following means:

- The security service at the gate ensures that the patient is registered and that he/she reaches the reception area promptly and safely.
- The receptionist ensures that patients are attended to promptly.
- A nurse is assigned to monitor the corridor in order to avoid overcrowding. This nurse answers questions and addresses concerns from the outpatients. He or she may forward complicated or difficult questions to the physicians.
- The nurse in the corridor makes sure that those patients who are waiting for laboratory results are seated comfortably in the reception area.
- Critical cases are prioritized to make sure that the door-to-needle time is as short as possible.

19.1.1 Standard Nursing Shifts

Typically, a hospital must be able to deliver health care 24 hours per day, 7 days per week. Nursing care is a vital component of this effort, and several nursing shift models have been developed to ensure optimum coverage. At BMC, nursing staff is divided into three shifts: the morning shift, the afternoon shift, and the night shift.

- The *morning shift* is scheduled for 30 h per week, usually 6 h per day, from 8:00–14:00.
- The *afternoon shift* is also scheduled for 30 h, 6 h per day, from 14:00–20:00.
- The *night shift* covers the 12 h from 20:00–8:00 the next morning.

This organized schedule ensures that nurses maintain a good equilibrium between professional and private activities. The nurses on duty get to know their patients, build a good nurse–patient relationship, and provide holistic care, all of which aid in minimizing errors when dispensing therapy.

19.1.2 Nursing Duties During a Shift and How the Outgoing Shift Hands Over to the Incoming Shift

Handing over the care of a patient to the next shift is a crucial aspect of quality care. The hospital health team strives for continuous improvement. Hand-over of a shift takes at least 30 min, and the information exchange should be as detailed as possible. Hospital hand-over includes joint bedside visits, reading of patient files, and good verbal communication between the incoming and the outgoing shift staff. The incoming nursing team is provided with the names of all the inpatients, their reasons for admission, treatment plans, changes made to their medications, their most troubling complaints, the anticipated required nursing care, and the goal of the entire health team, particularly the physicians. Hand-over is an important part of each nurse's shift, not only for information sharing but also to optimize time and resource management.

19.1.3 The Pharmacy: How to Dispense Prescribed Drugs to Outpatients

The majority of patients consulting at BMC are managed as outpatients. After the consultation and diagnostic work, the patient receives his or her medication and leaves the hospital. Patients presenting with clinical conditions needing inpatient care, however, are admitted as inpatients.

Every patient must consult with a physician and must obtain a prescription signed by the physician before medications may be dispensed from the pharmacy by a qualified person. Authorized dispensers include pharmacists, pharmacy auxiliaries, and other qualified health workers who are trained in proper storage, precise preparation, and use of prescribed medications, including dosages and intervals. As they are often the final link between the medication and the patient, their role is of vital importance.

Pharmacists and other dispensers should follow the procedures outlined below to ensure the proper delivery of medication to the patient.

1. The dispenser receives a signed, authenticated prescription from the physician via the corridor nurse. The prescription must contain the following details:
   (a) Patient's personal identification
   (b) Explanation of therapeutic appropriateness
   (c) Clearly written names and quantity of medications
2. The dispenser should verify that the prescriber has selected the correct drug, dosage, and quantity for the patient.
3. The dispenser correctly interprets the prescription or instructions on the prescription, including the following:
   (a) Check the name of the drug(s)
   (b) Check the dosage, administration, and duration of the treatment
   (c) Check the availability of the drug in the pharmacy
4. The dispenser verifies that the prescribed drug is available from the pharmacy and retrieves the drug from the storage area. This involves:
   (a) Checking the expiration date and verifying that the drug is undamaged
   (b) Checking and double-checking the drug product for accuracy of identity, strength, and galenic
5. The dispenser communicates the correct way to take the medication to the patient. This involves:
   (a) Proper labeling of the medicine bag with the drug name and dosage
   (b) Thorough explanation of the dosage and intervals, especially in cases of illiteracy
6. The patient understands the instructions from the dispenser. This involves the following:
   (a) The dispenser repeats the labeled instructions orally, in layman's terms if possible
   (b) The patient should repeat the instructions back to the dispenser
   (c) The dispenser emphasizes the need for compliance and provides appropriate warnings and cautions

(d) The dispenser gives special attention to the following patients:
   - Pregnant women
   - Those with visual or hearing impairment
   - Patients who are functionally illiterate
   - Children and elderly patients
   - Patients taking multiple medications
7. The patient confirms that they understand the instructions for therapy.
8. The dispenser keeps accurate records of the patient's data, medications given or dispensed, and date of the operation or transaction.

Prescribers and dispensers must collaborate in promoting correct dispensing. Teamwork is vital in order to ensure quality patient care. A good team spirit should be cultivated by all health care personnel.

Good communication within a functional team facilitates good relations between the health care deliverer and the patient, which leads to the following positive incomes:

1. *Patient's understanding of the treatment plan improves patient compliance and clinical outcome:* Good doctor–patient relations facilitate the clinical workup to obtain a correct diagnosis. A clear explanation to the patient of all processes is crucial to maintain a healthy therapeutic alliance. A patient who understands the diagnosis and treatment is much more likely to comply with the prescribed treatment regimen. Clear and comprehensive communication regarding a specific treatment plan improves patient compliance and understanding.
2. *Reduction of unnecessary prescriptions:* Efforts are made to avoid prescription of unnecessary auxiliary medication. Advice such as "eat five fruits each day," "drink three litters of clean water each day," or "walk at least 20 minutes, twice each day" may be more appropriate than prescribing loads of multivitamin tablets or unnecessary laxatives.
3. *Improved patient outcome after discharge:* Collaboration promotes clear explanations of how each drug should be taken, what side effects may occur, and what to do in case of adverse effects or no response to the drug.

The pharmacist/dispenser has a crucial role in this collaboration and in the health care system of the hospital in general. Additional duties may include communicating with physicians (to check a prescription or respond to a question) and ensuring patient compliance with treatment guidelines.

19.2 Patient Admission to the Hospital Wards and Inpatient Care

The general outlook of the patient is the major criterion when deciding between an inpatient or outpatient course of treatment. Hospitalization is indicated in the following instances:

- Severe disease conditions that require parenteral (non-oral) medications: severe malaria, pyelonephritis, endocarditis, and diabetic ketoacidosis.
- Mild disease conditions when oral intake of medications is compromised, such as in persistent or intractable vomiting.
- Mild disease conditions when medication compliance is anticipated to be poor.
- Patients with milder disease conditions when appropriate home care is temporarily unavailable.
- Cases of child abuse and domestic violence.
- Upon the patient's request when there are genuine home safety concerns.

19.2.1 Patient Admission to the Hospital Wards

After the consultation, if the physician decides to admit the patient, the following series of steps should be followed (Fig. 19.1).

The decision to admit a patient is a significant step in acute management of a patient. The decision is primarily made by the physician who

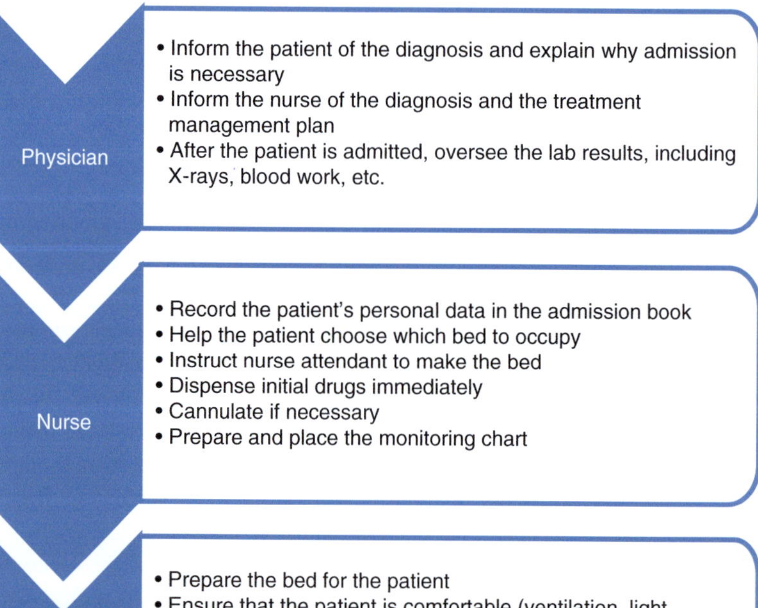

Fig. 19.1 Patient admissions procedure

consulted with the patient. Further elements supporting the decision to admit a patient may come from the nurses, laboratory technicians, and other health care workers, based on pertinent clinical or social factors. The nurse-in-charge is informed of the decision in writing, and she then informs the patient and his/her escort(s) of the decision to admit and the rules regarding treatment of admitted individuals. The nurse coordinates a speedy and harmonious admission process, including choosing and preparing the bed, placing appropriate intravenous lines, and preparing the chart for vital signs and medication.

Hospital admission is defined as the occupation of a hospital bed for therapeutic purposes extending overnight (Fig. 19.1). In certain cases, an overnight stay may not be needed. In such cases, a patient may occupy a hospital bed for therapeutic purposes for a given period during the day. The latter is referred to as *hospital detention.*

The hospital admission procedure requires a concerted health care team effort. The procedure is as follows:

1. Inform the patient and his/her escorts of the decision that he/she is to be admitted. Explain the various admission options. In correlation with availability, allow the patient and family to make an informed decision as to which bed the patient will occupy. Patients who require frequent observation should be assigned to a ward that is continuously supervised by the nursing staff and is readily accessible to the physician.
2. Prepare the room and/or bed for the patient.
3. Record the patient's personal data in the admission book: name, address, occupation, employment, and diagnosis at admission. Note clearly allergies to any drug or food as well as weight, height, and vital signs (blood pressure, temperature, respiration rate).
4. The patient is helped into the bed in the ward of his or her choice. The nurse should adjust the bed and instruct the patient on the use of the toilet and the bathroom. A bottle of water should be provided to each patient.
5. All questions asked by the patient in relation to the diagnosis at admission and the treatment procedure should be answered clearly and plainly. The nurse and the physician should thoroughly explain therapeutic procedures, and the patient's consent for all procedures should be obtained. Ample time for questions and explanations should be allocated.
6. Under supervision of the physician, nurses perform procedures such as sample collection, intravenous (iv) cannulation, feeding tube insertion, and urinary catheter placement. Efficient and timely administration of prescribed medications is also the responsibility of the nurse on duty.
7. Level of functioning, including activities of daily living, bathing, dressing, toileting, mobilizing continence, and feeding should be periodically assessed and documented by the assigned nurse. Precise data about the patient should be obtained and analyzed in order to customize and provide individualized care for the patient.
8. Based on the patient's evolving clinical condition, the patient's discharge is anticipated and planned.

Figure 19.1 contains a simplified flow chart of the admissions process.

19.2.2 Administration of Medication to Inpatients

Accuracy in preparing and administering medication is important. Nurses should keep in mind the "five right" guidelines for drug administration, which can be summed up by the abbreviation DDPRT:

- The right drug
- The right dose
- The right patient
- The right route
- The right time

Following the steps below will help to ensure that medications are administered without error. If iv medications are overly complicated, inform the physician promptly. An oral or alternative route will be suggested by the physician without delay.

1. Prepare medication for one patient at a time.
2. Calculate the correct drug dose and time at which the dose should be taken.
3. Prepare and arrange all the medications in a tray for administration.
4. Make sure that the patient has drinking water available for oral medications.
5. Take the medication to each patient at the specified time.
6. Explain the purpose of the medication and its action to the patient.
7. Administer the drugs properly.
8. Stay with the patient until the medication has been swallowed; ask the patient to open his or her mouth.
9. Assist the patient in retuning to a comfortable position.
10. Record on the treatment chart the actual time that each drug was administered.
11. Evaluate the patient's response to the medication.
12. Thank your patient. Show professional empathy.

19.2.3 Inpatient Monitoring and Vital Signs Measurement

While in the hospital, patients need to be regularly visited in their beds by hospital staff, according to the following schedule:

- By the physician twice per day (the morning round occurs at 9:00 and the afternoon round at 14:00).
- By the nurses at least once every 2 hours, and by a nurse attendant hourly (and more frequently if necessary).

Five vital signs are taken for each patient:

- Body temperature [degrees Celsius]
- Pulse [beats per minute]
- Respiratory rate [thoracic ampliations per minute]
- Blood pressure [mmHg]
- Oxygen saturation [percentage]

These vital signs are clinical indicators of an individual's general health status. The physiologic values correlate with the well-being of the patient. Because these values change along with a patient's condition, vital signs have important prognostic values, and they are used to monitor the efficacy of a dispensed therapeutic procedure both at admission and throughout the patient's stay.

Guidelines for taking vital signs are as follows:

- Vital signs should be taken initially, before consulting the physician.
- The patient's clinical condition should determine the frequency at which vital signs are measured.
- Nurses must collaborate with physicians to determine the frequency of vital sign assessment, and signs must be monitored frequently enough to detect changes and trends, so that good therapeutic decisions may be made.
- Nurses should be able to measure vital signs correctly, communicate findings appropriately, and initiate intervention as needed.
- Equipment should be functional and appropriate. The equipment used to measure vital signs must work properly to ensure accurate findings.
- The nurse must be familiar with the patient's medical history, therapies, and prescribed medications. Some illnesses or treatments cause predictable changes in vital signs.

19.3 Discharging an Inpatient from the Wards to His/ Her Home

During the morning rounds, the attending physician decides which patients are to be discharged (Fig. 19.2). Hospital staff members work together in a concerted team effort to enable patients to

Fig. 19.2 Patient discharge procedure

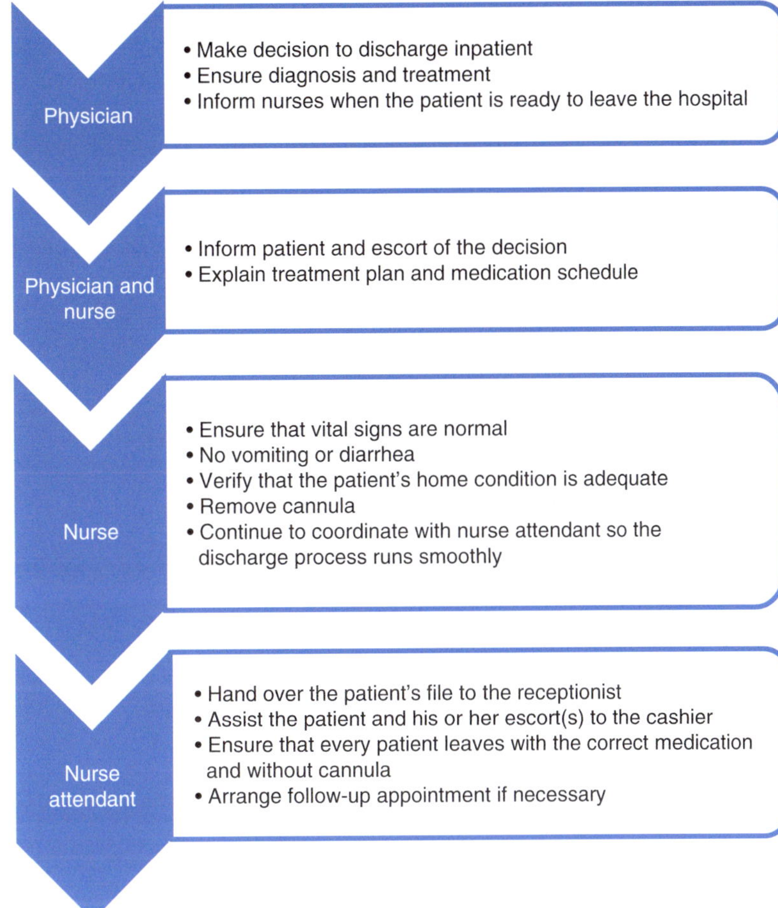

leave the hospital without delay. The chart below depicts the procedure.

The decision to discharge a patient is made by the physician in charge of the wards. This clinical decision is based on the general condition of the patient, in particular the vital signs, the ease with which medication can be further administered, the autonomy of the patient, and the adequacy of the social support at home.

Once the decision has been made, the doctor and the nurse inform the patient. The nurse coordinates the discharge procedure, so it runs smoothly. This process includes clearly communicating with the appropriate individuals, explaining the continued treatment scheme to be carried out at home, retrieving the medication, coordinating the payment of bills, and arranging for follow-up visits.

19.4 Medical Follow-Ups After Initial Ambulatory or Inpatient Patient Management

Follow-up appointments should be given where necessary. It is more effective to give patients a precise written appointment, for example, "Tuesday 21 June at 11 in the morning," rather than simply saying "next week" or "in two days' time."

19.5 Physiotherapy Services

Physiotherapy, also called physical therapy, is therapy for the preservation, enhancement, or restoration of movement and physical function impaired or threatened by disease, injury, or disability that utilizes therapeutic exercise, physical modalities (such as massage and electrotherapy), assistive devices, and patient education and training (Table 19.1 and Fig. 19.3). The 3 Rs for physiotherapy are as follows:

- *Re*education = recover functional deficits
- *Re*adjustment = compensate for functional deficit once situation is stabilized
- *Re*integration = return to participative life

A standard minimal-resource facility may provide physiotherapy services for clients with ambulatory problems or impaired physical processes secondary to cerebrovascular accidents (CVAs), arthritis, geriatrics, and other conditions (Fig. 19.4).

When professionally conducted, physiotherapy enables good recovery from a multitude of disease conditions, and importantly, it may reduce medication consumption (Table 19.2).

Table 19.1 Physiotherapy services

Method	Therapeutic goal	Indication/comments
Bandage and taping	• Analgesia • Facilitating healing by stabilizing muscles and reducing amplitudes of joint movements	• Osteoarticular contusions • Muscle tears • Hematomas
Respiratory training Ampliation of the thoracic cage to improve breathing pattern	• Inflate lung to prevent atelectasis and improve breathing patterns • To promote mucous secretion from the lungs • To increase cardiac tolerance to effort	• After severe pneumonia • After myocardial infarction • After stroke
Cardio Careful conditioning of the heart by short spans of adapted vigorous training interposed by relaxation	• Improve exercise tolerance	• Rehabilitation after mild to severe illness
Global muscular reconditioning • Tonification • Proprioceptive training • Coordination • Joint relaxation	• Analgesia • Improve muscle power • Improve endurance	• Convalescence after major illness or trauma • Malnutrition • Confinement-incarceration
Group therapy • Behavioral therapy • Sharing experience • Coaching	• Improve social skills • Obtain psychological comfort • Learn coping methods to live with a chronic condition	• Stroke • Chronic systemic diseases, e.g., diabetes, hypertension, and lower back pain • Mood disorder
Hydrotherapy • Swimming • Walking in water • Relaxing in water	• Improvement of amplitude of joint movements • Improvement of muscle power • Improve mood	• Scapulo-humeral pain (shoulder pain) • Knee injuries • Arthrosis of the knee and hip joint • Ankle contusions
Lymphatic drainage Physical draining of lymph from dependent areas by massage and or bandage	• To promote drainage of lymph and extravascular fluids from dependent areas, mainly lower limbs or in sacroiliac region in patients that are mainly in lateral decubitus	• Lymphedema • Cardiac insufficiency
Pelvic floor training	• To obtain better control of miction and defecation • Reduce dyspareunia • Reduce pelvic organ prolapses	• After childbirth • *Treatment of complications of female genital mutilations* • Recurrent PID
Postural hygiene	• Learn how to lift and carry loads • Learn how to sit for long hours without straining specific muscle groups	• Scoliosis • Lordosis • Prevention in professions like cashiers, cleaners, carpenters, masters, etc.

Table 19.1 (continued)

Method	Therapeutic goal	Indication/comments
Proprioceptive training	• Better gait • Prevent falls • Obtain autonomy by ambulating with ease and comfort	• Joint dysfunction due to wear and tear • Stroke
Tonification of paravertebral muscles	• Reduce back pain • Obtain better posture • Reduce incidence of fall	• Variable spondyloarthropathy • Post-traumatic back pain • Stroke
Tonification of specific muscle groups (isometric stretching)	• To reduce pain • Improve muscle power and joint functions: Glenohumeral joint, knee, ankle, elbow, wrist, interphalangeal joints, carpal and metacarpophalangeal joints, cervical spine	To the spine, knee, hip, angle, feet, hands Muscle injuries to: • Abductors • Adductors • M. Quadriceps femoris • M. Biceps rachis • M. Biceps femoris • Rotator cuff injuries
Ultrasound therapy	• Pain reduction • Improve joint function • Improve muscle function	• Acute and chronic pain of musculoskeletal origin • Nerve pain

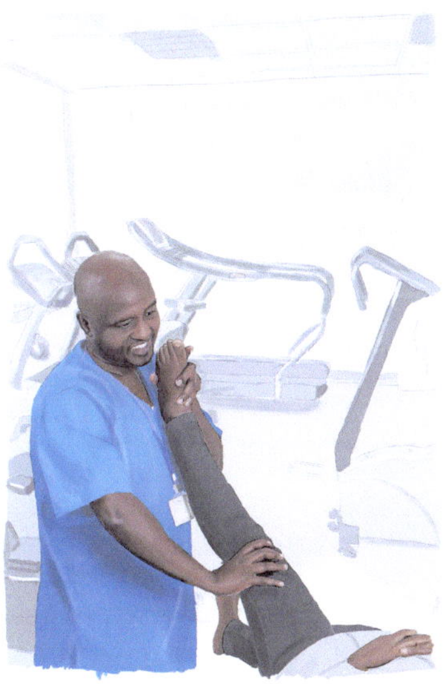

Physiotherapy

List of clinical conditions for which physiotherapy is required that are described in the text. For easy reference, the corresponding page on which the disease condition is described is in brackets.

Cardiovascular (p250)
Congenital (p250)
Neurological (p250)
Orthopedic (p250)
Post-surgical conditions (p250)
Post-traumatic convalescence (p250)
Rehabilitation after various conditions (p250)

Fig. 19.3 Physiotherapy is an essential therapeutic modality in a minimal resource facility. Note the key components, namely, the physiotherapist, physiotherapy bed, and essential instrumentation

- The physiotherapy service is operated 3 days a week by a highly trained physiotherapist.
- All scheduled physiotherapy cases should be booked for appointment by the receptionist. The contact numbers of the client should also be recorded, so that they can be reminded about the appointment date if necessary.
- Those patients who come to the hospital for a physiotherapy appointment should not be confused with the typical outpatient.
- A nurse or a receptionist should accompany the patient to the physiotherapy room.
- The physiotherapist should take the patient to the cashier at the end of the session.

- The physiotherapist should notify the receptionists if the patient needs to come back for another appointment, so that the receptionist can book the patient again.
- The physiotherapist should communicate to the doctor on the progress of the individual patients.
- Physiotherapy patients who present acute complaints should be referred to a physician for a consultation.
  - o Impairment: problem in body function or structure
    - – For example, patient has a motor deficiency

- o Activity limitation: difficulty encountered by an individual in executing a task or action
  - – For example, patient cannot climb stairs
- o Participation restriction: problem experienced by an individual in involvement in life situations
  - – For example, patient lost his/her job

19.5.1 Basic Requirements to Establish a Physiotherapy Unit

Within the hospital, establishing a physical therapy unit with a given budget is quite feasible. The main items are:

- *A dedicated health care worker* with some anatomic knowledge: the main muscle groups, skeletal system, and a good notion of the cardiovascular, respiratory, and the nervous system.
- *A quiet and accessible space:* preferably no stairs, measuring about 4 m by 4 m. The more space one has the better.
- *Office equipment*: desk, chair, notebook.

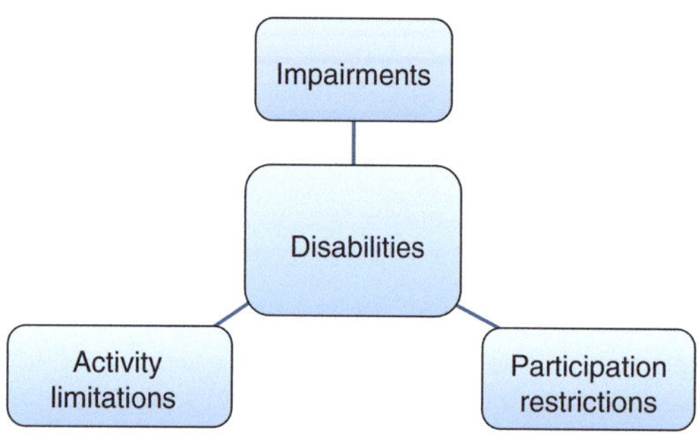

Fig. 19.4 Physiotherapy may be appropriate for several categories of disabilities

Table 19.2 Major medical conditions for which physiotherapy is prescribed

System	Examples of disease condition	Comment
Cardiovascular	• Aerobic exercise • Movements and physical exercise with sustained pulse rate	Maximal tolerated pulse = 220 − age
Congenital	Specific directed exercise	For pediatric cases, the parents should be involved. Care should be taken to avoid falls
Neurological	• Repeated specific physical exercise • Brain jogging • Memory exercise	The formal educational level and cultural background should be considered by the health care giver
Orthopedic	• Active and passive components • Muscle tonification • Stretching	Encourage physical activity; prescribe physiotherapy with the goal of muscle tonification
Postsurgical	• Gradual movement from the decubitus to supine position. Accompanied ambulation supine, with or without walking aid • Accentuate body part tonification: Limbs, thorax, abdomen or perineum	Surgeon should be consulted as often as needed
Post-traumatic	• Directed specified body part training	• Pain control may be needed • Great care must be taken when fractures are involved
Rehabilitative	• Planned physical exercise after prolonged severe illness	The general focus is to restore the patient's maximum physical autonomy

- *Devices for measuring body constants*: stethoscope, metric sphygmomanometer, thermometer, and metric measuring tapeline.
- *Basic physical therapy equipment*: treatment table (can be locally fabricated), mats, treatment room chair, a large mirror, various weights (0.5, 1.0, 2.0, and 5.0 kg), fixed exercise bicycle, wooden 10 cm steps (at least five steps, house made).
- *Educational material*: skeleton, anatomical posters (shoulder, hip, knee, muscle groups).

19.5.2 Scheduling Physiotherapy Sessions

Patients are scheduled for physiotherapy after being assessed by the physician. The physician formulates a prescription which contains the number of physical therapy sessions and the frequency at which they may be dispensed based on the therapeutic goals that are set (Table 19.1). Typically, initially, nine sessions are prescribed. The frequency at which these sessions are dispensed varies from one session per week to three session per week. A typical physical therapy session lasts for 45 minutes composed of passive and active exercise components depending on the pathology present.

References

1. Petty NJ. Principles of musculoskeletal treatment and management: a handbook for therapists (physiotherapy essentials) (English) 30. 2017.
2. Papadakis MA, McPhee SJ, Rabow MW. Current medical diagnosis and treatment. New York, NY: McGraw-Hill Education; 2019. https://accessmedicine.mhmedical.com/book.aspx?bookID=2449.
3. Preclinical and clinical lecture notes of the curriculum of medical studies, Faculty of Medicine, University of Lausanne, Course year 2015–2021.
4. Scientific-Units-Recommendations-Formulas (SURF) guidelines, Médecine Interne General, Philippe Furger en collaboration avec Thierry Fumeaux et le SURF-team. 2020.
5. Pocket Book of Hospital Care for Children. Guidelines for the management of, common, childhood illnesses, 2nd ed. World Health Organisation; 2013.
6. Essential med notes, 2020 Comprehensive medical references and review for the United States Medical Licensing Exam (USMLE) step II and the Medical Council of Canada Qualifying Exam (MCCQE) Part 1, 36th ed., Sara Mirali and Ayesh Seneviratne.
7. WHO model list of essential medicines, 20th list. World Health Organization; March 2017, Amended August 2017. https://apps.who.int/iris/bitstream/handle/10665/273826/EML-20-eng.pdf?ua=1.
8. The Gambia standard drug treatment guidelines, 2nd ed. Department of State for Health and Social Welfare, The Republic of the Gambia; 2001. http://apps.who.int/medicinedocs/documents/s22418en/s22418en.pdf.
9. Cornuz J, Pasche O, Kermode-Noppel T. Compas: Stratégies de prise en charge clinique, Médecine interne générale ambulatoire. Lausanne: Institute of Social and Preventive Medicine; 2010.
10. Diseases and conditions: comprehensive guides on hundreds of conditions. Mayo Clinic. https://www.mayoclinic.org/diseases-conditions.

Contents

20.1   **Organization of the Surgical Unit** 253
20.1.1 Personnel 254
20.1.2 Equipment 255
20.1.3 Consumables 255
20.1.4 Costing of Surgical Procedures 256

20.2   **The Surgical Procedure** 256
20.2.1 Preoperative Stage 256
20.2.2 Intraoperative Stage 257
20.2.3 Postoperative Stage 258
20.2.4 Blood Transfusion Unit in a Standard Minimal-Resource Facility 259

20.1 Organization of the Surgical Unit

Surgery is the branch of medicine that is concerned with diseases and conditions requiring or amenable to operative or manual procedures (Fig. 20.1).

During routine clinical practice, attending staffs often encounter clinical conditions that require surgical procedures to obtain a definitive cure. The type of procedure depends on the diagnosis. Such clinical cases may range from the drainage of abscesses requiring simple local anesthetics to more complex interventions that need to be performed under general anesthesia and last for several hours. The appropriate surgical unit is set up to meet all exigencies of the surgical procedure to be performed. Typically, surgical settings will fall into one of two categories: the emergency or the elective surgical care unit. Irrespective of the setting, all surgical units have a common organization, which is outlined below.

The most common general surgical cases include acute surgical care cases in the trauma setting, obstetrical cases, lump and bump excisions, and abdominal wall defect corrections in the nonemergency surgery setting.

Subspecialties such as neurosurgery and orthopedic and otolaryngeal surgery have been budding in recent years, mainly through the assistance of foreign medical specialists with a few Gambian medical personnel having trained overseas.

M. Touray, A. Touray, *Clinical Work and General Management of a Standard Minimal-Resource Facility*, Sustainable Development Goals Series, https://doi.org/10.1007/978-3-030-71032-3_20

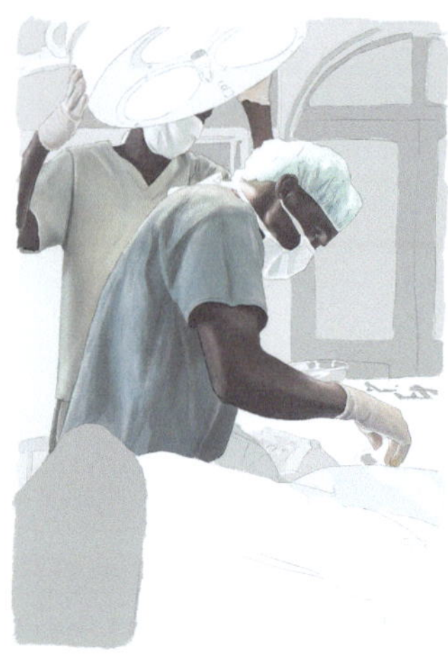

Fig. 20.1 Surgical unit in a standard minimal-resource facility. Note the key components, namely, the surgeon, his/her assistant, good light system, surgical table, and essential instrumentation

A functional surgical unit requires all of the following:

- Personnel
- Equipment
- Consumables
- Costing methodology for procedures
- Detailed plans outlining procedures performed at the facility

20.1.1 Personnel

Every surgical team requires the right personnel in the operating theatre in order to successfully carry out any procedure. These include:

- The patient
- Theatre matron
- Scrub nurse
- Runner nurse
- Orderly
- Surgeon
- Anesthetist

All participants are paid for their services, except the patient (without whom there would be no surgery). Before the commencement of any procedure, accurate verification of the patient's identity, the type of procedure, and the concerned body part is crucial. Verification can be achieved before administration of anesthesia by oral con-

firmation between the patient and the anesthetist, the scrub nurse, or any other member of the surgical team.

20.1.1.1 Theatre Matron

The theatre matron is often considered the *chef d'orchestre* or maestro of the surgical team, and he/she is responsible for coordination and making sure that everything is in place for a successful intervention (Fig. 20.1). His/her duties include:

- Responsibilities of running the theatre.
- Managing the booked cases.
- Taking care of equipment.
- Making sure that equipment is sorted according to cases.
- Making sure that equipment is available and in order for each planned surgery.
- Scrubbing in with the surgeon if the scrub nurse is not available, or running for the scrub nurse.
- Taking quarterly stock of equipment and taking responsibility for any lost equipment.

20.1.1.2 Scrub Nurse and Runner Nurse

The *scrub nurse* assists the surgeon to slip into his/her gown. He/she is an integral part of the procedure. This nurse should know the required surgical instruments/material for each procedure and should provide them to the surgeons in a timely and orderly fashion throughout the procedure.

The *runner nurse* provides a link between the scrub nurse and the nonsterile portions of the surgery. He/she provides additional material (swabs, sutures, etc.) for the procedure as and when needed. These two nurses may interchange roles from one procedure to another, as they are both qualified to assist the surgeon. Some other responsibilities include:

- Deputizing for the matron in his/her absence.
- Scrubbing in for cases (all cases require a scrub nurse and a runner to fetch things needed during the surgery).
- Running when the matron is scrubbed.

20.1.1.3 Orderly

The orderly is responsible for the transportation of the patient in and out of the theatre as well as for:

- Keeping the theatre clean before and after each case.
- Making sure that clean drapes and gowns are available for the surgeries.
- Doing any job requested by the matron, scrub nurse, or doctors.
- One of the already employed cleaners can be delegated for this job when cases are scheduled.

20.1.1.4 Surgeon

A surgeon is a medical specialist who practices surgery. The surgeon is the main participant in the surgical team and is responsible for the actual surgical procedure. Except in minor cases, two surgeons are often necessary to ensure the effective and timely execution of procedures. In the teaching hospital setting, the second surgeon is often replaced by a surgeon-in-training (surgical registrar or resident). Responsibilities of the surgeon include:

- Performing a "time-out" to ensure confirmation of the identity of the patient, the site of operation, the consent of the patient, the availability of the blood products if needed, and the procedure to be performed. A similar check is performed at the end of the procedure to make sure that all swabs, needles, and instruments used are accounted for and the specimen(s) correctly labeled.
- A surgical report of the procedure is written by the surgeon, mentioning any eventual difficulties or incidents encountered.
- After surgery, the surgeon gives clear written medical orders to the nurse-in-charge. Prior to that, the surgeon should be briefed about available medication at the facility. Medications prescribed by the surgeon that are not available at the facility should be purchased by the family prior to the operation.

20.1.1.5 Anesthetist

In our setting, the anesthetist is a specialized nurse responsible for the administration of anesthetics as well as analgesics during and after surgery. In the event of complications during surgery, he/she requires the assistance of an anesthesiologist, who is a medical doctor specialized in anesthesiology.

- The anesthesiologist is responsible for monitoring the vital signs such as cardiovascular and respiratory functions of the patient during procedures.

20.1.2 Equipment

Every surgical procedure requires the following equipment (Table 20.1). A robust maintenance schedule must be in place to ensure that all equipment is always in good working order:

- Anesthetic machine
- Oximeter
- Vital sign monitoring system
- Oxygen supply
- Theatre lights

20.1.3 Consumables

The following table lists the consumables that should be available in a surgical setting (Table 20.1).

Table 20.1 Consumables

Item	Description
Sutures	Ties: Vicryl 2/0, 0
	On needle absorbable: Vicryl (2/0, 0), vicryl rapid (3/0, 4/0), PDS (1/0)
	Non absorbable, for example, nylon 2/0, 3/0, 0, Prolene 03/0, 4/0, silk 2/0
Dressing materials	Gauze and plasters
Prep solutions	Savlon, Betadine, and Spirit
Sterile gloves	Size 6, 7, 7.5, 8 and 8–9
Scalpel blades	Range of sizes
Cannulas	For intravenous access, range of sizes
Drainage materials	Chest drains, corrugated drains and tube drains for abdominal surgeries
Nasogastric tubes	Long, thin, hollow tube which is passed through a nostril of the nose into the throat and down into the stomach. The tube can be used to feed a child if they are unable to take enough food by mouth or if they are not safely able to take food by mouth. Liquid foods pass through the tube into the stomach
Foley catheters	2-way: Sizes 12–18
	3-way: Sizes 18–22

20.1.4 Costing of Surgical Procedures

Costing procedures is a sensitive issue given the fragile prevailing economic condition of most patients. On one hand, attending surgeons would not perform without being paid. On the other hand, the hospital must obtain finances to maintain the surgical theatre and to remunerate the personnel. The administration consults directly with the medical director of the facility to determine cost for the patient and the renumeration of the attending surgeon and other participants.

As a guiding principle, the total cost to be borne by the patient can be shared using the 1/3–1/3–1/3 principle.

- 30% for the surgeon and his direct team.
- 30% theatre fees for the maintenance of the theatre and refill of consumables.

- 30% for the hospital that is arranging the consultations, providing the postsurgical nursing services and the follow-up.

In The Gambia, specific examples are as below:

- Minor cases: 2500–5000 GMD.
- Major cases: 10,000–15,000 GMD.
- Surgeons are remunerated at the rate of 1000–3000 GMD for minor cases and 6000–10,000 GMD for major cases.

20.2   The Surgical Procedure

The surgical procedure can be broken down into three stages:

1. Preoperative stage
2. Intraoperative stage
3. Postoperative stage

The WHO surgical checklist below is widely used and accepted in order to ensure safety before, during, and after surgical procedures (Fig. 20.2).

20.2.1 Preoperative Stage

This stage covers the period from the confirmation of a diagnosis to the beginning of the surgical procedure itself (Table 20.2).

An internist determines whether the medical condition of the patient can tolerate the surgical procedures. This is done in the setting of a preoperative consultation. This consultation is structured like any other medical consultation, consisting of history taking, thorough physical examination, and essential laboratory tests.

In the history, care is taken to thoroughly investigate the patient's previous surgical experience, their facility of wound healing, and personal and family history of coagulopathies.

During the physical examination, the presence of keloidal scars is noted and reported, and any

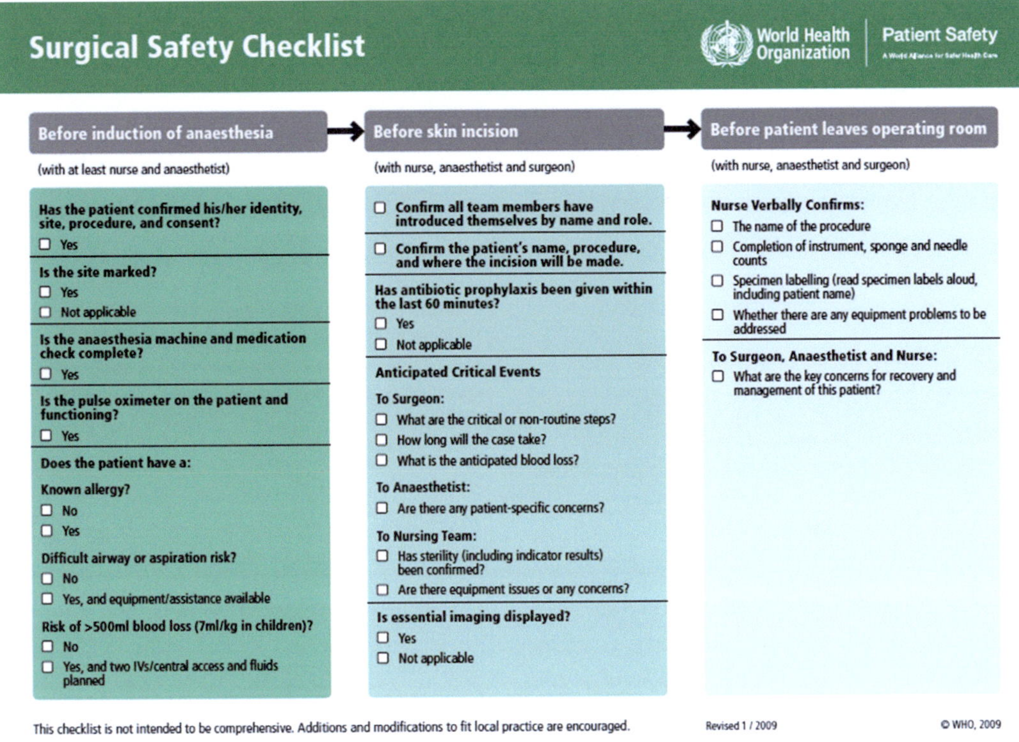

Fig. 20.2 The WHO surgical checklist

anomalies found during the cardiopulmonary examination are well documented and discussed with the surgical team.

Finally, paramedical examinations are performed to ensure the biologic fitness of the patient for the surgical procedure. Typically, the following paramedical investigations are carried out:

- Electrocardiogram (12-lane)
- FBC
- International normalized ratio (INR)
- Urine sticks (optional)
- Chest X-ray (optional)
- Directed echography (optional)

Following the paramedical examinations, surgical and anesthetic consultations are arranged with the patient to explain the procedure and the likely complications as well as the possible risks of anesthesia. The surgeon should explain the procedure to the patient and his/her family in simple, plain terms, and if possible, in the language that they understand best. Once the patient accepts the decision to go ahead with surgery, he/she assents to the procedure by marking a consent form with his/her signature or thumbprint.

The nursing staff is then responsible for ensuring that the following steps are carried out:

- The patient informs the nursing staff of possible dentures or prostheses that he/she may be wearing.
- Clean and possibly shave certain body parts before the operation.
- Inform the patient when to stop eating and drinking before the surgical procedure.
- The patient is given theatre gown or loose-fitting clothes on the day of the procedure.

20.2.2 Intraoperative Stage

This is a decisive stage of surgery. It includes:

- Administration of various anesthetic drugs.
- Adherence to established pathology-specific surgical protocols.

Table 20.2 Types of anesthesia

Method	Description/use	Comments
General anesthesia	*Intravenous:* Propofol, thiopentone sodium *or* *Inhalation:* Isoflurane, desflurane, medically inducing coma with loss of protective reflexes producing analgesia, amnesia, hypnosis, immobility	Usually 4 stages involved: • Stage 1. Induction • Stage 2. Excitement • Stage 3. Surgical anesthesia • Stage 4. Overdose *Cardiopulmonary monitoring is required:* • Continuous electrocardiography, continuous pulse oximetry • Blood pressure, and • Capnography
Regional anesthesia	• Fentanyl intravenous • Morphine sulfate, 10 mg ampoule, injected near a specific nerve or nerve bundle through a special needle or catheter to block sensation of pain from the area supplied by the nerve	It is most often used when procedure is confined to a specific region of the body or involves a large area of the body where systemic use of anesthetic might cause significant adverse side effects
Spinal block	• Procaine, levobupivacaine • Injecting of local anesthetic into the subarachnoid space generally through a fine needle, usually 9 cm (3.5 in)	Used either on its own or with sedation or general anesthetic in orthopedic surgery on pelvis, hip, or Caesarean section Contraindicated in bleeding disorders (thrombocytopenia or systemic anticoagulation)
Epidural anesthesia	*Bupivacaine* • Injected through a catheter placed into the epidural space. The injection can result in loss of sensation of pain, by blocking the transmission of signals through nerve fibers	Large doses may cause paralysis of the intercostal muscles and thoracic diaphragm and loss of sympathetic nerve input to the heart, which may cause dyspnea, a significant decrease in heart rate and blood pressure
Local anesthesia	• *Rapidocaine, lidocaine*, 1–5 ml instilled intramuscularly around the lesion • Wait 3–5 min for the anesthesia to set in before starting the procedure	Use before suturing, debriding, or cleaning wounds Suturing is done on wounds without loss of substance, preferably within 6 h of occurrence of the trauma

• Proper utilization of surgical equipment and consumables.
• Execution of specific surgical procedures adapted to the diagnosis in question.

20.2.2.1 Choice of Anesthesia

Below are the available methods of anesthesia. The procedure is performed by a qualified nurse anesthetist (Tables 20.2 and 20.3).

20.2.2.2 Major Surgical Diagnoses

The following tables list common diagnoses and recommended surgical procedures for conditions that are commonly encountered in a hospital setting (Tables 20.4, 20.5, and 20.6).

20.2.3 Postoperative Stage

Optimal recovery from surgery requires a multidisciplinary team working together, with persistent close monitoring of patient vitality and well-being.

Recovery can take place in a room adjacent to the theatre, in the patient's wardroom, or in an intensive care unit. Nurses are charged with the

Table 20.3 Anesthetics, preoperative medicines, and medical gases

1. General anesthetics and oxygen	
Inhalational medicines	
Halothane	Inhalation
Isoflurane	Inhalation
Nitrous oxide	Inhalation
Oxygen	Inhalation (medical gas)
Injectable medicines	
Ketamine	Injection: 50 mg (as hydrochloride)/ml in 10 ml vial
Propofol	Injection: 10 mg/ml; 20 mg/ml Thiopental may be used as an alternative depending on local availability and cost
2. Local anesthetics	
Bupivacaine	Injection: 0.25%; 0.5% (hydrochloride) in vial Injection for spinal anesthesia: 0.5% (hydrochloride) in 4 ml ampoule to be mixed with 7.5% glucose solution
Lidocaine	Injection: 1%; 2% (hydrochloride) in vial Injection for spinal anesthesia: 5% (hydrochloride) in 2 ml ampoule to be mixed with 7.5% glucose solution Topical forms: 2–4% (hydrochloride)
Morphine	Injection: 10 mg (sulfate or hydrochloride) in 1 ml ampoule

responsibility of closely monitoring patient recovery. Blood pressure, pulse, breathing pattern, and oxygen blood saturation are closely monitored. Common acute postsurgical complications may include nausea and vomiting, bleeding in the throat after tracheal intubation, pain at the surgical site, and thirst. These may be addressed with the help of the internist.

In minor cases, the patient is given food and water as soon as the effects of anesthesia have worn off. In some major cases, food intake is more progressive according to the instructions of the surgeon.

As a standard, patients are put on intravenous perfusions, analgesics, and antibiotics. Where judged necessary, thromboprophylaxis may be prescribed to prevent deep-vein thrombosis.

Special care is taken to prevent bed sores by using proper bedding and by moving the patient appropriately. As soon as the patient is able to ambulate, he/she is encouraged to start walking around in the presence of a nurse or family member.

Patients are discharged with clear instructions: For example, on special dietary restrictions, on how soon to resume normal day-to-day activities, and on incisional wound dressing. An appointment date for postoperative follow-up is provided as well as instructions for any adjuvant therapy that may be needed.

20.2.4 Blood Transfusion Unit in a Standard Minimal-Resource Facility

In collaboration with national health authorities, standard minimal-resource facilities are enabled to provide lifesaving blood transfusion services where and when needed. Below is an outline of a blood transfusing service (Table 20.7).

Table 20.4 Emergency surgical diagnoses and procedures

Diagnosis	Procedure	Comments
Appendicitis	Appendectomy: Open or laparoscopic	• Young patients • Early surgery after diagnosis to prevent serious complications (peritonitis)
Chest	Pneumothorax/hemothorax drained with chest tube	Ensure appropriate protection of injured body part
Closed abdomen hepatic rupture	Radiology studies to assess possible internal bleeding Clinical observation if hemodynamically stable Emergency surgery if instability	
Ingestion of caustic substances	Caustic injury to the esophagus and/or the stomach	Intentional ingestion or history of psychiatric disorder
Large bowel obstruction • Sigmoid volvulus • Cecal volvulus	Resection of sigmoid volvulus, colon cancer	Found mostly in older patients
Open wound, limbs	Wound exploration with local anesthetics Surgery in case of penetrating wound Plaster of Paris (POP) Surgery: osteosynthesis	
Peptic ulcer (perforated)	• Laparotomy • Suturing of the ulcer • Proton pump inhibitor (PPI) administration associated with antibiotics	• History of cigarette smoking and presence of *H. pylori* • Failed triple therapy?
Peritonitis	Laparotomy and peritoneal lavage with antibiotics Specific procedure depends on etiology	Most common causes are perforated hollow viscus: Peptic ulcer and appendicitis
Small bowel obstruction	Reduction of incarcerated hernia/postoperative adhesions resection Resection of sigmoid volvulus, colon cancer	Personal history of previous surgery or an inguinal hernia Prevention by repair of inguinal hernia
Soft-tissue infections	Incision, drainage and thorough lavage with abundant diluted Betadine solution	Debridement and regular wound dressing
Trauma, head	Surgical evacuation of epidural or subdural hematoma, otherwise trephination	Usually due to motor vehicle accidents and sports accidents
Visceral artery aneurysm	Initially characterization by ultrasonography and Doppler ultrasonography Arterioplasty	Urgent referral to the vascular surgery unit

Table 20.5 Common emergency room procedures/minor procedures

Procedure	Indications	Comments
Biopsy	For diagnostic purposes	Pathology studies to confirm diagnosis
Central venous line placement	Venous access for volume resuscitation, administration of vasopressors and inotropes	Invasive procedure (femoral vein is the preferred access route in case of emergencies)
Chest drain placement	Pleural effusion/empyema	Check for immune deficiencies. Institute appropriate antibiotherapy covering anaerobes
Creation of arteriovenous fistulae	End-stage kidney failure	Vascular access for hemodialysis
Debridement or amputation	Ulcers or diabetic foot	Ensure control of blood sugar levels by proper observance of medications
Dilation and curettage	In utero fetal death	History of miscarriage
Local and regional anesthesia	Ingrown toenails, amputations	
Local excision	Lipoma, nevus, basaliomas	Pathology studies to rule out cancer
Nasogastric tube placement	Prevention of vomiting	
Tracheal intubation	Unconscious patient or trauma with compromised airways	Evaluate Glasgow coma score
Tracheotomy	In cases where tracheal intubation is not feasible	Invasive procedure reserved for extreme emergencies
Urinary catheter placement	Measurement of urine output	Use for short durations to avoid urinary tract infection

Table 20.6 Elective surgical procedures

Diagnosis	Procedure	Comments
General		
Abdominal conditions • Mechanical obstruction • Cholecystectomy	Bowel obstruction Cholecystectomy for gallstones	Affects mostly obese middle-aged women Laparoscopic approach preferred over open surgery
Fissure	Surgical fissurectomy	Avoid constipation
Fistula • Ano-vesicular • Anovaginal	Fistulectomy	History of anal abscesses
Goiter	Lobectomy or total thyroidectomy	Lifetime hormone substitution therapy needed after total thyroidectomy
Hemorrhoids	Hemorrhoidectomy, hemorrhoidopexy	Avoid constipation (food fibers or laxatives) and spices
Hernia • Inguinal • Femoral • Umbilical • Incisional (postoperative)	Herniorrhaphy or mesh repair	Avoid or treat causes of increased abdominal pressure (constipation, chronic coughing, prostate hypertrophy)
Gynecology/obstetrics		
Breast lump	Lumpectomy, mastectomy	Check for family history of breast cancer
Cervical cancer	Radiation therapy, hysterectomy	
Complications during delivery	Caesarean section	
Postdelivery hemorrhage	Vessel ligation, hysterectomy	Leading cause of maternal mortality
Uterine myoma	Myomectomy, hysterectomy	
Oncology		
Colorectal cancer	Colectomy or lower anterior resection with lymphadenectomy	Affects mostly older patients above 50 years of age
Gastric cancer	Total or partial gastrectomy with lymphadenectomy	Presents as chronic gastrointestinal bleed and anemia
Liver cancer	Segmental resection or hepatectomy	History of Hepatitis B or C with liver cirrhosis
Esophageal cancer	Esophagectomy with lymphadenectomy	Presents as progressive dysphagia Poor prognosis due to late diagnosis
Urology		
Acute urinary retention	Placement of urinary catheter	History of prostate hypertrophy
Benign urogenital cases (hydrocele, epidydimal cysts, kidney stones)	Hydrocele repair, epidydimal cyst excision, orchiectomy, circumcision, vasectomy, nephrolithotomy, nephrectomy	
Obstructive prostate hypertrophy, prostate cancers	Prostatectomy	
Phimosis, cultural and religious practices	Circumcision	Ensure sterility of material

Table 20.7 Blood transfusion indications and procedure

Theme	Comments

Blood transfusion
Is the process of transferring whole blood or blood components from one person (donor) to another (recipient)
 	
Clinical benefits of blood transfusions
• Restoration of lost blood
• Improvement clotting time
• Improve the ability of the blood to deliver oxygen to the body's tissues
	Clinical background
	Blood transfusion is a routine medical procedure in which donated blood is provided through a narrow tube placed within a vein in the arm
	
	Indications of blood transfusion
	• Significant blood loss during surgery or injury
	• Severe anemias of any origin
	• Bleeding disorders
	
	Requirements for blood transfusion
	• Physician familiar with basics of hematology and allergy management
	• A trained laboratory technician familiar with the laboratory tests outlined below
	• A clinical diagnostic laboratory equipped facilities able to perform
	  • Full blood count
	  • ABO blood grouping
	  • Crossmatching
	  • Serologies screening for major blood-borne infectious diseases: HBV, HCV, HIV, syphilis, and malaria
	• Blood bags: Special plastic bags that can contain 450 ml of blood
	• Blood transfusion catheter
	
	Indication of blood transfusion
	• Significant blood loss during surgery or injury
	• Severe anemias of any origin
	• Bleeding disorders
	
	Components of blood
	• *Erythrocytes* (red cells) for gas exchange
	• *Leucocytes* (white cells) for defense
	• *Plasma* is the liquid part of blood containing several proteins
	• *Platelets* for proper clot formation
	
	Note: In a minimal-resource facility, erythrocytes are most commonly transfused. Patients can also receive whole blood, but whole blood transfusions are not common
	
	Potential complications associated with transfusion
	• Mild complications: Allergic reactions, which might cause hives and itching, and fever
	• Blood-borne infections: HIV or hepatitis B or C (rare)
	• Acute immune hemolytic reaction
	• Delayed hemolytic reaction
	• Graft versus host disease
	
	The procedure of transfusing packed erythrocytes
	• Determine blood type: A, B, AB, or O, and whether Rh-positive or Rh-negative
	• The donated blood is crossmatched for compatibility with recipient blood type
	• Exclude past history of transfusion complication by taking good medical history
	• The wide gauge intravenous transfusion catheter is placed in an appropriate vein
	• Perform proper identification check to ensure correctness of blood to be donated
	• With the patient in a comfortable recumbent position, the donated blood bag that has been stored in a plastic bag is transfused via intravenous catheter slowly for 1–2 h
	• Periodic monitoring of BP and respiratory pattern by attending nurse
	• The patient is instructed to report to nurse immediately if the patient develops fever, dyspnea, chills, unusual pruritus, chest or back pain, or a sense of uneasiness

(continued)

Table 20.7 (continued)

Theme	Comments
	Clinical notes • In some cases, 2 mg dexamethasone tab is administered to the patient to attenuate any presumptive allergic reaction • Based on the clinical situation, 20 mg furosemide may be given reduce fluid overload • Transfusion is generally considered if hemoglobin is less than 7 g/dL • Leukocyte reduction of donor blood is the removal of white blood cells by filtration. Most standard transfusion canula sets have an inbuilt filter which depletes the leucocytes as the transfusion proceeds. Leucocyte-depleted donor blood is generally better tolerated • Addition of riboflavin with subsequent exposure to UV light has been shown to be effective in inactivating pathogens (viruses, bacteria, parasites, and white blood cells) in blood products

Contents

21.1   **Local Factors that Must Be Considered When Adapting the WHO
        Essential Medicine List** 265

21.2   **The Pharmacy and the Medicine Dispenser** 266
21.2.1 Basic Knowledge Needed for Medicine Dispensing 267
21.2.2 Routes of Administration of Medicines 267
21.2.3 Medicines with Age or Weight Restrictions 267
21.2.4 The Art of Prescribing a Medication and the BMC-EML 269

Bibliography 269

According to WHO, "essential medicines are those that satisfy the primary health care needs of the population and they should be available within the context of functioning health systems at all times in adequate amounts, in the appropriate dosage forms, with assured quality, and at a price the individual and the community can afford."

To practice evidence-based medicine (EBM), Bijilo Medical Center (BMC) has adapted the WHO Essential Medicines List (EML). Based on local epidemiological factors, economic impacts, cultural reasons, and national regulatory laws, the EML has been adapted by BMC to accommodate local conditions, on one hand, and maintain the rigors of evidence-based medical practices of drug usage, on the other hand. To differentiate it from the WHO original document, the modified EML is called BMC-EML. Note that as the medi-cations necessarily differ in some respects between the documents, the numbering and order of the categories also vary.

21.1   Local Factors that Must Be Considered When Adapting the WHO Essential Medicine List

The WHO EML is exhaustive and well thought out. Nonetheless, based on a multitude of factors, pragmatic modifications are made to adapt the EML to specific local conditions. Some of the factors that must be considered when adapting the EML to a specific low-income region are listed and discussed below:

Epidemiological data: It is important to liaise with local health authorities and research

© The Author(s), under exclusive license to Springer Nature Switzerland AG 2021
M. Touray, A. Touray, *Clinical Work and General Management of a Standard Minimal-Resource
Facility*, Sustainable Development Goals Series, https://doi.org/10.1007/978-3-030-71032-3_21

institution if available to learn about prevalent microbes in the area of action. The strains and species of locally prevailing pathologic bacteria, fungi, and protozoa need to be considered when establishing the list of antimicrobial agents the facility has to purchase. A constant review of emergence of resistance to these elected antimicrobes should be exercised. Relevant changes should be effected periodically.

Economic factors: In most cases, the burden of the cost of drugs and supplies is borne by the patients. Due to the low-income nature of the region, the cost of medicine and supplies should be kept at a minimum. Costs of antibiotics, test kits, and other consumables vary greatly. Utmost care is used to select those with the best quality-price-benefit ratio for the patient—all these, bearing in mind the exigence of evidence-based medicine. Generics are favored wherever possible. We strongly discourage the unnecessary use of auxiliary medicine.

Cultural, religious and traditional sensitivity: To obtain a good clinical outcome, care givers and institutions pay special attention the prevailing local traditions. In the same light, the choice of medication and supplies reflects this important notion wherever possible. Specific examples may be the use of suppositories, choice of contraceptive medication and devices, blood transfusion medicine and methods, and various probes for ultrasound examination, just to mention a few.

Logistical considerations: Logistical challenges are myriad. Medicines may have to be imported from far. The sea, air, and road transportation need special planning. The cost around these operations may be significant. To ensure sustainability, efforts must be made to keep these costs at a minimum. The cold chain may be important. The shelf life of the medicine and supplies should not be overlooked. Consequently, to the extent possible, we opt for medicines with a long shelf life that do not need cooling and that are packaged in a nonfragile manner. Special arrangements are made for vaccines and a short list of medicines that must be transported and maintained at lower temperatures.

Legal obligations: Special attention must be paid to legal regulations around selected medicines and supplies. For example, morphine derivatives and radioactive material, need special attention when including in an adpated essential medcine list. The toxicity of material use for cleaning surfaces or for developing and fixing films also need special consideration. We consult with the relevant regulatory health authorities to obtain the essential certificates for the purchase and use of such medicines and supplies.

21.2 The Pharmacy and the Medicine Dispenser

In most low-income regions with a low density of healthcare personnel trained to prescribe medicines, the roles of a pharmacy in a healthcare facility and in the community are multiple and very important (Fig. 21.1). National regulatory authorities mandated to restrict the inappropriate acquisition of prescribed medicines are often overwhelmed.

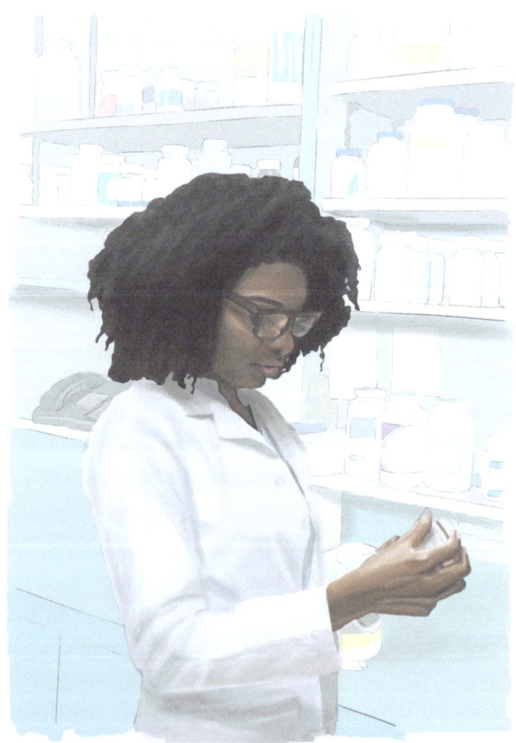

Fig. 21.1 The pharmacy is a crucial unit in a standard minimal-resource facility. The pharmacy constitutes a convivial place where patients receive their medicine. They obtain appropriate instructions on how to use these medications

Hence, to obtain a good clinical outcome for consulting patients, it is very important for healthcare facilities to establish an in-house pharmacy that is functional, well-staffed, and adequately supplied with essential drugs. We strive to prescribe medicines that are in the WHO Essential Medicine List. We make sure that patients obtain their prescribed medicines in our facility. The correct dispensing of prescribed medicine is an integral and critical part of healthcare.

It may be a challenge to recruit an already trained medicine dispenser often called "pharmacist." Most national healthcare systems provide courses with specific curricula to train medicine dispensers who are capable of adequately dispensing prescribed drugs. In the absence of such trained drug dispensers, it is common practice to train other healthcare workers (nurse attendants, laboratory assistants, or public health officers) to function as medicine dispenser. Such in-house training can be obtained on the job. It is the joint responsibility of the physician in charge and senior state-registered nurse to provide such in-house medicine dispensing training.

The uninterrupted supply of medicine and other medical consumables is another challenge that impacts directly on the quality of healthcare provided. A sustained availability of these essential supplies depends on financial factors, logistical issues, as well as the level of motivation and training of directly involved pharmacy staff: Proper stock records must be kept, and resulting statics are used to make bulk, yearly procurement of supplies. Unfortunately, to ensure quality control of the purchased medicine and supplies, we opt for overseas procurement. Specifically, we would put in our annual order in June, arrange for the transportation, and we would typically receive the goods in September of the same year. The shelf life of the purchased supplies needs to be monitored.

21.2.1   Basic Knowledge Needed for Medicine Dispensing

To be able to dispense prescribed medication to patients, the medicine dispenser must have a basic knowledge on the galenic form in which the medication is present, the mode of application, the indication for prescribing, and eventual side effects. It is the responsibility of the physician in charge or a senior experienced nurse to train the candidate drug dispenser. Below are some of the pertinent notions and vocabulary that must be very clear to the candidate medicine dispenser to be able to adequately dispense prescribed drugs to patients and their escorts.

21.2.2   Routes of Administration of Medicines

This refers to the way a medicine is administered to the patient (Tables 21.1, 21.2, and 21.3). The route needs to be understood by the drug dispenser, who should take time to explain it to the patient. In general, the routes of administration are either oral (by mouth) or parenteral (routes other than the mouth).

For simplicity, medicine administration routes can be summarized as follows:

- *Oral* route: medication is the provision of medication by mouth which will then be absorbed into the gastrointestinal lumen.
- *Topical* route (skin, eyes, ears)
- *Inhalation* route (nose, mouth)
- *Parenteral* route: any pathway of administering a medicine other than the oral (oro-gastro-enteral) pathway. Mainly by injections (intravenous, intramuscular, subcutaneous, intra spinal, intrathecal, etc.)
- *Vaginal* route
- *Anal* route
- *Sublingual* route

21.2.3   Medicines with Age or Weight Restrictions

Several biological and clinical factors of the patient have to be considered when administering medication (Table 21.4). Among these are:

- Age and weight (most important!)
- History of allergy

Table 21.1 Oral administration: principal dosage forms used to present medicines for oral administration

Galenic	Definition
Solid oral dosage form	• Refers to tablets or capsules or other solid dosage forms such as "melt" that are immediate-release preparations. It implies that there is no difference in clinical efficacy or safety between the available dosage forms, and countries should therefore choose between the form(s) listed depending on quality and availability • The term "solid oral dosage form" is never intended to allow any type of modified-release tablet
Tablets	Refers to a specific type of tablet: *Chewable* – tablets that are intended to be chewed before being swallowed *Dispersible* – tablets that are intended to be dispersed in water or another suitable liquid before being swallowed *Soluble* – tablets that are intended to be dissolved in water or another suitable liquid before being swallowed *Crushable* – tablets that are intended to be crushed before being swallowed *Scored* – tablets bearing a break mark or marks where subdivision is intended in order to provide doses of less than one tablet *Sublingual* – tablets that are intended to be placed beneath the tongue The term "tablet" is always qualified with an additional term (in parentheses) in entries where one of the following types of tablet is intended: Gastro-resistant (such tablets may sometimes be described as enteric-coated or as delayed release), prolonged release or another modified-release form
Capsules	Refers to hard or soft capsules The term may sometimes be modified to become enteric-coated, delayed release, or prolonged release
Granules	Preparations that are issued to the patient as granules to be swallowed without further preparation, to be chewed, or to be taken either in or with water or another suitable liquid The term "granules" without further qualification is never intended to allow any type of modified-release granules
Oral powder	Preparations that are issued to the patient as powder (usually as single dose) to be taken either in or with water or another suitable liquid
Oral liquid	Liquid preparations intended to be swallowed; that is, oral solutions, suspensions, emulsions, and oral drops, including those constituted from powders or granules, but not those preparations intended for oromucosal administration, for example, gargles and mouthwashes Oral liquids presented as powders or granules may offer benefits in the form of better stability and lower transport costs. If more than one type of oral liquid is available in the same market (e.g., solution, suspension, and granules for reconstitution), they may be interchanged and, in such cases, should be bioequivalent. It is preferable that oral liquids do not contain sugar and that solutions for children do not contain alcohol

Table 21.2 Parenteral administration: principal dosage forms of medicines

Term	Definition
Injection	Refers to solutions, suspensions, and emulsions, including those constituted from powders or concentrated solutions
Intravenous infusion	Refers to solutions and emulsions including those constituted from powders or concentrated solutions

Table 21.3 Other dosage forms: other routes through which medicines are administered

Route of administration	Term to be used
To the eye	Eye drops, eye ointments
Topical	For liquids: Lotions, paints For semi-solids: Cream, ointment
Rectal	Suppositories, gel or solution
Vaginal	Pessaries or vaginal tablets
Inhalation	Powder for inhalation, pressurized inhalation, nebulizer

- Drug interactions
- Ethnicity
- Eating habits
- Exposure to sunlight
- Sporting activity
- Gender

The medicine dispenser should have knowledge about the proper use of the medication and notions of age or weight limitation of certain medication. These notions are herein tabulated below.

Table 21.4 Medication age/weight restrictions

Medication	Restriction
Artesunate + pyronaridine tetraphosphate	>5 kg
Benzyl benzoate	>2 years
Betamethasone topical preparations	Hydrocortisone preferred in neonates
Cefazolin	>1 month
Ceftriaxone	>41 weeks corrected gestational age
Doxycycline	>8 years (except for serious infections, for example, cholera)
Fluoxetine	>8 years
Ibuprofen	>3 months (except iv form for patent ductus arteriosus)
Mefloquine	>5 kg or >3 months
Metoclopramide	Not in neonates
Silver sulfadiazine	>2 months
Tetracaine	Not in preterm neonates
Trimethoprim	>6 months
Xylometazoline	>3 months

21.2.4 The Art of Prescribing a Medication and the BMC-EML

In prescribing medication, effort is made to adhere to this established BMC-EML and to minimize the use of auxiliary medication (Fig. 21.1). For example, advice such as "eat five fruits per day" is more appropriate than prescribing expensive multivitamins for which there may be no scientific evidence of efficacy. In the same vein, BMC advises patients to "drink 3 liters of water per day and walk at least 20 min, 3×/day" instead of prescribing laxatives.

The prescription of anti-infectious agents, painkillers, anti-reflux medication, and other drug groups is guided by the same principles: providing adequate advice first and then prescribing medications only where absolutely indicated.

The BMC-EML (current at the time of publication) is provided in Chap. 22. It is required that all healthcare workers be thoroughly familiar with these medicines. However, formal prescription of medicines remains the responsibility of physicians.

Following the BMC-EML are ancillary reference tables listing medicines with age or weight restrictions, as well as principal dosage forms used in the EML.

Prescribing drugs is a medical act of both high therapeutic value and potential risk. When deciding upon a prescription, the practitioner should bear in mind that it should be: Effective, Rational, Adjusted, Secure, Monitored, and Economical (ERASME).

Bibliography

1. Papadakis MA, McPhee SJ, Rabow MW. Current medical diagnosis and treatment. New York, NY: McGraw-Hill Education; 2019. https://accessmedicine.mhmedical.com/book.aspx?bookID=2449.
2. Preclinical and clinical lecture notes of the curriculum of medical studies, Faculty of Medicine, University of Lausanne, Course year 2015–2021.
3. Scientific-Units-Recommendations-Formulas (SURF) guidelines, Médecine Interne General, Philippe Furger en collaboration avec Thierry Fumeaux et le SURF-team. 2020.
4. Pocket Book of Hospital Care for Children. Guidelines for the management of, common, childhood illnesses, 2nd ed. World Health Organisation; 2013.
5. Essential med notes, 2020 Comprehensive medical references and review for the United States Medical Licensing Exam (USMLE) step II and the Medical Council of Canada Qualifying Exam (MCCQE) Part 1, 36th ed., Sara Mirali and Ayesh Seneviratne.
6. WHO model list of essential medicines, 20th list. World Health Organization; March 2017, Amended August 2017. https://apps.who.int/iris/bitstream/handle/10665/273826/EML-20-eng.pdf?ua=1.
7. The Gambia standard drug treatment guidelines, 2nd ed. Department of State for Health and Social Welfare, The Republic of the Gambia; 2001. http://apps.who.int/medicinedocs/documents/s22418en/s22418en.pdf.
8. Cornuz J, Pasche O, Kermode-Noppel T. Compas: Stratégies de prise en charge clinique, Médecine interne générale ambulatoire. Lausanne: Institute of Social and Preventive Medicine; 2010.
9. Diseases and conditions: comprehensive guides on hundreds of conditions. Mayo Clinic. https://www.mayoclinic.org/diseases-conditions.

Adapted Essential Medicines List for a Standard Minimal-Resource Health Facility

22

Contents

22.1   **Essential Medicines for Neurological Conditions in a Standard Minimal-Resource Facility** 272

22.2   **Essential Medicines for Ear, Nose, and Throat (ENT) Conditions in a Standard Minimal-Resource Facility** 272

22.3   **Essential Medicines for Cardiology Conditions in a Standard Minimal-Resource Facility** 272

22.4   **Essential Medicines for Respiratory Conditions in a Standard Minimal-Resource Facility** 272

22.5   **Essential Medicines for Gastrointestinal Conditions in a Standard Minimal-Resource Facility** 272

22.6   **Essential Medicines Used in Urology and Nephrology Conditions in a Standard Minimal-Resource Facility** 280

22.7   **Essential Medicines Used in Gynecology-Obstetrics Conditions in a Standard Minimal-Resource Facility** 280

22.8   **Essential Medicines Used in Musculoskeletal Conditions in a Standard Minimal-Resource Facility** 283

22.9   **Essential Medicines Used in Dermatology and Allergic Conditions in a Standard Minimal-Resource Facility** 283

22.10   **Essential Medicines Used for Hematology Conditions in a Standard Minimal-Resource Facility** 283

22.11   **Essential Medicines Used in Infectious Disease Conditions in a Standard Minimal-Resource Facility** 283

22.12   **Essential Medicines Used in Endocrinology Conditions in Standard Minimal-Resource Facility** 292

22.13   **Essential Medicines Used in Ophthalmology Conditions in a Standard Minimal-Resource Facility** 292

22.14 **Essential Medicines Used in Psychiatry Conditions in a Standard Minimal-Resource Facility** 295

22.15 **Essential Medicines Used for Palliative Care in a Standard Minimal-Resource Facility** 295

Bibliography 298

22.1 Essential Medicines for Neurological Conditions in a Standard Minimal-Resource Facility

The following proposed list of medicines may be used to treat neurological and related disease conditions in a standard minimal-resource center (Table 22.1). The mechanism of action of the medicines is specifically directed against the variable etiologies: infectious, metabolic, toxic, congenital, traumatic, degenerative, and oncologic. Supportive agents may be included to facilitate rapid symptomatic relief.

Neurologic disease conditions affect the brain, spinal cord, nerves, and muscles. The medicines are classified based on their mechanism of action. It is noteworthy that the drugs mentioned below may affect mainly cellular function in the nervous system.

22.2 Essential Medicines for Ear, Nose, and Throat (ENT) Conditions in a Standard Minimal-Resource Facility

The following proposed list of medicines may be used to treat ear, nose, and throat disease conditions in a standard minimal-resource center.

The mechanism of action of the medicines is specifically directed against the variable etiologies:

- Infectious
- Allergic
- Metabolic
- Toxic
- Degenerative
- Hyper-prolific or neoplastic

- Congenital
- Traumatic

The medication uses in these disease conditions are outlined elsewhere in this chapter.

Supportive agents may be included to facilitate rapid symptomatic relief.

22.3 Essential Medicines for Cardiology Conditions in a Standard Minimal-Resource Facility

The following proposed list of medicines may be used to treat cardiovascular disease conditions in a standard minimal-resource center (Table 22.2). The mechanism of action of the medicines is specifically directed against the variable etiologies: infectious, metabolic, toxic, degenerative, congenital, traumatic, and neoplastic. Supportive agents may be included to facilitate rapid symptomatic relief (Table 22.3).

22.4 Essential Medicines for Respiratory Conditions in a Standard Minimal-Resource Facility

22.5 Essential Medicines for Gastrointestinal Conditions in a Standard Minimal-Resource Facility

The following proposed list of medicines may be used to treat gastroenterology disease conditions in a standard minimal-resource center (Table 22.4). The mechanism of action of the medicines is

Table 22.1 Essential medicines for neurological conditions in a standard minimal-resource facility

Medicine class	Generic name, galenic forms, indications, and notes
Nonsteroidal anti-inflammatory drugs (NSAIDs) inhibits cyclooxygenases (COX-1 and COX-2), thereby disrupting the production of prostaglandin, an important mediator of pain and inflammation *Effects of NSAIDs* • Reduces pain • Decreases fever • Prevents blood clots • Decreases inflammation *Common classes* • Salicylates • Propionic acid derivatives • Acetic acid derivatives • Enolic acid (oxicam) derivatives • Selective COX-2 inhibitors (coxibs) • Sulfonanilide	*Acetylsalicylic acid* • Suppository: 50–150 mg • Tablet: 100–500 mg • Indications: Antiplatelet, acute and chronic use, for use for rheumatic fever, juvenile arthritis, Kawasaki disease, Juvenile joint diseases, myocarditis • Note: Salicylism: Nausea, emesis, diarrhea, hyperthermia, tinnitus, hyperpnea (respiratory alkalosis); higher toxicity in children and the elderly (dehydration, hyperthermia, metabolic acidosis) *Ibuprofen* • Oral liquid: 200 mg/5 ml • Tablet: 200 mg, 400 mg, 600 mg • Note: Not for use in children less than 3 months of age • Analgesic, anti-inflammatory, and antipyretic properties *Naproxen* • Oral tabs: 500 mg, 250 mg • Analgesic, anti-inflammatory, and antipyretic properties *Adverse effects* • Increased risk of gastrointestinal ulcers and bleeding • Renal function impairment • Allergic reactions • Increase risk of cardiovascular events
Nonopioids Group of medicines including NSAIDs and acetaminophens	*Paracetamol* • Oral liquid: 120 mg/5 ml, 125 mg/5 ml • Suppository: 100 mg • Tablet: 100–500 mg • Note: Not recommended for anti-inflammatory use, due to lack of proven benefit to that effect. Better tolerated option than other NSAIDs (gastric tract symptoms) • Intoxication: Causes hepatic necrosis, renal tubular necrosis, hypoglycemia • Antidote: Acetylcysteine
Opioids analgesics Also known as narcotic analgesics, are pain relievers that act on the central nervous system. Common examples are morphine, oxycodone, and hydrocodone *Side effects* • Nausea, vomiting • Dizziness and sedation feelings of euphoria • Headache • Lethargy • Respiratory depression • Additivity • Dry mouth, constipation • Pruritus	*Codeine* • Tablet: 30 mg (phosphate) • Good p.o. bioavailability • Cough suppressant • Note: Abusive use and addiction *Fentanyl* • Transdermal patch: 12 µg/h, 25 µg/h, 50 µg/h, 75 µg/h, and 100 µg/h. for the management of cancer pain • Adverse effects: Muscle stiffness, no release of histamine *Morphine* • Granules (slow release, to mix with water): 20–200 mg (morphine sulfate) • Injection: 10 mg (morphine hydrochloride or morphine sulfate) in 1 ml ampoule, IM or iv • Oral liquid: 10 mg (morphine hydrochloride or morphine sulfate)/5 ml • Tablet (slow release): 10–200 mg (morphine hydrochloride or morphine sulfate) • Tablet (immediate release): 10 mg (morphine sulfate) • Alternatives limited to hydromorphone

(continued)

Table 22.1 (continued)

Medicine class	Generic name, galenic forms, indications, and notes
	Oxycodone • Extended use may cause a diminution of therapeutic effects, a need to increase opioid dose, and neurological complex modification leading to drug dependence
General anesthetics and oxygen Medicines that when administered can induce diminished consciousness with loss of protective reflexes	*Administered by inhalation* • Halothane • Isoflurane • Nitrous oxide • Oxygen *Administered by injections* • *Ketamine:* 50 mg (as hydrochloride)/ml in 10 ml vial, iv • *Propofol:* 10 mg/ml, 20 mg/ml, iv • Thiopental may be used as an alternative, depending on local availability and cost.
Local anesthetics Medicines used to induce the absence of sensation (especially pain) in a specific part of the body	*Bupivacaine* • Injection: 0.25%, 0.5% (hydrochloride) in vial, IM • Injection for spinal anesthesia: 0.5% (hydrochloride) in 4 ml ampoule to be mixed with 7.5% glucose solution *Lidocaine* • Injection: 1%, 2% (hydrochloride) in vial, IM • Injection for spinal anesthesia: 5% (hydrochloride) in 2 ml ampoule to be mixed with 7.5% glucose solution • Topical forms: 2–4% (hydrochloride) *Morphine* • Injection: 10 mg (sulfate or hydrochloride) in 1 ml ampoule • IM or iv
Anticonvulsants/antiepileptics	*Carbamazepine* • Oral liquid: 100 mg/5 ml • Tablet (chewable): 100 mg, 200 mg • Tablet (scored): 100 mg, 200 mg • Diazepam • Gel or rectal solution: 5 mg/ml in 0.5 ml, 2 ml, 4 ml tubes • Long-acting (>24 h) benzodiazepine *Lorazepam* • Parenteral formulation: 2 mg/ml in 1 ml ampoule, 4 mg/ml in 1 ml ampoule • Indication: Status epilepticus • Magnesium sulcate • Injection: 0.5 g/ml in 2 ml ampoule (equivalent to 1 g in 2 ml, 50% weight/volume); 0.5 g/ml in 10 ml ampoule (equivalent to 5 g in 10 ml, 50% weight/volume) • For use in eclampsia and severe preeclampsia and not for other convulsant disorders *Midazolam* • Solution for oromucosal administration: 5 mg/ml, 10 mg/ml • Ampoule: 1 mg/ml, 10 mg/ml • For buccal administration when solution for oromucosal administration is not available • Phenobarbital • Injection: 200 mg/ml (sodium) • Oral liquid: 15 mg/5 ml • Tablet: 15–100 mg • Side effects: Respiratory depression, tolerance, dependence

Table 22.1 (continued)

Medicine class	Generic name, galenic forms, indications, and notes
	Phenytoin • Injection: 50 mg/ml in 5 ml vial (sodium salt), iv • Oral liquid: 25–30 mg/5 ml • Solid oral dosage form: 25 mg, 50 mg, 100 mg (sodium salt) • Tablet (chewable): 50 mg • The presence of both 25 mg/5 ml and 30 mg/5 ml strengths on the same market could cause confusion in prescribing and dispensing, and should be avoided • Side effects: Nystagmus, diplopia, ataxia, gingival enlargement, acne, hirsutism, potential teratogen *Valproic acid (sodium valproate)* • Oral liquid: 200 mg/5 ml • Tablet (crushable): 100 mg • Tablet (enteric coated): 200 mg, 500 mg (sodium valproate) • Indications: Large spectrum, antimanic, antimigraine • Side effects: Reversible alopecia, thrombocytopenia, potential teratogen
Antiparkinsonism medicines	*Levodopa + carbidopa* Galenic forms: Tablet: 100 mg + 10 mg, 100 mg + 25 mg, 250 mg + 25 mg

Table 22.2 Essential medicines prescribed for cardiology conditions in a standard minimal-resource facility

Medicine class	Generic name, galenic forms, indications, and notes
Antianginal medicines Wide variety of medicines that are used in the management of angina, a cardiac pathology characterized by a narrowing of the coronary arteries. Retrosternal (chest pain) is the main symptom	*Bisoprolol* • Galenic forms • Tablet: 1.25 mg, 5 mg • Includes metoprolol and carvedilol as alternatives *Glyceryl trinitrate* • Tablet (sublingual): 500 µg *Isosorbide dinitrate* • Tablet (sublingual): 5 mg *Verapamil* • Tablet: 40 mg, 80 mg (hydrochloride).
Antiarrhythmic medicines • Medicines used to convert an irregular heartbeat (arrhythmia) to its normal rhythm • Prevent an arrhythmia • Control the heartbeat during an arrhythmia *Note*: Commonly antiarrhythmics work by slowing the heart rate or by stabilizing myocardium	*Bisoprolol* • Tablet: 1.25 mg, 5 mg • Includes metoprolol and carvedilol as alternatives *Digoxin* • Injection: 250 µg/ml in 2 ml ampoule, iv • Oral liquid: 50 µg/ml • Tablet: 62.5 µg, 250 µg *Epinephrine (adrenaline)* • Injection: 100 µg/ml (as acid tartrate or hydrochloride) in 10 ml ampoule, IM *Lidocaine* • Injection: 20 mg (hydrochloride)/ml in 5 ml ampoule, IM *Verapamil* • Injection: 2.5 mg (hydrochloride)/ml in 2 ml ampoule, iv • Tablet: 40 mg, 80 mg (hydrochloride) *Amiodarone* • Injection: 50 mg/ml in 3 ml ampoule (hydrochloride), iv • Tablet: 100 mg, 200 mg, 400 mg (hydrochloride)

(continued)

Table 22.2 (continued)

Medicine class	Generic name, galenic forms, indications, and notes
Antihypertensive medicines A medicine that reduces high blood pressure Classification according to their mechanism of action: • Diuretics • Calcium channel blockers • ACE inhibitors • Angiotensin II receptor antagonists • Adrenergic receptor antagonists • Vasodilators • Renin inhibitors • Aldosterone receptor antagonist • Alpha-2 adrenergic receptor agonists	*Amlodipine* • Tablet: 5 mg (as maleate, mesylate, or besylate) *Bisoprolol* • Tablet: 1.25 mg, 5 mg • Includes atenolol, metoprolol, and carvedilol as alternatives • Atenolol should not be used as a first-line agent in uncomplicated hypertension in patients >60 years *Enalapril* • Tablet: 2.5 mg, 5 mg (as hydrogen maleate) *Hydralazine* • Powder for injection: 20 mg (hydrochloride) in ampoule, iv • Tablet: 25 mg, 50 mg (hydrochloride) • Hydralazine is listed for use only in the acute management of severe pregnancy-induced hypertension • Hydralazine is used in the treatment of essential hypertension and is not recommended in view of the evidence of greater efficacy and safety of other medicines *Hydrochlorothiazide* • Oral liquid: 50 mg/5 ml • Solid oral dosage form 12.5 mg, 25 mg *Methyldopa* • Tablet: 250 mg • Methyldopa is listed for use only in the management of pregnancy-induced hypertension • Methyldopa is used in the treatment of essential hypertension and is not recommended in view of the evidence of greater efficacy and safety of other medicines *Losartan* • Tablet: 25 mg, 50 mg, 100 mg
Medicines used in the heart failure Mostly, a combination of medicines are used to treat a failing heart so as to encompass the various underlying etiologies *Classification* • ACE inhibitors and ARBs • Anti-arrhythmic • Anti-arrhythmic • Antibiotics • Anticoagulants • Beta-blockers • Diuretics • Vasodilators	*Bisoprolol* • Tablet: 1.25 mg, 5 mg • Includes metoprolol and carvedilol as alternatives • Digoxin • Injection: 250 μg/ml in 2 ml ampoule, iv • Oral liquid: 50 μg/ml • Tablet: 62.5 μg, 250 μg *Enalapril* • Tablet: 2.5 mg, 5 mg (as hydrogen maleate) *Furosemide* • Injection: 10 mg/ml in 2 ml ampoule, iv • Oral liquid: 20 mg/5 ml • Tablet: 40 mg • Hydrochlorothiazide • Oral liquid: 50 mg/5 mL • Solid oral dosage form: 25 mg *Losartan* • Tablet: 25 mg, 50 mg, 100 mg *Spironolactone* • Tablet: 25 mg *Dopamine* • Injection: 40 mg/ml (hydrochloride) in 5 ml vial, iv *Spironolactone* • Tablet: 25 mg

Table 22.2 (continued)

Medicine class	Generic name, galenic forms, indications, and notes
Antiplatelet medicines Class of medicines that decrease platelet aggregation and inhibit thrombus formation. These medications are effective in the arterial circulation, where anticoagulants have minimal effect	*Acetylsalicylic acid* • Tablet: 100 mg *Clopidogrel* • Tablet: 75 mg, 300 mg • Thrombolytic medicines *Streptokinase* • Powder for injection: 1.5 million IU in vial
Lipid-lowering agents HMG-CoA reductase inhibitors (statins). These agents inhibit the rate-limiting step in cholesterol biosynthesis by competitively inhibiting HMG-CoA reductase	*Simvastatin* • Tablet: 5 mg, 10 mg, 20 mg, 40 mg • For use in high-risk patients • Contraindications: Hypersensitivity, active liver disease, pregnancy, lactation

Table 22.3 Essential medicines prescribed for respiratory conditions in standard minimal-resource facility

Class of medicine	Generic name, galenic forms, indications, and notes
Antiasthmatic and medicines for chronic obstructive pulmonary disease Medicines used to influence the in- and out-flow of air into the bronchi and bronchioles by either directly increasing their caliber (bronchodilators) or reducing the inflammatory processes that underlies asthma and COPD	*Beclomethasone* • Inhalation (aerosol): 50 μg (dipropionate) per dose, 100 μg (dipropionate) per dose (as chlorofluorocarbon [CFC] free forms) *Budesonide* • Inhalation (aerosol): 100 μg per dose, 200 μg per dose • Budesonide + formoterol • Dry powder inhaler: 100 μg + 6 μg per dose, 200 μg + 6 μg per dose • Epinephrine (adrenaline) • Injection: 1 mg (as hydrochloride or hydrogen tartrate) in 1 ml ampoule *Ipratropium bromide* • Inhalation (aerosol): 20 μg/metered dose *Salbutamol* • Inhalation (aerosol): 100 μg (as sulfate) per dose • Injection: 50 μg (as sulfate)/ml in 5 ml ampoule, IM • Metered dose inhaler (aerosol): 100 μg (as sulfate) per dose • Respirator solution for use in nebulizers: 5 mg (as sulfate)/ml
Medicines acting on the upper airways and mucosa In general, medicines have the capacity to dissolve mucous in the bronchi and sinus (e.g., acetyl cysteine), reduce pain (local anesthetic), or have antibacterial activity	*Acetyl cysteine* • Powder for solution, 600 mg sachets *Acetic acid* • Topical: 2%, in alcohol *Budesonide* • Nasal spray: 100 μg per dose *Ciprofloxacin* • Topical: 0.3% drops (as hydrochloride) *Xylometazoline* • Nasal spray: 0.05%, not for children <3 months

Table 22.4 Essential medicines prescribed for gastrointestinal conditions in a standard minimal-resource facility

Class of medicine	Generic name, galenic forms, indications, and notes
Antiulcer medicines The mainstay of antiulcer management is: • Eradication of *Helicobacter pylori* (*H. pylori*) • Withdrawal of NSAIDs • Prescription of proton pump inhibitors	*Omeprazole* • Powder for injection: 40 mg in vial • Powder for oral liquid: 20 mg, 40 mg sachets • Solid oral dosage form: 10 mg, 20 mg, 40 mg *Ranitidine* • Injection: 25 mg/ml (as hydrochloride) in 2 ml ampoule, iv • Oral liquid: 75 mg/5 ml (as hydrochloride) • Tablet: 150 mg (as hydrochloride)
Antiemetic medicines Antiemetic drugs are used to treat nausea and vomiting caused by various factors including medications, motion sickness, infections, or gastroenteritis Antiemetic drugs • Modulate peristalsis (prokinetic) or • Block specific neurotransmitter	*Dexamethasone* • Injection: 4 mg/ml in 1 ml ampoule (as disodium phosphate salt), iv or IM • Oral liquid: 0.5 mg/5 ml, 2 mg/5 ml • Solid oral dosage form: 0.5 mg, 0.75 mg, 1.5 mg, 4 mg *Metoclopramide* • Injection: 5 mg (hydrochloride)/ml in 2 ml ampoule, iv • Oral liquid: 5 mg/5 ml • Tablet: 10 mg (hydrochloride) • Not in neonates *Promethazine* • Injection: 10 mg in 2 ml vial, iv or IM • Tablet: 10 mg
Anti-inflammatory medicines Reduce the inflammatory process by specifically blocking cox ½ pathway and prostaglandins production or by reducing the syntheses and activities of the specific immune mediators	*Sulfasalazine* • Retention enema • Suppository: 500 mg • Tablet: 500 mg *Hydrocortisone* • Retention enema • Suppository: 25 mg (acetate)
Laxatives Substances that loosen stools, increase bowel movements, used to treat and prevent constipation *Classification* • Bulk laxatives: Methylcellulose, wheat bran, ispaghula, psyllium, and sterculia • Stimulant laxatives: Bisacodyl, senna, glycerol • Osmotic laxatives: Magnesium hydroxide and poorly absorbed sugars such as lactulose or sorbitol • Stool softeners	*Senna* • Tablet: 7.5 mg (sennosides or traditional dosage forms) *Bisacodyl* • Tablet 5 mg *Lactulose* • Powder for solution, 10 mg
Medicines used in diarrhea: Oral rehydration Medicines that may reduce the frequency of pass stool and to increase the consistence of stool. In addition, medicines are used to replenish the lost liquid	*Oral rehydration salts* Powder for dilution in 200 ml, 500 ml, 1 L *Constitution* • Glucose: 13.5 g/L (75 mEq) • Sodium chloride (NaCl): 2.6 g/L (75 mEq or mmol/L) • Potassium chloride (KCl): 1.5 g/L • Trisodium citrate dihydrate*: 2.9 g/L • Osmolarity: 245 mOsm/L • Note: Special hygienic precautions should be taken under tropical conditions. Immediate use after dissolving is advised *Loperamide hydrochloride* Tablet 2 mg

Table 22.4 (continued)

Class of medicine	Generic name, galenic forms, indications, and notes
Solutions correcting fluid, electrolyte, and acid-base disturbances Replacement of fluid and electrolytes orally can be achieved by giving oral rehydration solutions which contain defined amounts of sodium, potassium, and glucose	*Oral rehydration salts* • Powder for solution: To be dissolved in indicated amount of water and taken orally in small continuous sips • Potassium chloride • Powder for solution: To be dissolved in indicated amount of water and taken orally in small continuous sips
Classification • Oral • Parenteral	*Glucose* • Injectable solution: 5% (isotonic), 10% (hypertonic), 50% (hypertonic), iv *Glucose with sodium chloride* • Injectable solution: 4% glucose, 0.18% sodium chloride (equivalent to Na + 30 mmol/L, Cl- 30 mmol/L), iv • Injectable solution: 5% glucose, 0.9% sodium chloride (equivalent to Na + 150 mmol/L and Cl- 150 mmol/L), 5% glucose, 0.45% sodium chloride (equivalent to Na + 75 mmol/L and Cl- 75 mmol/L), iv *Potassium chloride* • Solution: 11.2% in 20 ml ampoule (equivalent to K + 1.5 mmol/mL, Cl- 1.5 mmol/ml) • Solution for dilution: 7.5% (equivalent to K 1 mmol/ml and Cl 1 mmol/mL), 15% (equivalent to K 2 mmol/ml and Cl- 2 mmol/ml) *Sodium chloride* • Injectable solution: 0.9% isotonic (equivalent to Na + 154 mmol/L, Cl- 154 mmol/L), iv *Sodium hydrogen carbonate* • Injectable solution: 1.4% isotonic (equivalent to Na + 167 mmol/L, HCO_3–167 mmol/L), iv • Solution: 8.4% in 10 ml ampoule (equivalent to Na + 1000 mmol/L, HCO_3–1000 mmol/L) *Water for injection* • Used to dissolve injectable Galenic powders: 2 ml, 5 ml, 10 ml ampoules, iv or IM
Vitamins and minerals These are nutrients your body needs in small amounts for the various embolic processes to function normally. Vitamins cannot be synthesized by the body and most be ingested from exogenous sources	*Ascorbic acid* • Tablet: 50 mg • Calcium • Tablet: 500 mg (elemental) *Cholecalciferol* • Vitamin D3 • Oral liquid: 400 IU/ml • Solid oral dosage form: 400 IU, 1000 IU • Ergocalciferol can be used as an alternative *Ergocalciferol* • Vitamin D3 • Oral liquid: 250 µg/ml (10,000 IU/ml) • Solid oral dosage form: 1.25 mg (50,000 IU) *Iodine* • Capsule: 200 mg • Iodized oil: 1 ml (480 mg iodine), 0.5 ml (240 mg iodine) in ampoule (oral or injectable), 0.57 ml (308 mg iodine) in dispenser bottle

(continued)

Table 22.4 (continued)

Class of medicine	Generic name, galenic forms, indications, and notes
	Nicotinamide • Tablet: 50 mg • Synonyms: Niacin, vitamin B3
	Pyridoxine • Tablet: 25 mg (hydrochloride) • Synonym: Vitamin B6
	Retinol • Vitamin A • Capsule: 50,000 IU, 100,000 IU, 200,000 IU (as palmitate) • Oral oily solution: 100,000 IU (as palmitate)/ml in multidose dispenser • Tablet (sugar coated): 10,000 IU (as palmitate) • Water-miscible injection: 100,000 IU (as palmitate) in 2 ml ampoule
	Riboflavin • Tablet: 5 mg • Synonyms: Lactoflavin or vitamin B2
	Sodium fluoride • In any appropriate topical formulation
	Thiamine • Tablet: 50 mg (hydrochloride) • Synonym: Vitamin B1

specifically directed against the variable etiologies: infectious, metabolic, toxic, degenerative, and oncologic. Supportive agents may be included to facilitate rapid symptomatic relief.

22.6 Essential Medicines Used in Urology and Nephrology Conditions in a Standard Minimal-Resource Facility

The following proposed list of medicines may be used to treat urologic and nephrological disease conditions in a standard minimal-resource center. The mechanism of action of the medicines is specifically directed against the variable etiologies: infectious, metabolic, toxic, degenerative, and oncologic. Supportive agents may be included to facilitate rapid symptomatic relief.

The mechanism of action of the medicines is specifically directed against the variable etiologies:

• Infectious
• Allergic
• Metabolic
• Toxic
• Degenerative
• Hyper-prolific or neoplastic
• Congenital
• Traumatic

The medications used in these disease conditions are outlined elsewhere in this chapter.

Supportive agents may be included to facilitate rapid symptomatic relief.

22.7 Essential Medicines Used in Gynecology-Obstetrics Conditions in a Standard Minimal-Resource Facility

The following proposed list of medicines may be used to treat gynecology and obstetrics disease conditions in a standard minimal-resource center (Table 22.5). The mechanism of action of the medicines is specifically directed against the variable etiologies: infectious, metabolic, toxic, congenital, traumatic degenerative, and neoplastic. Supportive agents may be included to facilitate rapid symptomatic relief.

Table 22.5 Essential medicines prescribed for gynecologic/obstetrics conditions in a standard minimal-resource facility

Class of medicine	Generic name, galenic forms, indications, and notes
Ovulation inducers Medicines that facilitate the stimulation of the development of ovarian follicles to reverse anovulation or oligo-ovulation	*Background* • Ovulatory disorders may be identified in 18–25% of couples presenting with infertility • May present as oligomenorrhea: Menstruation that occurs at intervals of 35 days to 6 months • Spontaneous conception may be difficult • Ovulatory disorders can be treated by inducing a single follicle to develop and ovulate (mono-follicular development) • Alternatively, multiple follicles can be stimulated to develop and ovulate, as is done with assisted reproductive technologies (ART) • Appropriate clinical judgment as to which method to choose: Based on the underlying cause of anovulation, the efficacy, costs, risks, burden of treatment, and potential complications associated with chosen method *Etiology and suggested approach* • Hypogonadotropic amenorrhea: Pulsatile gonadotropin-releasing hormone (GnRH) • Oligo-ovulatory secondary to polycystic ovary syndrome: Letrozole • For obese women with PCOS, propose lifestyle changes and weight loss as an initial strategy to restore ovulatory cycles • Doses, regimens, and monitoring for clomiphene and letrozole use must be monitored • For women with primary ovarian insufficiency (premature ovarian failure), no ovulation induction strategy has been shown to be effective. For such women, in vitro fertilization (IVF) with donor oocytes has high success rates • For women with hyperprolactinemic anovulation, ovulation induction with dopamine agonist bromocriptine is suggested *Clomiphene* • Tablet: 50 mg (citrate): Initial course: 50 mg 1×/d, 5 d. Begin on or about the fifth day of cycle if progestin-induced bleeding is scheduled or spontaneous uterine bleeding occurs prior to therapy. Therapy may be initiated at any time in patients with no recent uterine bleeding
Abnormal uterine bleeding Medicines that influence abnormal uterine bleeding through different mechanism such as modification of the trophicity of the uterine mucosa (estrogen and progesterone) or impacting on coagulation (tranexamic acid) influence the uterine	*Medroxyprogesterone acetate* • Tablet: 5 mg • Suspension, intramuscular, as acetate • Depo-Provera: 150 mg/ml (1 ml) (contains methylparaben) • Depo-Provera: 400 mg/ml (2.5 ml) *Indications* *Abnormal uterine bleeding*: Treatment of abnormal uterine bleeding due to hormonal imbalance in the absence of organic pathology, such as fibroids or uterine cancer *Amenorrhea, secondary*: Treatment of secondary amenorrhea due to hormonal imbalance in the absence of organic pathology, such as fibroids or uterine cancer *Contraception* (104 mg/0.65 ml and 150 mg/ml injection): Prevention of pregnancy in women of childbearing potential *Endometrial hyperplasia prevention*: Prevention of endometrial hyperplasia in nonhysterectomized postmenopausal persons receiving daily oral conjugated estrogens 0.625 mg *Endometrial carcinoma* (400 mg/ml injection): Adjunctive therapy and/or palliative treatment of inoperable, recurrent, and/or metastatic endometrial carcinoma

(continued)

Table 22.5 (continued)

Class of medicine	Generic name, galenic forms, indications, and notes
	Endometriosis (104 mg/0.65 ml injection): Management of endometriosis-associated pain *Tranexamic acid (Cyklokapron)* • 500 mg Tabs • Posology: 2 × 2 taps/d
Oral hormonal contraceptives Medications containing synthetic versions of the natural female hormones estrogen and progesterone that are *taken by mouth* to prevent pregnancy *Mechanisms of action*: • Ovulation inhibition • Preventing sperm from penetrating through the cervix	*Ethinylestradiol + levonorgestrel* • Tablet: 30 µg + 150 µg *Ethinylestradiol + norethisterone* • Tablet: 35 µg + 1 mg *Levonorgestrel* • Tablet: 30 µg, 750 µg (pack of two), 1.5 mg *Classification* according to composition • Combined: Contains estrogen and progesterone • Progestin only: Contains only progesterone
Injectable hormonal contraceptives Medications containing synthetic versions of the natural female hormones estrogen and progesterone that *are injected* to prevent pregnancy	*Estradiol cypionate + medroxyprogesterone acetate* • Injection: 5 mg + 25 mg, IM • Medroxyprogesterone acetate *Injection (intramuscular): 150 mg/ml in 1 ml vial* • Injection (subcutaneous): 104 mg/0.65 ml in prefilled syringe or single-dose injection delivery system *Norethisterone enanthate* • Oily solution: 200 mg/ml in 1 ml ampoule
Implantable intrauterine contraceptive devices A small, often T-shaped birth control device, made out of plastic or copper, that is inserted into the uterus to prevent pregnancy The device could hormones with contraceptive activity Commonly called a coil *Mechanisms of action* • Timed release of hormones to hinder ovulation or sperm development • The ability of copper to act as a natural spermicide within the uterus • Use of nonhormonal, physical blocking mechanism	*Copper-containing device* • A gynecology consultation is mandatory • Patient education and active involvement in decision-making *Levonorgestrel-releasing intrauterine system* • Intrauterine system with reservoir containing 52 mg of levonorgestrel *Etonogestrel-releasing implant* • Single-rod etonogestrel-releasing implant, containing 68 mg of estrogen *Etonogestrel* • Levonorgestrel-releasing implant • Two-rod levonorgestrel-releasing implant, each rod containing 75 mg of levonorgestrel (150 mg total) *Classes of IUDs* • Nonhormonal: Copper-containing IUD • Hormonal: Progestogen-releasing IUD
Barrier methods Prevents pregnancy by stopping the male's sperm from coming into contact with the female's ovum	*Male condom* • Coital-dependent barrier contraceptive that does not interfere with fertility • Reduce the risk of pregnancy and transmission of many STIs, including HIV • Appropriate counseling encourages correct condom use and minimizes difficulties • Free handouts in some standard minimal facilities *Female condom* • Provides a physical barrier between the female and male genitalia and secretions during vaginal intercourse • Designed to protect against both pregnancy and STIs

Table 22.5 (continued)

Class of medicine	Generic name, galenic forms, indications, and notes
	Diaphragm • A reusable female contraceptive device consisting of a soft dome-shaped cup with a flexible rim that does not require a pelvic examination for fitting • Available in single-size and multisize options and are made of silicone or latex • Diaphragms do not protect against acquiring STIs and are used in conjunction with spermicide foam, gel, or cream
Intravaginal contraceptives	*Progesterone vaginal ring* • Progesterone-releasing vaginal ring containing 2.074 g of micronized progesterone • For use by women actively breastfeeding at least 4× per day

22.8   Essential Medicines Used in Musculoskeletal Conditions in a Standard Minimal-Resource Facility

The following proposed list of medicines may be used to treat musculoskeletal disease conditions in a standard minimal-resource center.

The mechanism of action of the medicines is specifically directed against the variable etiologies:

- Infectious
- Allergic
- Metabolic
- Toxic
- Degenerative
- Hyper-prolific or neoplastic
- Congenital
- Traumatic

The medications used in these disease conditions are outlined elsewhere in this chapter.

Supportive agents may be included to facilitate rapid symptomatic relief.

22.9   Essential Medicines Used in Dermatology and Allergic Conditions in a Standard Minimal-Resource Facility

The following proposed list of medicines may be used to treat dermatology and allergic disease conditions in a standard minimal-resource center

(Table 22.6). The mechanism of action of the medicines is specifically directed against the variable etiologies: infectious, metabolic, toxic, degenerative, and oncologic. Supportive agents may be included to facilitate rapid symptomatic relief.

22.10   Essential Medicines Used for Hematology Conditions in a Standard Minimal-Resource Facility

The following proposed list of medicines may be used to treat hematologic disease conditions in a standard minimal-resource center (Table 22.7). The mechanism of action of the medicines is specifically directed against the variable etiologies: infectious, metabolic, toxic, degenerative, and oncologic. Supportive agents may be included to facilitate rapid symptomatic relief.

22.11   Essential Medicines Used in Infectious Disease Conditions in a Standard Minimal-Resource Facility

The following proposed list of medicines may be used to treat infectious disease conditions in a standard minimal-resource center (Table 22.8). The mechanism of action of the medicines is specifically directed against the variable etiologies: viruses, bacteria, protozoa, helminths, and fungi.

Table 22.6 Essential medicines prescribed for dermatological and allergic conditions in a standard minimal-resource facility

Class of medicine	Generic name, galenic forms, indications, and notes
Dermatologic anti-infective medicines Agents that inhibit progression of disease process by disrupting the proliferator of viruses, bacteria, fungus, or parasites on the skin	*Tetracycline* • Ointment: 2% *Neomycin* • Ointment: 2% *Potassium permanganate* • Aqueous solution: 1:10,000 *Silver sulfadiazine* • Cream: 1% • >2 months *Miconazole* • Cream or ointment: 2% (nitrate) *Selenium sulfide* • Detergent-based suspension: 2% *Terbinafine* • Cream: 1% or • Ointment: 1% terbinafine hydrochloride
Dermatologic anti-inflammatory and antipruritic medicines A heterogenous group of medication consisting of classic AINS, antihistamines, and corticosteroids that are applied topically *Properties* • Analgesic • Anti-inflammatory • Soothing • Cooling • Antipruritus	*Betamethasone* • Cream or ointment: 0.1% (as valerate) • Hydrocortisone preferred in neonates *Diclofenac gel (Olfen gel)* • Gel, 11.6 mg diclofenac/g gel *Calamine lotion* • Hydrocortisone • Cream or ointment: 1% (acetate) *Common indications of topical AINS:* • Injuries to tendons, ligaments, muscles, and joints, for example, sprains, bruises, strains, or back pain after sports or accident • Localized forms of soft-tissue rheumatism, such as tendinitis (tennis elbow), shoulder-hand syndrome, bursitis, peri-arthropathies • Symptomatic therapy of osteoarthritis of small- and medium-sized, close-up joints such as finger joints or knees
Medicines affecting skin differentiation and proliferation	*Benzoyl peroxide* • Cream or lotion: 5% *Salicylic acid* • Solution: 5% *Urea* • Cream or ointment: 5%, 10%
Scabicides and pediculicides Medicine that disrupts the lifecycle (adult-egg proliferation cycle) by inhibiting the adult growth and reproduction systems	*Benzyl benzoate* • Lotion: 25% • >2 years *Permethrin* • Cream: 5% • Lotion: 1% *Ivermectin* • Tabs: 3 mg • *Dexamethasone:* Injection: 4 mg/ml in 1 ml ampoule (as disodium phosphate salt)

Table 22.6 (continued)

Class of medicine	Generic name, galenic forms, indications, and notes
Antiallergics and medicines used in anaphylaxis An acute, life-threatening, multisystem syndrome caused by the sudden release of mast cell mediators into the systemic circulation *Mechanism* Most often results from immunoglobulin E (IgE)-mediated reactions to foods, drugs, and insect stings, or other causes of degranulation of mast cells	*Epinephrine (adrenaline)* • Injection: 1 mg (as hydrochloride or hydrogen tartrate) in 1 ml ampoule, IM • Anaphylactic shock intramuscular treatment *Hydrocortisone* • Powder for injection: 100 mg (as sodium succinate) in vial, iv • Glucocorticoid • Indications: Hormonal substitution, organ rejection • Autoimmune disease • Decrease in glucose tolerance (note: Diabetic patients) • Side effects: Hypertension, muscle wasting, cutaneous atrophy (note: Wounds), osteoporosis, mood elevation (euphoria, insomnia, agitation) *Loratadine* • Oral liquid: 1 mg/ml, tablet: 10 mg *Prednisolone* • Oral liquid: 5 mg/mL, tablet: 5 mg, 25 mg

Table 22.7 Essential medicines prescribed for hematology conditions in a standard minimal-resource facility

Class of medicine	Generic name, galenic forms, indications, and notes
Antianemia medicines Therapeutic agent which increases either the number of red cells or the amount of hemoglobin in the blood	*Ferrous salt* • Oral liquid: Equivalent to 25 mg iron (as sulfate)/mL • Tablet: Equivalent to 60 mg iron *Ferrous salt + folic acid* • Tablet: Equivalent to 60 mg iron +400 μg folic acid (nutritional supplement for use during pregnancy) *Folic acid* • Tablet: 400 μg*, 1 mg, 5 mg • Periconceptual use for prevention of first occurrence of neural tube defects
Medicines affecting coagulation	*Enoxaparin*
Coagulation prevents bleeding and loss of blood from the circulatory system *Mechanism of clotting* • Following injury to the vessel wall, tissue factor is exposed on the surface of the damaged endothelium • The interaction between tissue factor and factor VII activates the *coagulation* cascade • This produces thrombin and culminates in the formation of an insoluble clot, the thrombus	• Injection: Ampoule or prefilled syringe; 20 mg/0.2 ml, 40 mg/0.4 ml, 60 mg/0.6 ml, 80 mg/0.8 ml, 100 mg/1 ml, 120 mg/0.8 mL, 150 mg/1 ml • Note: Alternatives are limited to nadroparin and dalteparin *Heparin sodium* • Injection: 1000 IU/ml, 5000 IU/ml, 20,000 IU/ml in 1 ml ampoule, iv *Tranexamic acid* • Injection: 100 mg/ml in 10 ml ampoule, iv *Warfarin* • Tablet: 1 mg, 2 mg, 5 mg (sodium salt)
Blood transfusion and blood components The process of transferring blood or blood products into one's circulation intravenously	*Background* • Standard minimal-resource facilities comply with guidelines established to safeguard the supply of safe blood components. The program may be coordinated through an appropriate tertiary center and is based on voluntary, nonremunerated blood donation • Assuring self-sufficiency and the security of the blood supply are important national goals to prevent blood shortages and meet the transfusion requirements of the patient population • All preparations should comply with WHO requirements

(continued)

Table 22.7 (continued)

Class of medicine	Generic name, galenic forms, indications, and notes
	Component of full blood Full blood freshly obtain from the vein of a healthy patient may be fractioned as below: • Fresh-frozen plasma • Platelets • Red blood cell concentrate • Whole blood *The practical procedure of blood transfusion in a minimal standard facility*
Human immunoglobulins (Ig) They are prepared from large pools of whole blood or apheresis-derived plasma. Ig preparations are concentrated, purified, filtered, and sterilized, making the risk of infectious disease transmission virtually zero	*Anti-D immunoglobulin* • Injection: 250 μg in single-dose vial, iv *Anti-rabies immunoglobulins* • Injection: 150 IU/ml in vial, IM *Anti-tetanus immunoglobulins* • Injection: 500 IU in vial, IM *Normal immune-globulin* • Intramuscular administration: 16% protein solution • Intravenous administration: 5%, 10% protein solution • Subcutaneous administration: 15%, 16% protein solution • Indicated for primary immune deficiency • Indicated for primary immune deficiency and Kawasaki disease

Table 22.8 Essential medicines prescribed for infectious disease conditions in a standard minimal-resource facility

Class of medicine	Generic name, galenic forms, indications, and notes
Antifilarials Medication that inhibits the growth and reproduction of filarial worms. The medication usually has no effect on the unhatched egg which may survive treatment and hatch in posttreatment period. Hence, a second dose usually 10 days after the initial dose	*Albendazole* • Tablet (chewable): 400 mg *Ivermectin* • Tablet (scored): 3 mg • Posology: 0.2 mg/kg unique dose on Day 0 to be repeated on Day 10
Antischistosomes and other antinematode medicines	*Praziquantel* • Tablet 600 mg
Antibacterial Medicines that inhibit proliferation of bacteria *Classifications* of antibiotic based on effect on growth • *Bacteriostatic*: Slow or inhibit the growth of bacteria • *Bactericidal*: Destroy bacteria by targeting the cell wall or cell membrane of the bacteria *Classification* of antibiotics based on synthesis *Folic acid synthesis inhibitors* • Sulfonamides: Sulfamethoxazole • Sulfadiazine • Dihydrofolate reductase inhibitors, e.g., trimethoprim	*Amoxicillin* Galenic forms • Powder for oral liquid: 125 mg (as trihydrate)/5 ml, 250 mg (as trihydrate)/5 ml • Solid oral dosage form: 250 mg, 500 mg (as trihydrate) • Powder for injection: 250 mg, 500 mg, 1 g (as sodium) in vial Indication: • Community-acquired pneumonia (mild to moderate) • Community-acquired pneumonia (severe) • Complicated severe acute malnutrition • Exacerbations of chronic obstructive pulmonary disease (COPD) • Lower urinary tract infections • Otitis media • Pharyngitis • Sepsis in neonates and children • Sinusitis • Uncomplicated severe acute malnutrition second choice • Acute bacterial meningitis

Table 22.8 (continued)

Class of medicine	Generic name, galenic forms, indications, and notes
Cell wall synthesis inhibitors • Penicillins • Cephalosporins • Carbapenems • Beta lactamase inhibitors *Protein synthesis inhibitors* • Tetracyclines: Tetracycline, doxycycline • Aminoglycosides: Gentamicin, neomycin • Aminophenols: Chloramphenicol • Macrolides: Erythromycin • Azithromycin, clarithromycin *DNA gyrase inhibitors* • Ciprofloxacin • Norfloxacin • Levofloxacin *Classification* of *bacteria* based on oxygen requirement • *Aerobes* require oxygen for growth • *Anaerobes* grow only in the absence of oxygen *Classification of bacteria* based on gram stain on the basis of their cell wall structure: • *Gram-positive:* Bacteria staining purple in gram-stained smear. They have thick layer of peptidoglycan • *Gram-negative:* Bacteria staining pink in gram-stained smear. Gram-positive bacteria, when dead may stain red. They have thick outer membrane • *Gram-variable:* The organisms is gram positive but appear gram negative or is gram negative but appear gram positive	*Amoxicillin + clavulanic acid* (co-amoxicillin) Galenic forms • Oral liquid: 125 mg amoxicillin +31.25 mg clavulanic acid/5 ml • 250 mg amoxicillin +62.5 mg clavulanic acid/5 ml • Tablet: 500 mg (as trihydrate) + 125 mg (as potassium salt) • Powder for injection: 500 mg (as sodium) + 100 mg (as potassium salt), 1000 mg (as sodium) + 200 mg (as potassium salt) in vial Indications • Community-acquired pneumonia (severe) • Complicated intra-abdominal infections (mild to moderate) • Exacerbations of COPD • Hospital-acquired pneumonia • Low-risk febrile neutropenia • Lower urinary tract infections • Sinusitis • Skin and soft-tissue infections • Bone and joint infections • Community-acquired pneumonia (mild to moderate) • Community-acquired pneumonia (severe) • Otitis media *Ampicillin powder for injection:* • 500 mg, 1 g (as sodium salt) in vial • Community-acquired severe pneumonia • Complicated severe acute malnutrition • Sepsis in neonates and children • Acute bacterial meningitis *Benzathine benzyl penicillin* • Galenic form: Powder for injection: 900 mg benzyl penicillin (= 1.2 million IU) in 5 ml vial, 1.44 g benzyl penicillin (= 2.4 million IU) in 5 ml vial • Indications: Syphilis *Benzyl penicillin* • Galenic form: Powder for injection: 600 mg (= 1 million IU), 3 g (= 5 million IU) sodium or potassium salt in vial Indications • Community-acquired pneumonia (severe) • Complicated severe acute malnutrition • Sepsis in neonates and children • Syphilis second choice • Acute bacterial meningitis *Cefalexin* Galenic forms • Powder for reconstitution with water: 125 mg/5 ml, 250 mg/5 ml (anhydrous) • Solid oral dosage form: 250 mg (as monohydrate) Indications • Often used in case of penicline allergy • Exacerbations of COPD • Pharyngitis • Skin and soft-tissue infections

(continued)

Table 22.8 (continued)

Class of medicine	Generic name, galenic forms, indications, and notes
Clinically significant bacterial groups: *Gram-positive cocci* *Aerobes:* Staphylococcus Streptococcus Enterococcus *Gram-positive rods (bacilli)* Aerobes: Bacillus species Anaerobes: Clostridium species *Gram-negative cocci* *Aerobes:* Neisseria species, moraxella species *Gram-negative rod* *Aerobes*: *Escherichia coli* Klebsiella, Proteus, Shigella, Salmonella, Vibrio species *Gram-negative coccobacilli* *Aerobes:* Haemophilus, Bordetella, Brucella, Legionella species	*Cefazolin* • Galenic form: Powder for injection: 1 g (as sodium salt) in vial. Indications: Also indicated for surgical prophylaxis • Bone and joint infections *Cefixime* Galenic form: • Capsule or tablet: 200 mg, 400 mg (as trihydrate) • Powder for oral liquid: 100 mg/5 ml Indication: • Acute invasive bacterial diarrhea/dysentery • *Neisseria gonorrhoeae* *Cefotaxime* • Galenic form: Powder for injection: 250 mg per vial (as sodium salt), iv Indication • Third-generation cephalosporin of choice for use in hospitalized neonates • Acute bacterial meningitis • Community-acquired pneumonia (severe) • Complicated intra-abdominal infections (mild to moderate) • Complicated intra-abdominal infections (severe) • Hospital-acquired pneumonia • Pyelonephritis or prostatitis (severe) • Bone and joint infections • Pyelonephritis or prostatitis (mild to moderate) • Sepsis in neonates and children *Ceftriaxone* Galenic form: • Powder for injection: 250 mg, 1 g (as sodium salt) in vial, iv Indications: • Acute bacterial meningitis • Community-acquired pneumonia (severe) • Complicated intra-abdominal infections (mild to moderate) • Complicated intra-abdominal infections (severe) • Hospital-acquired pneumonia • *Neisseria gonorrhoeae* • Pyelonephritis or prostatitis (severe) second choice • Acute invasive bacterial diarrhea/dysentery • Bone and joint infections • Pyelonephritis or prostatitis (mild to moderate) • Sepsis in neonates and children *Cloxacillin* Galenic forms • Capsule: 500 mg, 1 g (as sodium salt) • Powder for injection: 500 mg (as sodium salt) in vial, iv or IM • Powder for oral liquid: 125 mg (as sodium salt)/5 ml • Cloxacillin, dicloxacillin, and flucloxacillin are preferred for oral administration, due to better bioavailability Indications • *N. gonorrhoeae*

Table 22.8 (continued)

Class of medicine	Generic name, galenic forms, indications, and notes
	Ciprofloxacin Galenic forms • Oral liquid: 250 mg/5 ml (anhydrous) • Solution for iv infusion: 2 mg/ml (as hyclate) • Tablet: 250 mg (as hydrochloride) Indications • Acute invasive bacterial diarrhea/dysentery • Low-risk febrile neutropenia • Pyelonephritis or prostatitis (mild to moderate) • Cholera • Complicated intra-abdominal infections (mild to moderate) *Clarithromycin* Galenic forms • Solid oral dosage form: 500 mg • Powder for oral liquid: 125 mg/5 ml, 250 mg/5 ml • Powder for injection: 500 mg in vial, iv Indication: • Erythromycin may be an alternative • Clarithromycin is also listed for use in combination regimens for eradication of *H. pylori* in adults • Community-acquired pneumonia (severe) second choice • Pharyngitis *Clindamycin* Galenic forms • Capsule: 150 mg (as hydrochloride) • Injection: 150 mg (as phosphate)/ml, iv • Oral liquid: 75 mg/5 ml (as palmitate) Indication: Bone and joint infections *Doxycycline* *Galenic forms* • Oral liquid: 25 mg/5 ml, 50 mg/5 ml (anhydrous) • Solid oral dosage form: 50 mg, 100 mg (as hyclate) • Powder for injection: 100 mg in vial, iv Indications • Use in children <8 years only for life-threatening infections when no alternative exists • *C. trachomatis*, cholera • Community-acquired pneumonia (mild to moderate) • Exacerbations of COPD *Gentamicin* Galenic forms • Injection: 10 mg, 40 mg (as sulfate)/ml in 2 ml vial, iv Indications • Community-acquired pneumonia (severe) • Complicated severe acute malnutrition • Sepsis in neonates and children • *Neisseria gonorrheae* *Metronidazole* Galenic forms • Injection: 500 mg in 100 ml vial, iv • Oral liquid: 200 mg (as benzoate)/5 ml • Suppository: 500 mg; 1 g • Tablet: 200–500 mg

(continued)

Table 22.8 (continued)

Class of medicine	Generic name, galenic forms, indications, and notes
	Indications • *Clostridium difficile* infection • Complicated intra-abdominal infections (mild to moderate) • Complicated intra-abdominal infections (severe) • Trichomonas vaginalis • Complicated intra-abdominal infections (mild to moderate) *Nitrofurantoin* Galenic forms • Oral liquid: 25 mg/5 ml • Tablet: 100 mg Indication: Lower urinary tract infections *Sulfamethoxazole + trimethoprim** Galenic forms • Injection: 80 mg + 16 mg/ml in 5 ml ampoule; 80 mg + 16 mg/ml in 10 ml ampoule iv • Oral liquid: 200 mg + 40 mg/5 mL • Tablet: 100 mg + 20 mg; 400 mg + 80 mg; 800 mg + 160 mg Indication • Lower urinary tract infections second choice • Acute invasive diarrhea/bacterial dysentery
Antifungal medicines Treat fungal infections by acting on the synthesis of • The fungal cell membrane, • Cell wall components, • Membrane permeability, • Nucleic acids and, • Attachment to the mitotic spindle function of the fungi during cell division *Classification* • Azoles • Imidazole: Clotrimazole, Econazole, Miconazole, Oxiconazole, Ketoconazole • Triazoles: Fluconazole • Allylamine: Terbinafine (Lamisil)	*Clotrimazole* Galenic forms • Vaginal cream: 1%, 10% • Vaginal tablet: 100 mg, 500 mg *Fluconazole* Galenic forms • Capsule: 50 mg • Injection: 2 mg/ml in vial, iv • Oral liquid: 50 mg/5 mL *Griseofulvin* • Oral liquid: 125 mg/5 mL • Solid oral dosage form: 125 mg, 250 mg *Nystatin* • Lozenge: 100,000 IU • Oral liquid: 50 mg/5 ml; 100,000 IU/ml • Pessary: 100,000 IU • Tablet: 100,000 IU; 500,000 IU.
Antiviral medicines *Antiherpes medicines*	*Acyclovir* Galenic presentation • Oral liquid: 200 mg/5 ml • Powder for injection: 250 mg (as sodium salt) in vial, iv • Tablet: 200 mg
Antimalarial medicines *For curative treatment*	*Amodiaquine* Galenic presentation • Tablet: 153 mg or 200 mg (as hydrochloride) • To be used in combination with artesunate 50 mg *Artemether* • Oily injection: 80 mg/ml in 1 ml ampoule • For use in the management of severe malaria • Artemether + lumefantrine • Tablet: 20 mg + 120 mg • Tablet (dispersible): 20 mg + 120 mg • Note: Not recommended in the first trimester of pregnancy or in children below 5 kg

Table 22.8 (continued)

Class of medicine	Generic name, galenic forms, indications, and notes
	Artesunate Galenic presentation • Injection: Ampoules, containing 60 mg anhydrous artesunic acid with a separate ampoule of 5% sodium bicarbonate solution, IM • Note: For use in the management of severe malaria • Rectal dosage form: 50 mg, 100 mg, 200 mg capsules (for pre-referral treatment of severe malaria only; patients should be taken to an appropriate health facility for follow-up care) • Tablet: 50 mg • Note: To be used in combination with either amodiaquine, mefloquine or • sulfadoxine + pyrimethamine *Artesunate + amodiaquine* • Galenic forms: Tablet: 25 mg + 67.5 mg, 50 mg + 135 mg, 100 mg + 270 mg • Note: Other combinations that deliver the target doses required, such as 153 mg or 200 mg (as hydrochloride) with 50 mg artesunate, can be alternatives *Artesunate + mefloquine* Galenic forms • Tablet: 25 mg + 55 mg, 100 mg + 220 mg • Artesunate + pyronaridine tetraphosphate • Tablet: 60 mg + 180 mg • Granules: 20 mg + 60 mg • Note: >5 kg *Dihydroartemisinin + piperaquine phosphate* • Galenic forms: Tablet: 20 mg + 160 mg, 40 mg + 320 mg • Note: >5 kg *Doxycycline* • Capsule: 100 mg (as hydrochloride or hyclate) • Tablet (dispersible): 100 mg (as monohydrate) • Note: For use only in combination with quinine *Mefloquine* • Galenic form: Tablet: 250 mg (as hydrochloride) • Note: To be used in combination with artesunate 50 mg *Quinine* Galenic forms • Injection: 300 mg quinine hydrochloride/ml in 2 ml ampoule, iv or IM • Tablet: 300 mg (quinine sulfate) or 300 mg (quinine bisulfate) • Note: For use only in the management of severe malaria; should be used in combination with doxycycline *Sulfadoxine + pyrimethamine* • Galenic forms: Tablet: 500 mg + 25 mg • Note: Only in combination with artesunate 50 mg

(continued)

Table 22.8 (continued)

Class of medicine	Generic name, galenic forms, indications, and notes
Antimalarial prophylaxis	*Doxycycline* Solid oral dosage form: 100 mg (as hydrochloride or hyclate) >8 years *Mefloquine* • Galenic form: Tablet: 250 mg (as hydrochloride) • Note: >5 kg or >3 months *Proguanil* • Galenic form: Tablet: 100 mg (as hydrochloride) • Note: For use only in combination with chloroquine.
Antiseptics	*Chlorhexidine* Solution: 5% (digluconate) *Ethanol* Solution: 70% (denatured) *Povidone iodine* Solution: 10% (equivalent to 1% available iodine)
Disinfectants	*Alcohol based* • Hand rub • Solution: Containing ethanol 80% volume/volume • Solution: Containing isopropyl alcohol 75% volume/volume *Chlorine base compound* • Powder: (0.1% available chlorine) for solution • Chloroxylenol • Solution: 4.8%.

Supportive agents may be included to facilitate rapid symptomatic relief.

22.12 Essential Medicines Used in Endocrinology Conditions in Standard Minimal-Resource Facility

The following proposed list of medicines may be used to treat endocrinologic and related disease conditions in a standard minimal-resource center (Table 22.9). The mechanism of action of the medicines is specifically directed against the endogenous synthesis of hormones in the case of pathologic over hyperactivity of an endocrine gland. In instances of hypoproduction, synthetic home is used to supplement the deficit. Supportive agents may be included to facilitate rapid symptomatic relief.

22.13 Essential Medicines Used in Ophthalmology Conditions in a Standard Minimal-Resource Facility

The following proposed list of medicines may be used to treat ophthalmologic and related disease conditions in a standard minimal-resource center (Table 22.10). The mechanism of action of the medicines is specifically directed against the variable etiologies: infectious, metabolic, toxic, degenerative, and oncologic. Supportive agents may be included to facilitate rapid symptomatic relief.

Table 22.9 Essential medicines prescribed for endocrinology conditions in a standard minimal-resource facility

Class of medicine	Generic name, galenic forms, indications, and notes
Oral antidiabetics Therapeutic agent administered by mouth to reduce and maintain blood sugar level at physiological levels	*Gliclazide* • Tablet: Solid oral dosage form: (controlled-release tablets) 30 mg, 60 mg, 80 mg • Note: Only for adults, not suitable for type 1 diabetes, or during pregnancy and breast feeding
Substances classes • Biguanide: Derivatives (metformin) • Glitazone • Sulfonylureas, e.g., Glibenclamide • Glinide • DPP-4 inhibitors • Alpha-glucosidase inhibitor • SGLT-2 inhibitors	*Glibenclamide* (Daonil) • Tablet: 5 mg • Note: Not suitable for above 60 years, high susceptibility to hypoglycemia • To be given with care to professional automobile driver *Metformin* • Tablet: 500 mg (hydrochloride)
Insulin and other medicines used for diabetes Insulin is a peptide hormone that regulates the uptake of glucose in body cells. It has a lowering effect of blood sugar and plays an essential role in the treatment of diabetes mellitus	*Insulin injection (soluble)* • Injection: 40 IU/ml in 10 ml vial, 100 IU/ml in 10 ml vial, IM • Intermediate-acting insulin • Injection: 40 IU/ml in 10 ml vial, 100 IU/ml in 10 ml vial (as compound insulin zinc suspension or isophane insulin), IM.
Thyroid hormones and antithyroid medicines *Note* • Thioamides are often started in patients with graves' hyperthyroidism to attain a euthyroid state rapidly in preparation for thyroidectomy • Patients who want to avoid or defer ablative therapy with radioiodine or surgery can continue the thioamides for prolonged periods • Approximately 20–30% of patients achieve permanent remission.	*Levothyroxine* • Galenic form: Tablet: 25 µg, 50 µg, 100 µg (sodium salt) *Oral dosing:* • *Adults (healthy)* who have been hypothyroid for only a few months: Initial: 1.6 mcg/kg/d; adjust dose by 12.5–25 mcg/d every 4–6 weeks as needed. Usual doses are ≤200 mcg/d (range: 100–125 mcg/d [70 kg adult]); doses ≥300 mcg/d are rare (consider poor compliance, malabsorption, and/or drug interactions) • *Adults >50 years* of age without evidence of coronary heart disease: Lower starting doses (e.g., 50 mcg/d) may be preferred • *Adults with cardiac disease*: Initial: 12.5–25 mcg/d; adjust dose by 12.5–25 mcg increments at 6- to 8-week intervals as needed • *Adults with severe longstanding hypothyroidism*: Initial: 12.5–25 mcg/d; adjust dose by 12.5–25 mcg/d every 2–4 weeks as appropriate • *Pregnant patients*: Dosage requirements may increase during pregnancy in patients with preexisting disease. If new-onset hypothyroidism occurs, initiate therapy with 1.6 mcg/kg/d (for severe hypothyroidism) or 1 mcg/kg/d (for mild hypothyroidism [TSH < 10 milliunits/L]) followed by appropriate dosage adjustments every 4 weeks *Propylthiouracil:* Note d osage range • Indication: Hyperthyroidism: • Children: Oral: Initial: 15 mg/d • Adults: Oral: Initial: 20–60 mg/d given in 2–3 divided doses; maintenance: 5–15 mg/d or alternatively 20–60 mg/d when receiving concurrent thyroid replacement therapy.

(continued)

Table 22.9 (continued)

Class of medicine	Generic name, galenic forms, indications, and notes
Hormones and antihormones A hormone is a chemical substance produced by special glands in the body and directly secreted into and transported by the blood stream to target organs where controls and regulates the activity of certain cells or organs *Hormones* have diverse biological effects and are essential for every activity of life, including • The processes of digestion metabolism • Growth • Reproduction • Mood control	*Dexamethasone-sone* Galenic forms • Injection: 4 mg/ml in 1 ml ampoule (as disodium phosphate salt), iv • Oral liquid: 2 mg/5 ml • Indication: Acute lymphoblastic leukemia *Hydrocortisone-sone* • Galenic forms: Powder for injection: 100 mg (as sodium succinate) in vial • Indication: Acute lymphoblastic leukemia *Methylprednisolone* • Galenic forms: Injection: 40 mg/ml (as sodium succinate) in 1 ml single-dose vial or 10 ml multidose vials; 80 mg/ml (as sodium succinate) in 1 ml single-dose vial, iv • Indications: Acute lymphoblastic leukemia *Prednisolone or prednisone* Galenic forms • Oral liquid: 5 mg/ml • Tablet: 5 mg, 25 mg Indications: • Chronic lymphocytic leukemia • Diffuse large B-cell lymphoma • Hodgkin's lymphoma • Follicular lymphoma • Acute lymphoblastic leukemia • Burkitt's lymphoma • *Note:* Prednisone is the preform of the active molecule that gets activated to prednisolone, the active form of the molecule in the liver. In cases of liver diseases, it is advisable to use prednisolone instead of prednisone *Tamoxifen* • Galenic forms: Tablet: 10 mg, 20 mg (as citrate) • Indications: Early-stage breast cancer, metastatic breast cancer
Adrenal hormones and synthetic substitutes	*Fludrocortisone* • Tablet: 100 µg (acetate) *Hydrocortisone,* synthetic glucocorticoid • Tablet: 5 mg, 10 mg, 20 mg • Solution for injection: 100 mg/ml *Dexamethasone,* synthetic glucocorticoid • Tablet: 4 mg • Solution for injection: 2 mg/ml.
Androgens	*Testosterone* Injection: 200 mg (enanthate) in 1 ml ampoule

Table 22.10 Essential medicines prescribed for ophthalmology conditions in a standard minimal-resource facility

Class of medication	Generic name, galenic forms, indications, and notes
Anti-infective agents	*Acyclovir* • Ointment: 3% w/w • Indication: Herpetic infections *Azithromycin* • Solution (eye drops): 1.5% • Indications: Large spectrum, may be used when the patient is allergic to penicillin • Class: Macrolide *Erythromycin* • Class macrolide • Ointment: 0.5% • Infections due to *C. trachomatis* or *N. gonorrhoeae* • Indication: Gram-negative infections • Tetracycline • Eye ointment: 1% (hydrochloride) • Indication: Purulent eye infections • Indications: Large spectrum, may be used when the patient is allergic to penicillin *Gentamicin* • Solution (eye drops): 0.3% (sulfate) • Class: Aminoside
Anti-inflammatory agents	*Prednisolone* • Solution (eye drops): 0.5% (sodium phosphate)
Local anesthetics	*Tetracaine* • Solution (eye drops): 0.5% (hydrochloride) • Not in preterm neonates
Miotics and antiglaucoma medicines	• *Acetazolamide* • Tablet: 250 mg • Pilocarpine • Solution (eye drops): 2%, 4% (hydrochloride or nitrate) • Side effects: Miosis, myopia • Timolol • Solution (eye drops): 0.25%, 0.5% (as hydrogen maleate)

22.14 Essential Medicines Used in Psychiatry Conditions in a Standard Minimal-Resource Facility

The following proposed list of medicines may be used to treat psychiatric and related disease conditions in a standard minimal-resource center (Table 22.11). The mechanism of action of the medicines is specifically directed to influence the affected neural pathway. It is noteworthy that the medicine acts on neural mechanisms to influence behavior. Supportive agents may be included to facilitate rapid symptomatic relief

22.15 Essential Medicines Used for Palliative Care in a Standard Minimal-Resource Facility

The following proposed list of medicines may be used to treat palliative conditions in a standard minimal-resource center (Table 22.12). The mechanism of action of the medicines is specifically directed to influence the mental state, respiration, pain, and transit so as to assure maximum comfort. Supportive agents may be included to facilitate rapid symptomatic relief.

Table 22.11 Essential medicines prescribed for psychiatry conditions in a standard minimal-resource facility

Class of medication	Generic name, galenic forms, indications, and notes
Psychotic disorders Antipsychotic agents are the primary medication for schizophrenia and related psychotic disorders. Psychosis signifies a nonspecific syndrome characterized by delusions (false beliefs), hallucinations (false sensory perceptions not shared by others), loss of contact with reality and bizarre behavior	*Antipsychotic medications* • Agents to treat agitation, hallucinations, schizophrenia, mania *Chlorpromazine* • Injection: 25 mg (hydrochloride)/ml in 2 ml ampoule, IM • Oral liquid: 25 mg (hydrochloride)/5 ml • Tablet: 100 mg (hydrochloride) • Class: First-generation neuroleptic *Fluphenazine* • Injection: 25 mg (decanoate or enanthate) in 1 ml ampoule, IM *Haloperidol* • Injection: 5 mg in 1 ml ampoule, IM • Tablet: 2 mg, 5 mg *Risperidone* • Solid oral dosage form: 0.25–6.0 mg • Side effect: Increases prolactin levels *Indication of antipsychotic*: May be used to treat • Acute psychosis from any cause • Chronic psychotic disorders such as schizophrenia • Acute agitation • Bipolar mania
Depressive disorders Antidepressants are medicines that treat depression	*Amitriptyline* • Tablet: 25 mg, 75 mg (hydrochloride) *Fluoxetine* • Solid oral dosage form: 20 mg (as hydrochloride) *Classification of antidepressants medicines* • Selective serotonin reuptake inhibitors (SSRIs) • Serotonin and norepinephrine reuptake inhibitors (SNRIs) • Tricyclic antidepressants (TCAs), for example, amitriptyline • Monoamine oxidase inhibitors (MAOIs) • Atypical antidepressants *Neurotransmitters* influenced by antidepressant medicine • *Dopamine* modulates decision-making, motivation, arousal, and the signaling of pleasure and reward • *Norepinephrine* influences alertness and motor function and helps regulate blood pressure and heart rate in response to stress • *Serotonin* regulates mood, appetite, sleep, memory, social behavior, and sexual desire
Bipolar disorders	*Carbamazepine* • Tablet (scored): 100 mg, 200 mg • Lithium carbonate • Solid oral dosage form: 300 mg • Valproic acid (sodium valproate) • Tablet (enteric-coated): 200 mg, 500 mg (sodium valproate).
Anxiety disorders	*Diazepam* Tablet (scored): 2 mg, 5 mg
Obsessive compulsive disorders	*Clomipramine* • Capsule: 10 mg, 25 mg (hydrochloride).
Psychoactive substance use	*Nicotine replacement therapy* • Chewing gum: 2 mg, 4 mg (as polacrilex) • Transdermal patch: 5–30 mg/16 h, 7–21 mg/24 h

Table 22.12 Essential medicines prescribed for palliative care conditions in a standard minimal-resource facility

Medication group	Generic name, galenic forms, indications, and notes
Medicines used in end-of-life care A heterogenous group of medicines that satisfy the palliative care needs of an individual. Care is symptomatic and supportive *Major symptoms occurring in end-of-life anorexia* • Anxiety • Constipation • Delirium • Depression • Diarrhea • Dyspnea • Fatigue • Nausea and vomiting • Pain • Respiratory tract secretions	*Scope of palliative care and medication* • Provides relief from pain and other distressing symptoms • Affirms life and regards dying as a normal process • Intends neither to hasten or postpone death • Integrates the psychological and spiritual aspects of patient care • Offers a support system to help patients live as actively as possible until death • Offers a support system to help the family cope during the patient's illness and in their own bereavement • Uses a team approach to address the needs of patients and their families, including bereavement counseling, if indicated • Will enhance quality of life, and may also positively influence the course of illness • Is applicable early in the course of illness, in conjunction with other therapies that are intended to prolong life, such as chemotherapy or radiation therapy, and includes those investigations needed to better understand and manage distressing clinical complications *Amitriptyline* • Tablet: 10 mg, 25 mg, 75 mg • Tricyclic antidepressant *Dexamethasone* • Injection: 4 mg/ml in 1 ml ampoule (as disodium phosphate salt), iv • Oral liquid: 2 mg/5 ml • Tablet: 2 mg, 4 mg, corticoid, co-analgesic specially used for bone pain *Diazepam* • Injection: 5 mg/ml, IM or iv • Oral liquid: 2 mg/5 ml • Rectal solution: 2.5 mg, 5 mg, 10 mg • Tablet: 5 mg, 10 mg • Long-acting (>24 h) antiepileptic drug (status epilepticus), myorelaxant, sedative • Note: Hypoventilation, hypotension *Fluoxetine* • Solid oral dosage form: 20 mg (as hydrochloride) • Note: SSRI discontinuation syndrome: Irritability, nausea, electric-like shock feeling, insomnia, profuse sweating (not to be mistaken with dependence) *Haloperidol* • Injection: 5 mg in 1 ml ampoule, IM • Oral liquid: 2 mg/ml • Solid oral dosage form: 0.5 mg, 2 mg, 5 mg • Typical incisive antipsychotic, sedative • Side effects: Sedation, constipation, orthostatic hypotension, extra pyramidal effects • Hyoscine butyl bromide (Buscopan) • Injection: 20 mg/ml, iv *Hyoscine hydrobromide* • Injection: 400 μg/ml, 600 μg/ml, iv • Transdermal patches: 1 mg/72 h *Lactulose* • Oral liquid: 3.1–3.7 g/5 ml • Osmotic laxative agent *Loperamide* • Solid oral dosage form: 2 mg • Nonanalgesic opiate, antidiarrheic

(continued)

Table 22.12 (continued)

Medication group	Generic name, galenic forms, indications, and notes
	Metoclopramide • Injection: 5 mg (hydrochloride)/ml in 2 ml ampoule, iv • Oral liquid: 5 mg/5 ml • Solid oral form: 10 mg (hydrochloride) • Antiemetic, laxative • Side effects: Nausea and emesis *Midazolam* • Injection: 1 mg/ml, 5 mg/ml, IM • Solid oral dosage form: 7.5 mg, 15 mg • Oral liquid: 2 mg/ml • Short-acting benzodiazepine
Antineoplastic medication Agents that inhibit the maturation and proliferation of malignant cells Chemotherapy, aimed at destruction of malignant cells using a variety of agents that directly affect cellular growth and development *Synonym* Chemotherapeutic agents	*Methotrexate* • *Powder for injection:* 50 mg (as sodium salt) in vial • *Tablet:* 2.5 mg (as sodium salt) • Early-stage breast cancer • Gestational trophoblastic neoplasia • Osteosarcoma • Acute lymphoblastic leukemia • Acute promyelocytic leukemia *5-fluorouracil* • *Injection:* 50 mg/ml in 5 ml ampoule, iv • Early-stage breast cancer • Early-stage colon cancer • Early-stage rectal cancer • Metastatic colorectal cancer • Nasopharyngeal cancer
Diagnostic agents: *Radio contrast media*	*Barium sulfate* Aqueous suspension

Bibliography

1. https://www.who.int/selection_medicines/committees/expert/19/applications/PalliativeCare_8_A_R.pdf.
2. https://www.hepatitis.va.gov/hbv/post-vaccination-testing.asp.
3. Papadakis MA, McPhee SJ, Rabow MW. Current medical diagnosis and treatment. New York, NY: McGraw-Hill Education; 2019. https://accessmedicine.mhmedical.com/book.aspx?bookID=2449.
4. Preclinical and clinical lecture notes of the curriculum of medical studies, Faculty of Medicine, University of Lausanne, Course year 2015–2021.
5. Scientific-Units-Recommendations-Formulas (SURF) guidelines, Médecine Interne General, Philippe Furger en collaboration avec Thierry Fumeaux et le SURF-team. 2020.
6. Pocket Book of Hospital Care for Children. Guidelines for the management of, common, childhood illnesses, 2nd ed. World Health Organisation; 2013.
7. Essential med notes, 2020 Comprehensive medical references and review for the United States Medical Licensing Exam (USMLE) step II and the Medical Council of Canada Qualifying Exam (MCCQE) Part 1, 36th ed., Sara Mirali and Ayesh Seneviratne.
8. WHO model list of essential medicines, 20th list. World Health Organization; March 2017, Amended August 2017. https://apps.who.int/iris/bitstream/handle/10665/273826/EML-20-eng.pdf?ua=1.
9. The Gambia standard drug treatment guidelines, 2nd ed. Department of State for Health and Social Welfare, The Republic of the Gambia; 2001. http://apps.who.int/medicinedocs/documents/s22418en/s22418en.pdf.

10. Cornuz J, Pasche O, Kermode-Noppel T. Compas: Stratégies de prise en charge clinique, Médecine interne générale ambulatoire. Lausanne: Institute of Social and Preventive Medicine; 2010.

11. Diseases and conditions: comprehensive guides on hundreds of conditions. Mayo Clinic. https://www.mayoclinic.org/diseases-conditions.

Immunization and Vaccines 23

Content

Bibliography 310

Immunization is the process of protecting an individual from an infectious disease by introducing a substance (vaccine) into the body that makes the individual to produce antibodies in the blood, which will prevent the subsequent development of the disease. Vaccine is a biologic preparation of killed microorganisms, living attenuated organisms, or living fully virulent organisms that is administered to produce or artificially increase immunity to a particular disease (Fig. 23.1).

Immunization is one of the most effective preventive health measures (Table 23.1). Vaccination programs directly benefit the immunized child. They also indirectly benefit unimmunized persons through community ("herd") immunity. Community immunity occurs when the portion of the population that is immune to the infection is large enough to decrease the risk of transmission (Tables 23.2 and 23.3). Community immunity protects children who are too young for immunization and persons with contraindications to vaccines. It relies on the majority of the population receiving routinely recommended immunizations.

The vaccination schedule is recommended and regulated by the national health department based on local epidemiological factors (Table 23.1). A standard minimal resource facility may supply vaccines regularly, and a cold chain is strictly maintained. Both infants and adults are immunized at BMC by trained healthcare providers (Table 23.4).

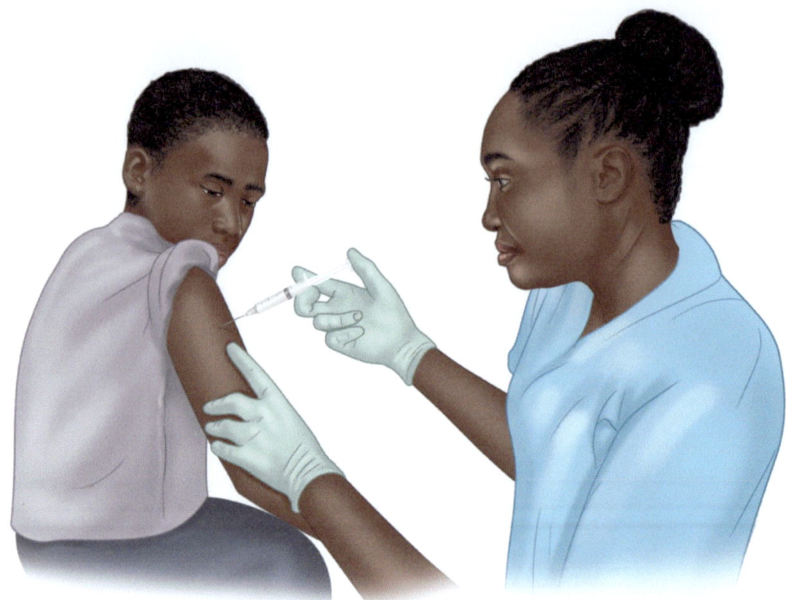

Fig. 23.1 Vaccination services is a significant activity in a standard minimal-resource facility. A well-trained healthcare provider equipped with a glove, a syringe, and skin disinfectant are the key needs to effect vaccination. Adequate transportation and storage of vaccines is important

Table 23.1 Diagnostic agents and vaccines

Diagnostic agents	Vaccination schedule, disease background
Tuberculin skin test (TST) testing for tuberculous vaccination or infection	*Tuberculin-purified protein derivative (PPD)* • Injection: SC, 5 units (0.1 ml) • Adult dosing • Tuberculin skin test: Intradermal: 5 units (0.1 ml) *Tuberculin skin test interpretation*: Criteria for positive TST read at 48–72 h: *Induration ≥5 mm*: • Patients with HIV infection (or risk factors for HIV infection, but unknown status) • Recent close contact to person with known active TB. Patients with chest X-ray consistent with prior TB • Patients with organ transplants • Immunosuppressed patients (receiving the equivalent of prednisone ≥15 mg/day for ≥1 month) *Induration ≥10 mm:* • Patients with clinical conditions that increase risk of TB infection • iv drug users • Mycobacteriology laboratory workers • Children <4 years of age, or infants, children, and adolescents exposed to adults at high risk *Induration ≥15 mm*: • Patients who do not meet any of the above criteria (no risk factors for TB) *Note:* A two-step test is recommended when testing will be performed at regular intervals (e.g., for healthcare workers). If the first test is negative, a second TST should be administered 1–3 weeks after the first test was read
Hepatitis B post vaccination testing An immune assay that quantifies the serum concentration of antibodies against HBsAg (HBsAb) in an individual	*Background* • Postvaccination testing is needed for certain groups who are at especially high risk for HBV infection • The purpose of postvaccination testing is to confirm if patients have achieved adequate immune response as measured by hepatitis B surface antibody • Perform testing 1–2 months after final dose of the HBV vaccine series • Persons with HBsAb concentrations of >100 IU/ml are considered immune

Table 23.1 (continued)

Diagnostic agents	Vaccination schedule, disease background
	Indications for postvaccination testing • Infants born to HBsAg+ women • Infants born to women whose HBsAg status remains unknown • Healthcare personnel and public safety workers at risk for blood or body fluid exposure • Hemodialysis patients • Individuals living with HIV • Immunocompromised persons such as hematopoietic stem-cell transplant patients or persons receiving chemotherapy • Sex partners of HBsAg+ persons
Varicella A detailed medical history may suffice to establish whether an individual had varicella disease (chicken pox) or not	Serological testing to check immunity before or after varicella vaccination is not routinely recommended because immunity following vaccination is often not detectable using currently available blood tests
Rubella also known as German measles or three-day measles is an infection caused by the rubella virus. This disease is often mild with half of people not realizing that they are infected	Immunity to rubella is not ensured and should be determined by laboratory testing for all women of childbearing age, regardless of birth year

Table 23.2 Vaccination recommendations for all

Vaccine	Notes, vaccine formulations, and schedules
BCG (bacillus Calmette–Guérin [BCG]) vaccine	*About the vaccine* • BCG is a live strain of *Mycobacterium bovis* developed for use as an attenuated vaccine to prevent tuberculosis (TB) and other mycobacterial infections • The vaccine was first administered to humans in 1921 and remains the only vaccine against TB in general use • Newborns and infants are the demographic group with the greatest potential benefit from BCG vaccination, and this intervention has been adopted for prevention of TB worldwide • BCG vaccination is appropriate for infants and children ≤5 years with a high risk of exposure to individuals with active pulmonary TB *Vaccination schedule* • BCG vaccination should be administered to healthy neonates as soon as possible after birth • Immunization of BCG-naïve school-age children (aged 7–14) not previously vaccinated has also been shown to confer partial protection against TB
Diphtheria, tetanus, and/or pertussis vaccines	*About the vaccine* • Routine immunization against diphtheria, tetanus, and pertussis during childhood provides protection against these diseases into adolescence • WHO recommends diphtheria, tetanus, and pertussis immunization during infancy for all children worldwide? Infants <12 months of age, particularly those <4 months of age, have a higher incidence and highest case fatality than any other age group • Routine infant and childhood immunization prevent morbidity and mortality • Diphtheria, tetanus, and pertussis immunizations for children 6 weeks through 6 years of age include DTaP vaccine and DTwP vaccine

(continued)

Table 23.2 (continued)

Vaccine	Notes, vaccine formulations, and schedules
	Vaccination schedule • DTaP vaccine is routinely recommended for infants and children at ages 2 months, 4 months, 6 months, 15–18 months, and 4 through 6 years • Booster doses are required beginning at age 11 years • DTaP vaccine is an inactivated vaccine. It is administered IM
Hemophilus influenzae type B vaccine	*Vaccination schedule* *Pediatric dosing for primary immunization* • *Infants 6 weeks to 6 months:* Minimum age for first dose is 6 weeks • INFANRIX DTPa-IPV + Hib susp injection • IM: 0.5 ml per dose for a total of 3 doses administered as follows: 2, 4, and 6 months of age *Note*: The number of doses for completion of Hib series is dependent upon products including some combination formulations (3 doses: ActHIB) *Adult dosing for dosing* • Immunization: IM • Adults who have not received the childhood Hib series and who are at increased risk for invasive Hib disease due to sickle cell disease, anatomic/functional asplenia, or splenectomy • Schedules are in general as follows: One dose (0.5 ml); may use any of the Hib conjugate vaccines • Reference to local modifications is highly recommended
Hepatitis B vaccine	*About the vaccine* • Injection is intramuscular, and the vaccine is inactivated *Vaccination schedule* • First dose within 24 h of birth, second dose at 1–2 months, third and final dose at age 6–12 months
HPV vaccine Human papilloma virus derived antigen used to vaccinate boys and girls during early adolescence	*About the vaccine* 9-valent HPV vaccine (Gardasil-9) is a noninfectious recombinant vaccine prepared from the purified virus-like particles (VLPs) of the major capsid (L1) protein of HPV types 6, 11, 16, 18, 31, 33, 45, 52, and 58 *Vaccination schedule* • Human papilloma virus vaccines, generally recommended for boys and girls of age 10 and above • Age below 15: Two doses at least 1 month apart • Above age 15, three doses as follows: 0, 1 month, and then 6 months
Measles, mumps, and rubella (MMR) combined vaccine	*About the vaccine* This combination vaccine includes live virus vaccines against measles, mumps, and rubella; it is an important tool for preventing serious illness due to these infections • The *measles virus* causes an acute infection characterized by fever, cough, coryza, conjunctivitis, rash, and enanthem, which may be followed by severe complications, including encephalitis. Adults with measles are at an increased risk of mortality compared with older children, and measles in pregnancy is associated with premature labor and spontaneous abortion • The *mumps virus* causes an acute infection characterized by parotid swelling. Mumps infection is usually self-limited but may be associated with complications, including orchitis and oophoritis, aseptic meningitis, and encephalitis. The most serious complications of mumps arise more frequently in adults than in children, including neurologic complications • The *rubella virus* causes a generally mild acute infection with a characteristic rash that can affect both children and adults. Fetal rubella infection can cause significant birth defects; immunity among adults (particularly women of childbearing age) is essential for elimination of the most important consequences of rubella: Congenital rubella syndrome, miscarriage, and fetal death

Table 23.2 (continued)

Vaccine	Notes, vaccine formulations, and schedules
	Vaccination schedules • *Children*: Routine immunization with MMR vaccine is recommended for children at 12–15 months and 4–6 years of age The second dose of MMR can be given as early as 28 days after the first dose, provided that both doses are given at ≥12 months of age • *Adults*: In general, immunity to measles and mumps may be presumed for adults born before 1957; healthcare workers are an exception
Pneumococcal vaccine	*Vaccination schedules* • One dose is recommended for adults: 65 years or older, regardless of previous history of vaccination with pneumococcal vaccines. PPSV23
Poliomyelitis vaccine	Immunization against poliovirus infection represents one of the world's great medical achievements *Vaccination schedules* *Adult dosing* • Immunization: IM, SubQ • *Previously unvaccinated*: Administer 0.5 ml per dose for a total of 3 doses given as follows: Two 0.5 ml doses administered at 1- to 2-month intervals, followed by a third dose 6–12 months later. If <3 months, but at least 2 months are available before protection is needed, 3 doses may be administered at least 1 month apart. If administration must be completed within 1–2 months, give 2 doses at least 1 month apart. If <1 month is available, give 1 dose • Completely vaccinated and at increased risk of exposure: One 0.5 ml dose *Pediatric dosing* • Immunization: IM, SubQ • *Primary immunization:* Infants and children 6 weeks to 47 months: Administer three 0.5 ml doses at 2, 4, and 6–18 months • *Booster dose:* Children 4–6 years: 0.5 ml as a single dose; administered ≥6 months after previous dose. Minimum interval between booster and previous dose is 6 months. The final (booster) dose should be given at ≥4 years, regardless of the number of previous doses
Rotavirus vaccine (Rotarix)	*About the vaccine* • Rotavirus is the most common cause of severe, acute gastroenteritis in infants and children worldwide • Rotavirus is a double-stranded RNA virus in the Reoviridae family. The outer capsid contains two proteins that define rotavirus • Vaccines so far licensed include pentavalent human-bovine rotavirus recombinant vaccine (RV5, PRV, RotaTeq), and attenuated human rota virus vaccine (RV1, HRV, Rotarix) is a monovalent vaccine derived from the most common human rotavirus serotype combination (G1P)

Table 23.3 Vaccination recommendations for certain regions

Vaccine	Clinical notes, vaccination schedules
Japanese encephalitis (JE) vaccine (Ixiaro)	*About the vaccine* • Japanese encephalitis virus (JEV), a mosquito-borne flavivirus, is the most important cause of viral encephalitis in Asia • JEV is transmitted in an enzootic cycle involving mosquitoes and vertebrate-amplifying hosts, primarily pigs and wading birds • Humans are incidental and dead-end hosts in the JEV transmission cycle, as they do not develop sufficiently high viremia to infect feeding mosquitoes • The most commonly recognized clinical presentation of JEV infection is acute encephalitis • Milder forms of disease, such as aseptic meningitis or nonspecific febrile illness with headache, also occur. Seizures (usually generalized tonic-clonic) are very common, especially among children • JE is diagnosed serologically by detection of JEV-specific immunoglobin (Ig)M antibody in cerebrospinal fluid (CSF) or serum by an enzyme-linked immunosorbent assay • There is no specific antiviral treatment for JE • Treatment consists of supportive care with emphasis on control of intracranial pressure, maintenance of adequate cerebral perfusion pressure, seizure control, and prevention of secondary complications • One JE vaccine is available: An inactivated Vero cell culture-derived vaccine (JE-VC; IXIARO) *Vaccination schedule* *Adult dosing* *Primary immunization* • Adults ≤65 years: IM: 0.5 ml/dose; a total of 2 doses given on days 0 and 7 *or* days 0 and 28. Series should be completed at least 1 week prior to potential exposure *Booster dose:* • IM: 0.5 ml/dose; given ≥11 months after primary immunization series completed, with ongoing or expected reexposure to Japanese encephalitis virus • IM: For IM injection. Do not inject iv, SubQ, or intradermally
Yellow fever vaccine (YF vax)	*About the vaccine* • Yellow fever is a mosquito-borne viral hemorrhagic fever with a high case-fatality rate • Clinical manifestations include hepatic dysfunction, renal failure, coagulopathy, and shock. The disease is endemic in tropical regions of South America and sub-Saharan regions in Africa • Yellow fever is the prototype member of the family Flaviviridae, a group of small (40–60 nm), enveloped, positive-sense, single-stranded RNA viruses that replicate in the cytoplasm of infected cells • An infected female mosquito inoculates approximately 1000 to 100,000 virus particles intradermally during blood feeding • Virus replication begins at the site of inoculation, probably in dendritic cells in the epidermis, and spreads through lymphatic channels to regional lymph nodes • The virus reaches other organs via the lymph and then the bloodstream, seeding other tissues. Large amounts of virus are produced in the liver, lymph nodes, and spleen and are released into the blood • During the viremic phase (days three to six), infection may be transmitted to blood-feeding mosquitoes' yellow fever is characterized by hepatic dysfunction, renal failure, coagulopathy, and shock • Other organ damages include renal and focal injury to the myocardium • The hemorrhagic diathesis in yellow fever is due to decreased synthesis of vitamin K-dependent coagulation factors by the liver, disseminated intravascular coagulation, and platelet dysfunction • The late phase of the disease is characterized by circulatory shock • The underlying mechanism may be cytokine dysregulation, as in the sepsis syndrome • The primary transmission cycle involves monkeys and daytime biting mosquitoes (*Aedes* species in Africa, *Haemagogus* species in South America)

Table 23.3 (continued)

Vaccine	Clinical notes, vaccination schedules
	The treatment of yellow fever • Consists of supportive care; there is no specific antiviral therapy available • Supportive care includes maintenance of nutrition, prevention of hypoglycemia, nasogastric suction to prevent gastric distention and aspiration, treatment of hypotension by fluid replacement and vasoactive drugs if necessary, administration of oxygen, management of metabolic acidosis, treatment of bleeding with fresh-frozen plasma, dialysis if indicated by renal failure, and treatment of secondary infections *Available vaccines* • A live-attenuated vaccine against yellow fever was developed in 1936 (yellow fever 17D vaccine) • The international certificate of immunization is valid for 10 years; a booster 0.5 ml dose is required every 10 years for the certificate to be reissued
Tick-borne encephalitis vaccine	*About the vaccine* • Tick-borne encephalitis is an acute viral illness caused by two closely related viruses of the family Flaviviridae: These viruses, which are endemic to forested areas, are transmitted by ticks • In addition to humans, they infect small mammals and, to a lesser extent, birds • The disease is characterized by abrupt onset of fever, severe headache, nausea and vomiting and severe back pain often associated with focal epilepsy and flaccid paralysis, especially of the shoulder girdle. Such paralysis may be permanent • The envelope glycoprotein of the TBE virus induces neutralizing and hemagglutination-inhibition antibodies and is the most important antigen for providing protection from disease *Vaccination schedule* • *Children:* Rapid immunization schedule is days 0, 7, 21 • *Adults:* Single dose booster is available
Cholera vaccine	*About the vaccine* • Cholera is an acute secretory diarrheal illness caused by toxin-producing strains of the gram-negative bacterium *Vibrio cholerae* • Cholera primarily affects resource-limited settings where there is inadequate access to clean water sources, as infection is most frequently acquired by the ingestion of food or water contaminated with *V. cholerae* • Cholera is endemic in approximately 50 countries, mostly in Africa and Asia • Infection with *V. cholerae* may have varying clinical outcome, ranging from asymptomatic intestinal colonization to severe diarrhea • Mild cases of *V. cholerae* infection causes simple watery diarrheal illness • Severe cholera is marked by rapid loss of fluid and electrolytes • Significant hypovolemia and electrolyte abnormalities, which can occur within a few hours of symptom onset, are the most important sequelae of severe cholera • Abdominal pain, nausea, and vomiting are other common symptoms, particularly in the early phases of disease • Most cases of cholera are presumptively diagnosed, based on consistent clinical manifestations *Treatment of cholera* • Aggressive volume repletion is the mainstay of treatment for cholera. Replacement fluids can be given orally • Antibiotics can shorten the duration of diarrhea, reduce the volume of stool losses, and lessen the duration of *V. cholera* shedding • Antibiotics are usually given orally. The antibiotic options for cholera include macrolides, fluoroquinolones, and tetracyclines • Adequate nutrition in patients with cholera is important to prevent malnutrition and facilitates recovery of normal gastrointestinal function • In addition, children with acute diarrhea may benefit from zinc and vitamin A supplementation • A clean water supply and appropriate sanitation are the cornerstones of cholera prevention • In addition, two oral cholera vaccines that are available internationally have demonstrated protective efficacy of 60–80% in areas at high risk of outbreak

(continued)

Table 23.3 (continued)

Vaccine	Clinical notes, vaccination schedules
	For residents in endemic areas • WHO recommends the inclusion of oral cholera vaccines in cholera control programs in endemic areas, in conjunction with other prevention and control strategies • WHO also recommends that oral cholera vaccines be considered as part of an integrated control program in areas at risk of a cholera outbreak • Two internationally licensed oral cholera vaccines are available, administered in two or three doses, depending on age
Meningococcal meningitis vaccine	*About the vaccine* • Can help prevent *meningococcal* disease, which is any type of illness caused by Neisseria meningitidis bacteria *Vaccination schedules* • The *vaccine* is usually given to babies at 1 year of age. A second dose is given when they are 3 years and 4 months old
Rabies vaccination	*About the vaccine* • Rabies is a feared human infection, with the highest case fatality rate of any infectious disease, caused by a number of different species of neurotropic viruses of the family Rhabdoviridae • Lyssaviruses are first amplified near the site of inoculation and subsequently enter local motor and sensory nerves. Viruses then migrate centrally in a retrograde direction within the axoplasm of peripheral nerves until reaching the spinal cord and brain • Almost all cases of rabies are transmitted from rabid animals through a bite • The average incubation period is one to 3 months • The prodrome: Malaise, anorexia, irritability, low-grade fever, sore throat, headache, nausea, and vomiting • There may also be specific neurologic signs and symptoms at the site of virus entry that are suggestive of rabies infection, including paresthesia, pain, and pruritus • An acute neurologic syndrome of either encephalitic or paralytic rabies follows the prodrome and typically lasts for 2–7 days • Manifestations may include hyperactivity, persistent fever, fluctuating consciousness, painful pharyngeal or inspiratory spasms, autonomic stimulation (hypersalivation), hydrophobia, and seizures. Paralytic rabies is characterized by quadriparesis and sphincter involvement • The differential diagnosis varies, depending on whether the patient presents with encephalitic or paralytic rabies *Vaccination schedules* *Adult dosing* • *Preexposure vaccination*: IM: A total of 3 doses, 1 ml each, on days 0, 7, and 21 or 28 • *Booster vaccination* (for persons with continuous or frequent risk of infection): IM: 1 ml based on antibody titers • *Immunocompetent*: IM: 4 doses (1 ml each) on days 0, 3, 7, 14 • *Immunocompromised*: IM: 5 doses (1 ml each) on days 0, 3, 7, 14, 28. Coadministration of immune globulin is indicated
Typhoid vaccine (Vivotif) *Synonym* Enteric fever	*About the vaccine* • More common in children and young adults than in older patients. Humans are the only reservoir for *S. enterica* serotype Typhi • Chronic *Salmonella* carriage is defined as excretion of the organism in stool or urine >12 months after acute infection • Chronic carriers represent an infectious risk to others, particularly in the setting of food preparation • Enteric fever usually presents with abdominal pain, fever, and chills approximately 5–21 days after ingestion of the causative microorganism • Clinical presentation relative bradycardia, pulse-temperature dissociation, and hypopigmented skin lesions on the trunk and abdomen • Hepatosplenomegaly, intestinal bleeding, and perforation may occur, leading to secondary bacteremia and peritonitis • Laboratory findings may include anemia, leucopenia, leukocytosis, and abnormal liver function tests • The diagnosis of enteric fever is made presumptively in patients with protracted fever without alternative explanation

Table 23.3 (continued)

Vaccine	Clinical notes, vaccination schedules
	Vaccination schedules *Adult dosing oral:* • *Primary immunization*: One capsule on alternate days (day 1, 3, 5, and 7) for a total of 4 doses; all doses should be complete at least 1 week prior to potential exposure • *Reimmunization* (with repeated or continued exposure to typhoid fever): Repeat full course of primary immunization every 5 years *IM*: Initial: 0.5 ml given at least 2 weeks prior to expected exposure Reimmunization (with repeated or continued exposure to typhoid fever) *Pediatric dosing* • Children ≥6 years: *Oral:* Refer to adult dosing • Children ≥2 years and adolescents: IM
Influenza vaccine (Fluarix)	*Vaccination schedules* • Influenza seasons vary in their timing and duration from year to year *Adult dosing* • In general, vaccination should begin soon after the vaccine becomes available
Varicella vaccine (Varilrix)	*About the vaccine* • VZV is one of eight herpesviruses known to cause human infection and is distributed worldwide • VZV infection causes two clinically distinct forms of disease: Varicella (chickenpox) and herpes zoster (shingles). Primary VZV infection results in the diffuse vesicular rash of varicella, or chickenpox • Endogenous reactivation of latent VZV results in a localized skin infection known as herpes zoster or shingles • Transmission occurs in susceptible hosts via contact with aerosolized droplets from nasopharyngeal secretions of an infected individual or by direct cutaneous contact with vesicle fluid from skin lesions • Primary varicella infection in children is generally a mild disease compared to more severe presentations in adults or immunocompromised patients of any age • Chickenpox is highly contagious. Transmission occurs in susceptible hosts via contact with aerosolized droplets from nasopharyngeal secretions of an infected individual or by direct cutaneous contact with vesicle fluid from skin lesions • The clinical manifestations of varicella develop within 15 days after the exposure and include a prodrome of fever, malaise, or pharyngitis, followed by the development of a generalized vesicular rash • Complications of varicella in children can include bacterial superinfection, while pneumonia is more common in adults • Patients with a history of underlying malignancy, steroid use, or immunosuppressive therapy, HIV infection, or solid organ transplantation are susceptible to disseminated varicella, due to impaired cellular immunity *Varicella immunization schedule* *SubQ:* • Two doses of 0.5 ml separated by ≥4 weeks (4–8 weeks apart per ACIP) • It is recommended that all children and adults without evidence of immunity receive 2 doses of the vaccine; those who received only 1 dose of a varicella-containing vaccine should receive a second dose

Table 23.4 Sera and immunoglobulins

Reagent	Formulation, clinical notes
Human immunoglobulins	*Anti-D immunoglobulin* *Injection:* 250 µg in single-dose vial, iv *Anti-rabies immunoglobulins* *Injection:* 150 IU/ml in vial, IM Anti-tetanus immunoglobulins *Injection:* 500 IU in vial, IM *Normal immune-globulin* *Intramuscular administration:* 16% protein solution *Intravenous administration:* 5%; 10% protein solution *Subcutaneous administration:* 15%; 16% protein solution Indicated for primary immune deficiency Indicated for primary immune deficiency and Kawasaki disease *Anti-venom immunoglobulin* • Injection. Exact type to be defined locally, IM • Antivenom remains the primary treatment for any patient with serious snake envenomation and should be used whenever available • High rates of adverse reactions occur for some antivenoms, but they may be lifesaving • Antivenoms consist of animal immunoglobulins developed against whole venom • Antivenoms vary with respect to the number of venoms against which they are raised, hence they may be monovalent polyvalent • Indications. When deciding whether to administer antivenom, clinicians who are unfamiliar with the management of snakebite should seek expert consultation with a physician experienced in management of snakebites in the region • Diphtheria antitoxin • Injection: 10,000 IU; 20,000 IU in vial, IM

Bibliography

1. https://www.who.int/biologicals.
2. Preclinical and clinical lecture notes of the curriculum of medical studies, Faculty of Medicine, University of Lausanne, Course year 2015–2021.
3. Scientific-Units-Recommendations-Formulas (SURF) guidelines, Médecine Interne General, Philippe Furger en collaboration avec Thierry Fumeaux et le SURF-team. 2020.
4. Pocket Book of Hospital Care for Children. Guidelines for the management of, common, childhood illnesses, 2nd ed. World Health Organisation; 2013.
5. Essential med notes, 2020 Comprehensive medical references and review for the United States Medical Licensing Exam (USMLE) step II and the Medical Council of Canada Qualifying Exam (MCCQE) Part 1, 36th ed., Sara Mirali and Ayesh Seneviratne.
6. WHO model list of essential medicines, 20th list. World Health Organization; March 2017, Amended August 2017. https://apps.who.int/iris/bitstream/handle/10665/273826/EML-20-eng.pdf?ua=1.
7. The Gambia standard drug treatment guidelines, 2nd ed. Department of State for Health and Social Welfare, The Republic of the Gambia; 2001. http://apps.who.int/medicinedocs/documents/s22418en/s22418en.pdf.
8. Cornuz J, Pasche O, Kermode-Noppel T. Compas: Stratégies de prise en charge clinique, Médecine interne générale ambulatoire. Lausanne: Institute of Social and Preventive Medicine; 2010.
9. Diseases and conditions: comprehensive guides on hundreds of conditions. Mayo Clinic. https://www.mayoclinic.org/diseases-conditions.

Content

References 319

Laboratory Medicine and Pathology supports clinicians by performing testing services for diagnostic and therapeutic evaluations (Fig. 24.1). In a standard minimal facility, a basic laboratory staffed by a qualified laboratory technician who works under the supper of an experienced physician is a necessity.

A wide range of tests may be conducted under controlled scientific conditions in the laboratory. The tests are conducted using biological fluids from presenting patients: blood, urine, sputum, feces, or skin.

The staff may constitute of the following:

- Chief laboratory technician
- Assistant laboratory technician
- Laboratory trainee

A minimum space of 12-m square, well-lit, and ventilated with at least three points of wall electric supply may be needed. The standard equipment needed are:

- Microscope with 10×, 40×, and 100× lens
- Centrifuge
- Hematology machine (e.g., Huma count)

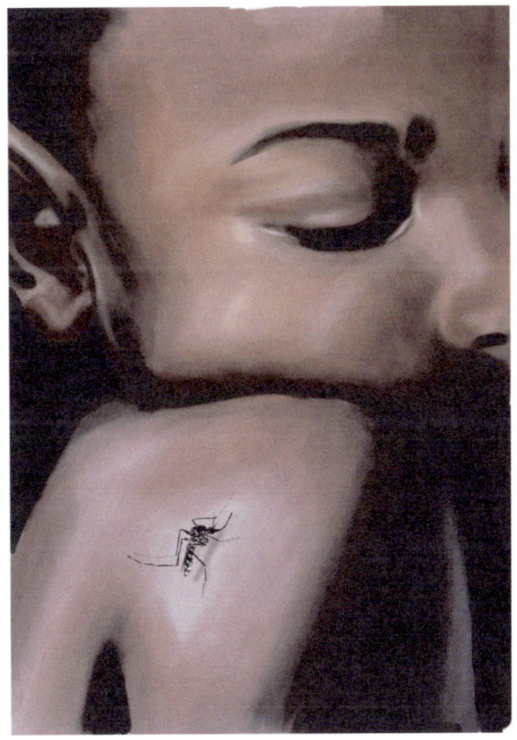

Fig. 24.1 A female anopheles mosquito after a full blood meal. Malaria and other vector-borne disease continues to be a major clinical diagnostic challenge

- Biochemistry machine, dry chemistry-based machines are preferred
- Pipettes
- Test tube racks
- Test tubes
- Erlenmeyer flasks
- Beakers
- Bunsen burner
- Syringes
- Graduated cylinder
- Thermometer
- Stopwatch
- Neubauer counter
- Balance scale

Services delivered by the clinical diagnostic laboratory are essential in providing quality healthcare. Based on medical history and physical examination, the healthcare giver orders pertinent laboratory examinations to confirm a suspected diagnosis. The laboratory tests conducted should have direct impact on the management plan of the patient in question. This is in line with the WHO dictum, "To test is to treat."

Before ordering the laboratory workups (Tables 24.1 and 24.2), the caregiver should explain in simple terms the tests to be done, their importance, and their impact on the management plan. The laboratory technician should explain the procedure to the patient and reassure the patient about sample taking, for example, venipuncture and urine and feces collection. Once the laboratory tests are done, the caregiver take time to explain the results to the patient.

Doing laboratory tests for every suspected disease condition is not necessary. Very often, the medical history and physical findings are sufficient to make a diagnosis and introduce an appropriate treatment plan. For example, a 21-year-old man, heavily exposed to mosquito bites in

Table 24.1 Essential hematology laboratory tests in a standard minimal-resource facility

Hematology	Reference values and comments

Hemoglobin
Hemoglobin (Hb) is the concentration of hemoglobin in whole blood, in grams per deciliter (g/dL)
• An increased Hgb may reflect a polycythemia (reactive or neoplastic) or be due to dehydration. A decreased Hb reflects anemia
	133–177 g/L
	• The laboratory uses the hematocrit (or packed cell volume, PCV) formula to calculate Hb = 0.56 × Hct
	• When interpreting the results, think of common causes of acute anemia:
	  – Blood loss through bleeding (gynecology, digestive, hemoptysis)
	  – Deficiency conditions (iron, folic acid, vitamin B12)
	  – Chronic infectious conditions. Hemoglobinopathies. Drugs induced

Hematocrit The hematocrit (Hct) is the packed spun volume of blood made up of red blood cell count (RBC), expressed as a percentage of total blood volume. It can be measured or calculated as Hct = (RBC × MCV)/10	0.40–0.52 i/i • Corpuscular cell volume is used to calculate the hemoglobin level • 0.56 × Hct = Hb • Very useful in grading anemia and for evaluating the response of anemic patients to substation therapies • An increased Hct can reflect polycythemia (reactive or neoplastic); if calculated, an increased Hct may reflect a normal number of RBC with an elevated MCV
MCH Mean corpuscular hemoglobin (MCH) is the average hemoglobin content in an RBC. It is calculated as MCH (pg/red cell) = Hgb (g/dL) × 10 ÷ RBC (millions/microL). A low MCH indicates decreased hemoglobin content per cell and is reflected in hypochromia on the peripheral blood smear. This may be seen in iron deficiency and disorders of globin synthesis	7–34 pg MCH is used to determine whether the anemia is hypochromic, hence determines whether iron substitution is indicated

Table 24.1 (continued)

Hematology	Reference values and comments
Mean corpuscular hemoglobin concentration (MCHC) The average hemoglobin concentration per RBC, in grams/dl. It is calculated as MCHC (g/dL) = Hgb (g/dL) × 100 ÷ Hct (percent). Low and high MCHC values are helpful in classifying anemias	310–360 g/L Used to determine whether the anemia is hypochromic, hence determines whether iron substitution is indicated Very low MCHC values are typical of iron deficiency anemia, and very high MCHC values typically reflect spherocytosis or RBC agglutination. Examination of the peripheral blood smear is helpful in distinguishing these findings
Mean corpuscular volume (MCV) is the average volume (size) of the patient's RBCs. It can be measured or calculated as above. Anemia can be classified based on whether the MCV is low, normal, or elevated	81–99 fl Indicates whether the anemia is macrocytic or microcytic, hence suggests whether folic acid substation is necessary. Bone marrow. Used to determine whether the condition is hyporegenerative
Reticulocyte Represents the immature red cells. Reticulocytes normally survive in the circulation for 1 day; after this time, they lose their reticulum (RNA) and become mature red blood cells. Under steady-state conditions, reticulocytes will represent approximately 1% of total circulating RBC	20–120 g/L Determine whether the regenerative activity of the anemia is hyporegenerative. Gives good indication of the synthetic activity of the bone marrow Under normal physiologic conditions, the lifespan of a red cell in the body is 120 days
Thrombocytes The platelet count is the number of platelets per microliter of blood (or number of platelets × 10^9/L). An elevated platelet count (i.e., thrombocytosis, also called thrombocythemia) may be seen in reactive and neoplastic conditions. A decreased platelet count (i.e., thrombocytopenia) may reflect platelet destruction, sequestration, or ineffective thrombopoiesis	150–350 g/L Thrombocytes are important components in coagulation. Useful in differential diagnosis of hemorrhagic conditions, petechia, and hypercoagulation conditions. Petechia may be seen in pathologic conditions associated with low platelet count Examination of the peripheral blood smear is helpful in distinguishing among possible causes
White blood cells/leukocytes The WBC is the number of WBCs per microL of blood (or number of WBCs × 10^9/L). An elevated WBC (i.e., leukocytosis) may be seen in neoplastic and non-neoplastic conditions. If the WBC is elevated, enumeration of the WBC differential and review of the peripheral blood smear is used along with clinical evaluation to determine the cause	4.0–10.00 G/L Useful biologic determinant of inflammatory and infectious status. Very often used to determine whether to initiate empiric antibiotherapy. Equally useful to determine the response of an infectious disease condition to an empirically instituted antibiotherapy

August, presents with chills, headache, and a fever of 39 °C. In such a case, a treatment for malaria may be introduced without waiting for a blood film confirmation for malaria. However, the caregiver should take time to give a thorough explanation to the patient.

Basic clinical diagnostic tests in the areas of hematology, biochemistry, microbiology, and immunology are essential. These can be established with minimal resources. Below are the basic tests needed in general (Tables 24.3, 24.4, 24.5, and 24.6).

Table 24.2 Essential biochemistry laboratory tests in a standard minimal-resource facility

Biochemistry	Reference values and comments
Glucose The amount of glucose in the blood *Terminology* • Blood sugar level • Glycemia • Fasting blood sugar • Random blood sugar	3.9–5.8 mmol/L Diagnosis and follow-up of diabetes. Determine iatrogenic glycemic status, for example, hypoglycemia induced by quinine Evaluation of a patient with altered level of consciousness, state of confusion
Glycated hemoglobin (HbA1C) • Hemoglobin formed in new red blood cells enters the circulation with minimal glucose attached • Red cells are freely permeable to glucose. As a result, glucose becomes irreversibly attached to hemoglobin at a rate dependent upon the prevailing blood glucose concentration	4.5–6.0% • Determines the patient's glycemic profile for the last 3 months • The average amount of A1C changes in a dynamic way and indicates the mean blood glucose concentration over the lifespan of the red cell • The A1C reflects mean blood glucose over the entire 120-day lifespan of the red blood cell • HbA1C correlates best with mean blood glucose over the previous 8 − 12 weeks
Creatinine Creatinine, a nitrogen-containing metabolite, is freely filtered across the glomerulus and is neither reabsorbed nor metabolized by the kidney	62–106 μmol/L Evaluates the kidney function. Kidney insufficiency may be caused by various infectious conditions, hypertension, diabetes, volume depletion-dehydration, drug toxicity, rhabdomyolysis
Urea Blood urea nitrogen (BUN) is generally less useful than the serum creatinine	BUN is used to evaluate renal function. It is generally less useful than the serum creatinine, because BUN can change independently in the regulation of systemic and renal hemodynamics
Uric acid Serum or plasma urate concentrations exceeding 400 μmol	<420 μmol/L High uric acid levels may be correlated with gout and gout-related arthropathies. Dietary advice may suffice. Alternatively, Zyloric may be prescribed
Cholesterol	<5.80 mmol/L Important in evaluating cardiovascular and cerebrovascular event risks
Sodium	136–150 mmol/L *Hyponatremia:* Polydipsia due to psychosis, low dietary solute intake, impaired urine dilution, thiazide-diuretic-induced hyponatremia, hypovolemic hyponatremia, hypervolemic hyponatremia (heart failure and cirrhosis), syndrome of inappropriate anti-diuretic hormone (ADH) secretion, CNS disturbances, malignancies, drugs (e.g., fluoxetine and sertraline), hypothyroidisms, adrenal insufficiency *Hypernatremia:* There are three mechanisms by which hypernatremia can occur: Unreplaced water loss, water loss into cells, and sodium overload
Potassium	3.6–5.0 mmol/L *Hyperkalemia:* Acute and chronic kidney disease, pseudo hyperkalemia, metabolic acidosis, insulin deficiency, increased tissue catabolism, reduced aldosterone secretion

Table 24.2 (continued)

Biochemistry	Reference values and comments
Liver function tests Blood tests used to help diagnose and monitor liver disease or damage *The liver function panel* • Alanine transaminase (ALT) • Aspartate transaminase (AST) • Alkaline phosphatase (ALP) • Albumin and total protein • Bilirubin • Gamma-glutamyl transferase (GGT) • L-lactate dehydrogenase (LD) • Prothrombin time (PT)	The pattern of liver test abnormalities may suggest that the underlying cause of the patient's liver disease is primarily the result of • Hepatocyte injury (elevated aminotransferases) • Cholestasis (elevated alkaline phosphatase) • Isolated hyperbilirubinemia • The magnitude of the liver test abnormalities and the ratio of the AST to ALT may make certain diagnoses more or less likely. ALT is a more specific marker of hepatic injury compared with AST • Abnormalities may also be acute or chronic, based on whether they have been present for more (chronic) or less (acute) than 6 months *Indications* • Screen for liver infections, such as hepatitis • Monitor the progression of a disease, such as viral or alcoholic hepatitis, and determine how well a treatment is working • Measure the severity of a disease, particularly scarring of the liver (cirrhosis) • Monitor possible side effects of medications
AST An enzyme that catalyzes metabolism of amino acids. Like ALT, AST is normally present in blood at low levels. An increase in AST levels may indicate liver damage, disease, or muscle damage Also known as • Aspartate aminotransferase • ASAT • Previously called GOT: Glutamate oxalate aminotransferase	10–50 U/L Evaluates hepatic cell injury. May be due to infections (HBV, HCV, parasites), drug toxicities, or traumatic assaults
ALAT An enzyme in the liver that is involved in conversion of proteins into energy for the liver cells Also known as • Alanine aminotransferase • GPT (glutamate pyruvate aminotransférase	10–50 U7l Evaluates hepatic cell injury. May be due to infections (HBV, HCV, parasites), drug toxicities, or traumatic assaults
Bilirubin (total) Produced during the normal breakdown of red blood cells, passes through the liver and is excreted in stool as bile giving stoll its characteristic yellowish color	Hyper-hemolysis or obstruction of the bile drainage system
Lipase	Lipase is mainly synthesized and stored as granules in the pancreatic acinar cells. There are several lipases in the human body, including lingual, pancreatic, lipoprotein, intestinal, gastric, and hepatic lipase. Activity of all the lipases is inhibited by bile acids. The activity of *pancreatic lipase* depends upon the presence of another enzyme, collapse, which facilitates attachment to triglyceride droplets and prevents bile salts from deactivating pancreatic lipase. One of the commonly used assays for pancreatic lipase takes advantage of this property; bile acids and collapse are added to the assay to inhibit all lipases other than pancreatic lipase, thus providing a specific assay for pancreatic lipase

(continued)

Table 24.2 (continued)

Biochemistry	Reference values and comments
Amylase	The main function of amylase is to cleave starch into smaller polysaccharides at the internal 1–4 alpha linkage in the process of digestion. The main sources of amylase in humans are the pancreas and salivary glands, but it can be found in other tissues in small quantities Patients with acute pancreatitis typically have an acute threefold elevation of amylase and/or lipase. However, enzyme elevations may not be as significant in patients with acute or chronic pancreatitis and alcoholic pancreatitis. Pancreatic enzymes may be elevated following trauma to the pancreas, postendoscopic retrograde cholangiopancreatography, or pancreatic ductal obstruction or surgery

Table 24.3 Essential serology laboratory tests in a standard minimal-resource facility

Serology-immunology	Reference values and comments
HBsAg	Negative Positive serology indicates active ongoing hepatitis
Syphilis (VDRL) A sexually borne disease caused by infection with Treponema pallidum. It is a sexually transmitted disease (STD)	Negative Latent chronic infection of Treponema pallidum. Useful in evaluating elderly patients with subacute onset of cognitive deficiency *Diagnosis and monitoring* • The TPPA test or TPHA test is used for *screening*. It becomes positive 2 weeks after infection • FTA Abs test is used to confirm the diagnosis • The VDRL test is used for monitoring the course of the therapy that is starting and being performed
HIV Several rapid tests presently available: "Determine" is the most commonly used • *HIV RNA detection:* Early HIV infection is characterized by markedly elevated HIV RNA levels, easily detectable with the HIV RNA (viral load) assays commonly used for monitoring of HIV disease • *HIV antigen detection*: The p24 antigen is a viral core protein that appears in the blood as the viral RNA level rises following HIV infection	Negative *Serological studies:* • After infection with HIV, the time at which antibodies against HIV antigens can be detected in the serum depends upon the sensitivity of the serologic test • Routine screening for HIV uses a two-tiered approach via an initial enzyme-linked immunosorbent assay (ELISA) that only detects the presence of antibodies, followed by a confirmatory Western blot if the initial ELISA is positive • Fourth-generation HIV tests are distinguished from antibody-only tests by their ability to detect both HIV antibodies and HIV p24 antigens. Combined HIV antigen/antibody tests can detect HIV-1 and HIV-2 infections
Thyroid panel These are tests that evaluate thyroid gland function	All patients with primary hyperthyroidism have a low TSH. The serum TSH concentration alone cannot determine the degree of biochemical hyperthyroidism; serum free T4 and T3 are required to provide this information

Table 24.3 (continued)

Serology-immunology	Reference values and comments
TSH	0.27–4.20 mU/L *If TSH is low* and only serum T3 is high (with normal free T4 concentration), the patient most likely has *Graves' disease or an autonomously* functioning thyroid adenoma. This pattern is more common in regions of marginal iodine intake. Another possibility is exogenous T3 ingestion. T3-hyperthyroidism can also be seen in patients taking antithyroid drugs *If TSH is low*, free T4 is high, and T3 is normal, the patient may have *hyperthyroidism with concurrent nonthyroidal illness*, amiodarone-induced thyroid dysfunction, or exogenous T4 ingestion. Patients who ingest exogenous T4 (levothyroxine) may have high serum T4 and T3 concentrations, but the T3/T4 ratio is lower than that in most patients with Graves' hyperthyroidism and toxic adenoma(s), whose T3/T4 ratio usually exceeds 20 (ng/mcg)
T4	9.75–21.30 pmol/L Levothyroxine
T3	4.0–8.3 pmol/L Liothyronine

Table 24.4 Essential urine laboratory tests in a standard minimal-resource facility

Urine	Reference values and comments
Urine sticks	The urine dipstick provides a rapid semiquantitative assessment of urinary characteristics on a series of test pads embedded on a reagent strip. Most dipsticks permit the analysis of core urine parameters: • Heme • Leucocyte esterase • Nitrite • Albumin • Glucose • Urobilinogen • Ketones
Urine microscopy *Classification* • Red cells • White cells • Epithelial cells • Casts • Crystals • Microorganisms	*Urine sediment examination procedure* • 10 ml of urine is centrifuged at 3000 rpm for 5 min • Pour most of supernatant out • Resuspended the pellet with gentle shaking of the tube • Use a pipette to place 50 μL (or a small drop) of resuspended sediment on a glass slide, followed by application of a coverslip • Report microscopy on standard laboratory sheet
Pregnancy test	*Test background and procedure* • Detection of human chorionic gonadotropin (hCG) in blood or urine is the basis of all pregnancy tests • The hCG is secreted into the maternal circulation after implantation, which occurs approximately 6 days after ovulation • This is the earliest that hCG can be detected with an ultrasensitive test *Note*: The ovulation to implantation interval has been observed to vary by up to 6 days in naturally conceived pregnancies. Late implantation has been associated with an increased risk of pregnancy loss

(continued)

Table 24.4 (continued)

Urine	Reference values and comments
Microalbuminuria A test to detect very small levels of a blood protein (albumin) in your urine *Indications:* To evaluate kidney disease in: • Type 1 diabetes • Type 2 diabetes • High blood pressure	*Test background and procedure* • 24-h urine collection is the gold standard for the detection of moderately increased albuminuria • The dipstick assessment is least sensitive and specific for determination of albuminuria • May be moderately increased in cardiovascular disease, diabetes, and nephrotic syndrome • Gives good indication of the state of nephropathy *Results and interpretation* Results of the microalbumin test are measured as milligrams (mg) of protein leakage over 24 h. Generally: • Less than 30 mg is normal • Thirty to 300 mg may indicate early kidney disease (microalbuminuria) • More than 300 mg indicates more advanced kidney disease (macroalbuminuria)

Table 24.5 Essential fecal laboratory tests in a standard minimal-resource facility

Fecal tests	Reference values and comments
Fecal occult blood a laboratory test used to examine stool samples for the presence of microscopic amounts (occult) of blood	Negative *Clinical background* • Testing for occult blood is stool-based done with fecal occult blood or immunochemical tests *Note:* Fecal immunohistochemical testing detects only human globin and therefore does not detect upper gastrointestinal bleeding (since the globin is digested in transit)
Helicobacter pylori (H. pylori) Test to detect *H. pylori* colonization of the gastrointestinal tract	Negative *Stool antigen assay*: • Detects bacterial antigen indicates an ongoing *H. pylori* infection • Is used to establish the initial diagnosis of *H. pylori* and to confirm eradication • Stool antigen testing is the most cost-effective in areas of low to intermediate prevalence of *H. pylori*
Fecal calprotectin Measurement of the calprotectin in the stool	>50 µg/g *Clinical background* • Calprotectin is a zinc- and calcium-binding protein that is derived mostly from neutrophils and monocytes • It can be detected in tissue samples, body fluids, and stools, making it a potentially valuable marker of neutrophil activity • Fecal calprotectin levels are increased in intestinal inflammation and is useful for distinguishing inflammatory from noninflammatory causes of chronic diarrhea • Elevated fecal calprotectin indicates the migration of neutrophils to the intestinal mucosa, which occurs during intestinal inflammation, including inflammation caused by inflammatory bowel disease
Shigella An infectious disease caused by a group of bacteria called *Shigella*	Negative *Clinical background and procedure* • Shigella infection (shigellosis) is an intestinal disease caused by a family of bacteria known as shigella • The main sign of shigella infection is bloody diarrhea and fever • Transmission is fecal-oral through direct contact with the bacteria in the stool: For example, childcare setting restaurants through contaminated food and drinks • Agar-based test to detect shigella species in feces. Useful for screening food handlers. Purchasable SS-Agar

Table 24.6 Essential tumor marker laboratory tests in a standard minimal-resource facility

Tumor markers	Reference values and comments
Alpha-fetoprotein (AFP)	*Clinical background and procedure* • Serum AFP concentration is a commonly marker for HCC • AFP is a glycoprotein that is normally produced during gestation by the fetal liver and yolk sac • Serum concentration can be elevated in patients with HCC
Carcino-embryonic antigen (CEA)	<2.5 ng/ml *Clinical background and procedure* • CEA is a protein found in many types of cells but associated with tumors and the developing fetus • Benign conditions that can increase CEA include smoking, infection, inflammatory bowel disease, pancreatitis, cirrhosis of the liver, and other benign conditions. Benign disease does not usually cause a CEA increase over 10 ng/ml • Useful as a tumor marker for intestinal cancer • Cancers that elevate CEA are mainly in the colon and rectum • Others include cancer of the pancreas, stomach, breast, lung, and certain types of thyroid and ovarian cancer • Levels over 20 ng/ml before therapy are associated with metastasis
Prostate-specific antigen PSA (total)	<0.4 ng/L *Clinical background and procedure* • PSA is a glycoprotein that is expressed by both normal and neoplastic prostate tissue • PSA is consistently expressed in nearly all prostate cancers • The absolute value of serum PSA is useful for determining the extent of prostate cancer and assessing the response to prostate cancer treatment • The use of PSA as a screening method to detect prostate cancer is common, although controversial • *Note:* PSA values may be influenced by bicycling, sexual activity, and strenuous bowel movement

References

1. Papadakis MA, McPhee SJ, Rabow MW. Current medical diagnosis and treatment. New York, NY: McGraw-Hill Education; 2019. https://accessmedicine.mhmedical.com/book.aspx?bookID=2449.

2. Preclinical and clinical lecture notes of the curriculum of medical studies, Faculty of Medicine, University of Lausanne, Course year 2015–2021.

3. Scientific-Units-Recommendations-Formulas (SURF) guidelines, Médecine Interne General, Philippe Furger en collaboration avec Thierry Fumeaux et le SURF-team. 2020.

4. Pocket Book of Hospital Care for Children. Guidelines for the management of, common, childhood illnesses. 2nd ed: World Health Organisation; 2013.

5. Essential med notes, 2020 Comprehensive medical references and review for the United States Medical Licensing Exam (USMLE) step II and the Medical Council of Canada Qualifying Exam (MCCQE) Part 1, 36th ed., Sara Mirali and Ayesh Seneviratne.

6. WHO model list of essential medicines, 20th list. World Health Organization; March 2017, Amended August 2017. https://apps.who.int/iris/bitstream/handle/10665/273826/EML-20-eng.pdf?ua=1.

7. The Gambia standard drug treatment guidelines, 2nd ed. Department of State for Health and Social Welfare, The Republic of the Gambia; 2001. http://apps.who.int/medicinedocs/documents/s22418en/s22418en.pdf.

8. Cornuz J, Pasche O, Kermode-Noppel T. Compas: Stratégies de prise en charge clinique, Médecine interne générale ambulatoire. Lausanne: Institute of Social and Preventive Medicine; 2010.

9. Diseases and conditions: comprehensive guides on hundreds of conditions. Mayo Clinic. https://www.mayoclinic.org/diseases-conditions.

10. https://www.uptodate.com.

11. https://www.who.int/biologicals.

Hospital Administration and Management

Contents

25.1	**Administration of a Standard Minimal-Resource Facility**	322
25.1.1	Costing Hospital Products and Services	323
25.1.2	Hospital Equipment and Material Inventory	323
25.1.3	Organization of the Reception	323
25.1.4	Accountancy, the Cashier, and Bookkeeping	324
25.1.5	Security of the Facility	324
25.2	**Stationery**	325
25.3	**Hospital Stock Management**	325
25.4	**Hospital Rules and Regulations**	325
25.4.1	Hospital Rules	326
25.4.2	Hospital Staff Regulations	326
25.5	**Continuous Training Sessions and Staff Meetings**	327
25.6	**Job Descriptions, Primary Staff Responsibilities, and Employment Procedures**	327
25.6.1	Medical Staff Job Descriptions in a Standard Minimal-Resource Facility	327
25.6.2	Paramedical Staff	329
25.6.3	Administrative Staff	331
25.7	**Hospital Maintenance Unit in a Standard Minimal-Resource Facility**	333
25.7.1	Electricity	333
25.7.2	Plumbing	333
25.7.3	Construction	334
25.7.4	Carpentry	334
25.7.5	Gardening	334
25.7.6	Housekeeping and Laundry	334
25.8	**Appendix: Checklists of Hospital Chores and Duties by Classified Department and Position**	334
25.8.1	Routine Hospital Chores	335
25.8.2	Human Resource Management Checklist	336
25.8.3	Facility Management Checklist	337
25.8.4	Nursing Team Management Checklist	337
25.8.5	Groundsman Management Checklist	338
25.8.6	Housekeeping Management Checklist	338

© The Author(s), under exclusive license to Springer Nature Switzerland AG 2021
M. Touray, A. Touray, *Clinical Work and General Management of a Standard Minimal-Resource Facility*, Sustainable Development Goals Series, https://doi.org/10.1007/978-3-030-71032-3_25

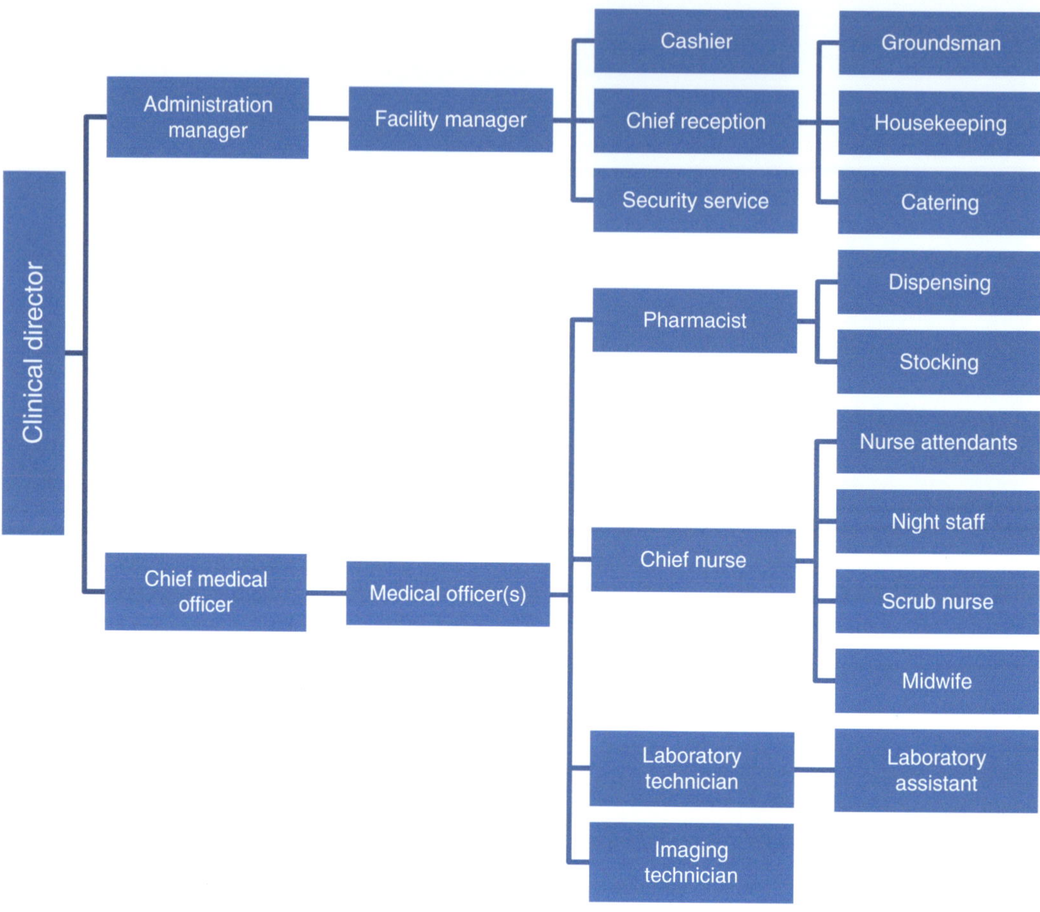

Fig. 25.1 Sample organization chart of a standard minimal-resource facility

The establishment and sustainability of a standard minimal-resource healthcare facility requires concerted efforts from multiple disciplines encompassing both clinical and nonclinical domains. Consistent performance and reevaluation of executive duties are mandatory. These constitute the basic principles of quality control, and they significantly affect patient outcome (Fig. 25.1).

The management and administration of a standard minimal-resource facility is structured to promote efficiency through orderly, transparent, responsible, and qualitative teamwork. This atmosphere of cohesive teamwork is guided by the spirit of "doctoring together." Every team player is equally important.

25.1 Administration of a Standard Minimal-Resource Facility

The administration is responsible for the day-to-day affairs of the medical facility. All changes and amendments are approved by the administration, and all department heads refer issues to the administration. The most important tasks of the administration are resource management (both human and material) and public relations.

The administration is the final check in guaranteeing that generated revenue is accurately recorded and properly handled (Fig. 25.2). To this end, administrative staff members must consistently check the payments transferred from the cashier against the balance sheets each day.

contact other health institutions to make sure that the decision made is in the best interest of all concerned parties.

25.1.2 Hospital Equipment and Material Inventory

Every 3 months, an inventory of hospital equipment is taken:

- Review the inventory list provided by the equipment manager.
- Complete the inventory.
- Make necessary changes.
- Notify the equipment management that the inventory is complete.

25.1.3 Organization of the Reception

It is the responsibility of the receptionists to ensure that the reception area is properly organized and that all incoming patients are satisfied with hospital services, including informing the laundry department if any cleaning needs to be done. To work smoothly, this organization requires staff with good interpersonal skills, the ability to manage a smooth patient flow, and excellent filing maintenance and retrieval skills. Reception staff should make sure that the facility and the employees are tidy and approachable at all times. They must maintain a high level of professionalism, using good communication tools and providing quick services to patients on an equal basis without discriminating for any reason.

The two receptionists should make sure that one of them will always be available at the reception. A good working relationship and close coordination is crucial to facilitate mutual understanding and ensure seamless coverage of the front desk. They should be able to take initiative and notify the administration of any needed changes. All patient concerns and questions should be addressed correctly, and patients should be comfortable while waiting to be seen. The receptionist should coordinate the flow of

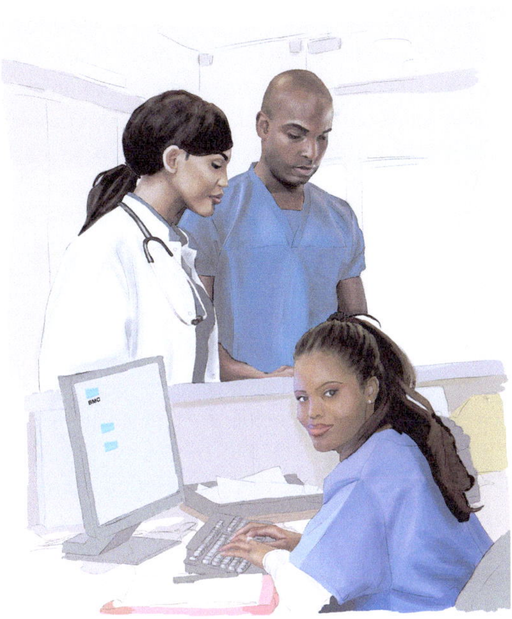

Fig. 25.2 Hospital administration

The administration takes all necessary measures in tracking missing revenue and solving complex financial issues, and he or she is responsible for utilizing the revenue for the hospital's benefit.

25.1.1 Costing Hospital Products and Services

The hospital management team is responsible for making decisions regarding the costing of products and services. These decisions should be based on the following factors:

- Hospital needs and national standards
- Patient condition and circumstances
- Demand for the products and services

When costing of products and services needs to be updated or changed, the administration or management shall consult all affected hospital staff, and the outcome of the discussion should be weighed on a balance of probabilities. The management may also wish to

patients from the reception to the consultation room based on patients' arrival times, but they should be knowledgeable enough to give priority to emergency cases.

For patients who have been seen previously, the receptionist must retrieve their files. To facilitate file retrieval, an affiliation card can be issued that provides the patient's biographical data and file number. If a power outage occurs, the file number on the affiliation card can be used to retrieve the old file. To avoid unnecessary duplication, the receptionist should promptly and properly refile all patient records after their consultations.

Because the receptionist is as important as any other professional in the hospital in providing good patient care, he or she should be well groomed and properly dressed in a hospital uniform. A high level of professionalism should be maintained at all times.

The most important function is communicating with incoming patients, so good communication tools must be used at all times. Quick service without any delay should be provided to all patients regardless of their time of arrival or reason for visiting the hospital.

25.1.4 Accountancy, the Cashier, and Bookkeeping

Revenue generated by the hospital must be received and tracked by the administration in order to reinvest these funds into needed areas. Financial transactions should be recorded and double-checked along two separate avenues, first at the cashier's office where patients settle their bills and then at the Administration office. Here the accountant or administrator rechecks the revenue received in each transaction and confirms its accuracy against the balance sheet.

The cashier is on the front lines. He or she collects the revenue that the hospital generates.

Before exiting the medical facility, all outpatients are taken to the cashier room. Here, they receive an account of charges and an explanation of acceptable methods of payment. The cashier ensures that the correct bill is given to each patient and that the patients fully understand the modes of payment. Upon receipt of payment, the cashier issues a receipt to the patient. Each patient's prescription form is also collected and kept by the cashier.

At the end of each shift, the cashier records all the revenue generated on a balance sheet bearing the names of the patients, their ticket numbers, the services rendered, and modes of payment. This data, including the prescription form, is passed on to the administration office.

In addition to handling financial transactions during his or her shift, the cashier is responsible for collecting the revenue generated during isolated shifts (nights and weekends) from ancillary staff. He or she should verify that such revenue is correct and properly documented before passing it on to the administration.

Cashiers should do their best to address the financial concerns of patients without referring such complaints to the clinical staff. If patients' financial situations are extremely complicated, however, the administration should be informed.

25.1.5 Security of the Facility

BMC collaborates with a private security company that provides security guards for both day and night shifts. The security guards rotate on a regular basis and are responsible for addressing the myriad security needs of the hospital. They are entrusted with the patient tickets and must issue ticket numbers to all incoming patients. Security staff are responsible for making sure that the visiting times are adhered to. They should make sure that no hospital property leaves the hospital without the prior permission of the management. They are responsible for recording the arrival times of the hospital staff, ensuring that every staff member signs in under his or her name, and returning the sign-in sheet to the administration each day. They are entrusted with several keys and must make sure that every staff member who takes a key from the key box signs for it. On a daily basis, security staff should also write a hand-over report that includes the names and signatures of recipients of keys, the time when each key was taken, and the time when it was returned.

25.2 Stationery

The hospital utilizes a wide range of stationery on a regular basis to aid in maintaining quality, consistency, and efficiency. To ensure continuity and maintenance of high standards, the proper handling of the stationery is a key priority. All stationery flows through and is managed by the administration, and supplies are distributed from the main store based on documented needs. Staff requesting new supplies of any kind must present a documented record of the previous stationery and how it was used.

Hospital units are responsible for making sure that stationery supplied to their units is properly managed. The units must also monitor stock levels so that supplies are always available, and they must request new supplies from the administration before the existing stock is exhausted. Examples of many of these forms may be found in Appendix A (Table 25.1).

25.3 Hospital Stock Management

Hospital stock management requires a thorough understanding of the medical facility's stock, mix as well as the usage demands and customary flow of inventory. Demand for hospital stock is generated by internal factors—hospital needs, prescriptions, and patient conditions—and supplies are restocked by means of purchase order requests. To maintain supplies at an optimum level, the stock management chain follows the following sequence:

- The facility manager determines the need for new supplies.
- Administration requests that new stock be added to inventory, either from the central medical stores or abroad.
- Arrival of all new stock is recorded; it must be counter-checked and signed for by heads of all hospital units: the administration, the facility manager, the physician, and the head or chief nurse. New stock is kept at the main store.
- It is the responsibility of the administrator and the facility manager to regularly monitor the hospital stock levels.
- The dispenser/pharmacist, accompanied by the administrator, must collect weekly supplies from the main store. The dispenser/pharmacist must record and sign for all the supplies that he or she takes from the store.
- Because the intake of new supplies is determined by the rate at which the previous inventory was depleted, the dispenser must provide a weekly report to the administrator listing all items dispensed from the pharmacy during the previous week.

25.4 Hospital Rules and Regulations

To ensure quality care for the patients and their escorts, provide a conducive working atmosphere for all employees. To abide by laws and ethics regulating healthcare, BMC established the following rules and regulations. Each employee is provided a copy of this document at the time of hiring. After being informed about the content, the employee signs a copy, which is archived in his or her personal employment file and is kept in the administrative office.

Table 25.1 Forms generated by the administration and stocked in the stationery office in a standard minimal-resource facility

Document/form	Comment
Consent forms	Consent forms are supplied by the main store and are then kept at the pharmacy and issued based on demand. All staff are advised in the proper use of these forms; all completed consent forms must remain confidential and must be kept on file in the patient's record
Job application forms	Job application forms must be stocked at the administration office at all times. No staff member should be employed or interviewed without properly filing a job application form. Completed forms are filed in the administration office and should only be accessible to the administrator
Laboratory request forms	Like all stationery, laboratory request forms are kept at the main store, and a supply is allocated to the pharmacy based on demand. The pharmacist in turn gives them to the laboratory technician based on demand, and the newly supplied laboratory forms must be documented by the pharmacist and signed for by the recipient (i.e., the laboratory technician). The technician must avoid the misuse of laboratory forms at all times and must correctly document laboratory results on the forms
Prescription forms	Prescription forms are kept by the administration, and a supply of new forms is issued to the receptionist when used forms are returned to the administration. The receptionists temporarily store the prescription forms and issue them to the prescribers based on demand. All patients must be issued a detailed prescription during their consultation, and this form should be used by the cashier to calculate the bill. The cashier must take these prescriptions together with the revenue earned to the administration at the end of each shift
Surgical consent forms	These are stored at the administration office and retrieved as needed
X-ray request forms	These forms are also kept at the pharmacy and are issued to the prescribers on request. Completed request forms must be properly filed in the radiology unit

25.4.1 Hospital Rules

1. Any person entering the hospital building must first report to Gate Security.
2. Only one escort is permitted to enter the hospital with a patient.
3. The taking of sand into the wards is not permitted.
4. Only one visitor per patient is permitted onto the ward at any time.
5. Always put rubbish in the bins provided.

25.4.2 Hospital Staff Regulations

The following list is taken from the BMC rules for hospital staff. It may be modified as necessary to suit the needs of other healthcare facilities.

1. Hospital property (equipment, furniture, tools, appliances, vehicles, etc.) may not be taken off the hospital premises without written authorization.
2. Prayer should occur only in designated areas. During working hours, patient care must take priority. In life-threatening situations (road traffic accident [RTA], dyspnea, suspicious myocardial infarction [MI], epilepsy, high fever), caregivers are expected to attend the patients unconditionally.
3. The correct uniform must be worn by staff as supplied. It is the responsibility of each staff member to maintain good personal hygiene and ensure that his or her uniform is clean. Proper flat shoes (not slippers) must be worn while on duty.
4. All members of staff are obliged to attend the weekly staff meeting on time.
5. All theft will be reported to the police immediately, and the appropriate action will be taken.
6. All professional misconduct will be reported to the registry of the corresponding professional medical board.
7. Personnel seeking medical care should do so by consulting the hospital doctor. A written record of this consultation must be kept. A

fee will be charged, and management will determine the appropriate staff discount, up to a maximum of 50%. Extended family members must pay full charges.

8. It is unprofessional for members of staff to recline on the beds in the wards or on the chairs in reception or over the desks. Free time should be used to the hospital's benefit—for example, ensuring that the work area is clean and tidy, and all records are up to date.

9. Mobile phones are to be switched off during working hours.

10. Staff is reminded that they must keep noise levels to a minimum, and they are asked to advise patients and visitors to do the same.

11. Personal visitors during working hours are not acceptable.

12. The management of the hospital can ask for visitation (physical search) of staff members and their belongings before they leave the hospital.

13. Days of leave must be approved by the management in advance, with a minimum of 2 days' notice.

14. Sporadic visitation of staff before leaving the hospital may be done.

15. To facilitate harmony and quality care, absence from work should be avoided. Sickness should be promptly communicated to the hospital management. A backing medical certificate (excused duty, or ED) will be requested. Failure to produce an ED certificate from a registered medical practitioner will result in no pay for the missed time period.

16. In appreciation of services provided by individual employees, several privileges are accorded by the hospital. These include partial payment on the fifteenth day of each month, taking time off for personal reasons, etc. The hospital reserves the right to withhold these privileges from individuals if needed.

25.5 Continuous Training Sessions and Staff Meetings

The hospital should organize regular meetings, continuing education programs, and seminars. At BMC, general hospital meetings are held every Wednesday to discuss key issues confronting the hospital and its staff.

Seminars are held in the nursing room every Tuesday and Thursday, so that the staff may refresh their knowledge of medical practice. The topics range from clinical practice to hospital issues.

Daily briefings are held to discuss patient issues and confront practice obstacles.

25.6 Job Descriptions, Primary Staff Responsibilities, and Employment Procedures

Due to staff turnover, growth, and evolving needs, every healthcare facility may have a procedure for taking applications and filling open staff positions. A standard minimal-resource facility recognizes the need to continually strengthen its health team and warmly welcomes all applicants who would like to join its team of dedicated staff. All interested candidates must compose a detailed application letter in their own handwriting, and the application must include any relevant documents that support their application. Suitably qualified applicants will then be contacted and asked to complete the job application form. After completing the form, the candidate will be called for an interview to assess their suitability for the post. When a candidate is hired, he or she will undergo a probationary period. At the end of this period, both parties shall decide whether a contract agreement should be signed or not.

25.6.1 Medical Staff Job Descriptions in a Standard Minimal-Resource Facility

25.6.1.1 Physician

1. Provide quality healthcare to every patient who comes to the facility.

2. Consult with patients and record details on the patient's record card. Note the following on this card: medical history, physical findings, suggested paramedical workup, diagnosis, and treatment.

3. Insist on proper record keeping and ensure that previous medical records are retrieved.
4. Explain to the patients in simple terms the findings, diagnosis, and treatment plan.
5. Perform the following procedures where necessary: veno-puncture/cannulation, abscess incision and drainage, ulcer management with dressings.
6. Participate in minor surgical procedures (e.g., suturing lacerations, redressing ingrown toenails).
7. Arrange follow-up consultations with patients.
8. Ensure that proper hygiene of the working area is maintained.
9. Attend and actively participate in patient briefings each morning.
10. Visit inpatients regularly: morning rounds at 9:00, regular visits to inpatients as needed, afternoon rounds at 14:00.
11. Supervise the discharging of patients and make sure that they obtain the correct prescribed medication before leaving.
12. Abide by approved international clinical guidelines.

25.6.1.2 Surgeon

Surgeons undertake most of the responsibilities of a physician, plus the additional task of carrying out major surgical procedures.

25.6.1.3 Trained Nurse (SRN, SEN, and CCN)

1. Join the doctors during daily rounds. Take notes of treatment and medication according to the doctors' instructions.
2. Verify abnormal vital signs taken by nurse attendants, and report findings to the physician.
3. Administer first aid to patients as required.
4. Coordinate dressing of wounds. Inform the doctor of the state of the wounds. Arrange an appropriate dressing schedule based on the physician's advice.
5. Be prepared to visit and provide care to patients at home if needed.
6. For all admitted patients:
   (a) Place cannulae when necessary.
   (b) Prepare the bed.
   (c) Keep patients informed and ensure that they are comfortable.
   (d) Ensure that patients have cool water at their disposal at all times during their stay.
   (e) Avoid bedsores during the patient's stay by ensuring that the sheets are clean and dry and, if necessary, by changing the patient's position regularly (especially when the patient is unconscious or paralyzed).
   (f) Check on all the patients' conditions on a regular schedule (one to 2 h, depending on the patients' needs). Inform the doctors of the state of all patients.
   (g) Administer medication as prescribed by the doctors.
   (h) Change linen regularly. Remove used linen from the beds for washing.
   (i) Waste management concerning sharp articles and/or objects soiled with biological fluids is accomplished with the assistance of the Ministry of Health. We obtain secured yellow boxes from the latter. These boxes are kept in designated areas of the hospital (the nursing room, the dressing area, the surgical area, and the delivery room). When full, the boxes are remitted to the Ministry of Health for incineration.

25.6.1.4 Nurse Attendant

1. Join the doctors during daily rounds. Take notes of treatment and medication according to the doctors' instructions.
2. Ensure smooth patient flow: collect the patient's file at the reception and accompany the patient to the consultation room.
3. Take vital signs of every new patient on arrival in the nursery or the consultation room and inform the senior nurse of the patient's temperature and blood pressure (adults only).
4. Assist patients after their consultation according to the doctors' instructions.
   (a) Outpatients: to the laboratory for testing and/or to the cashier.

(b) Inpatients: to the laboratory for testing and/or the nursing room for preparation for admission.

5. Administer first aid to patients as required.

6. Assist the nurses when dressing wounds:
   (a) Provide appropriate materials and prepare the dressing tray.
   (b) Follow the nurses' instructions during the dressing.
   (c) Clean all materials after the dressing is complete.

7. For all admitted patients:
   (a) Prepare the bed.
   (b) Ensure that patients are comfortable and have cool water at their disposal at all times during their stay.
   (c) Assist the nurses when administering medication.
   (d) Change linen regularly. Remove used linen from the beds for washing.
   (e) Ensure that treatment areas are kept clean and tidy; thoroughly clean sink and work surfaces as required for a sterile environment.
   (f) Verify regularly that wards, private rooms, and toilets are clean and hygienic. Whenever necessary, notify housekeepers of areas in need of attention.
   (g) Maintain patients' personal hygiene, including washing, cleaning up vomit, and emptying urinals.
   (h) Assist patients on their way out. Ensure that all patients leave with their correct medication.

25.6.2 Paramedical Staff

25.6.2.1 Laboratory Technician

1. Carry out all laboratory procedures as requested by the doctors, passing the results of the tests to the correct doctor.

2. Keep patients informed and comfortable during the procedures.

3. Direct patients to the waiting area during tests. When finished, call them to the consultation room to discuss their results with the doctor.

4. Record every laboratory test done in the laboratory record book.

5. Ensure that the laboratory is kept clean and tidy at all times. Clean the sink area thoroughly every morning.

6. Clean, dry, and stock all reusable laboratory material.

7. Check stock regularly and advise the doctor of laboratory materials that require restocking.

25.6.2.2 Radiographer

1. Collect the radiography request from the caring nurse or nurse attendant.

2. Inform each patient of his or her prescribed procedure.

3. Ensure that pregnant women are not unduly exposed to X-rays.

4. Perform the prescribed X-ray examination.

5. Ensure appropriate cleanliness of the radiography unit.

6. Ensure the availability of all supplies needed: X-ray films, developer, and fixer chemicals.

7. Report any malfunctioning equipment.

25.6.2.3 Pharmacist

The pharmacist is a certified drug dispenser. Per definition, this individual has completed a six-month drug dispensing course at the EFSTH and has worked under supervision at the EFSTH or one of its affiliated institutions. He or she is responsible for the following:

1. Procurement: ensuring that high-quality drugs are available at all times.

2. Distribution: moving the drugs safely to wherever they will be dispensed; making sure that storage and transport conditions do not adversely affect the drugs.

3. Verification of the accuracy of prescriptions: pharmacists and dispensers are often responsible for making sure that prescription errors are corrected by the physician.

4. Drug monitoring: dispensers are responsible for monitoring the rate at which certain drugs are prescribed. They should notify the prescribers when drug inventory is low or the

stock is about to expire, so that prescriptions can be modified accordingly.

5. Dispensing medicine according to the doctors' instructions. Writing down the name and schedule on the package.
6. Explaining clearly to patients how and when to take their medication; asking them to repeat the instructions as verification.
7. Recording all medication prescribed in the stock record book or the computer database.
8. Checking the main stock regularly and advising the administrator when new medicine and materials are required.
9. Before medication runs out in the pharmacy, collecting a supply from the main stock. Recording this in the request book.
10. Checking shelves monthly for expired medications and remove them from the pharmacy area. Notifying the doctor or administrator.
11. Ensuring that the pharmacy room is kept clean and tidy, thoroughly cleaning the work surfaces as required for a hygienic environment.

25.6.2.4 Ambulance Service

To facilitate rapid transfer of patients from or to our facility, a 24-h ambulance service is contracted. Generally, a physician or qualified nurse will determine whether a patient needs specific therapy that is not provided at BMC. If that is found to be the case, the physician formulates a transfer note and orders the transfer of the patient to an appropriate facility.

The ambulance driver is informed by the chief nurse, and a medical escort in the person of a nurse or nurse attendant is provided. Occasionally, the hospital is asked to pick up patients from their home to be brought to BMC for treatment. Finally, the ambulance service is involved in transporting patients from any facility to the airport for overseas treatment.

25.6.2.5 Drug Dispenser

Drug dispensers generally have no formal training in pharmacology or pharmacy management, as opposed to the pharmacist, who has undergone outside training beforehand. Drug dispensers are usually motivated individuals identified and trained in-house to dispense medication, although they are not qualified to assume the full role and duties of a trained pharmacist. They may perform the following:

1. Dispense medicine according to the doctor's prescription and instructions.
2. Write down the name and schedule on the medicine bag for the patient.
3. Explain clearly to patients how and when to take their medication; mention possible side effects.
4. Ask the patient to repeat the instructions to be sure that the instructions are understood.
5. Record all medication prescribed in the stock record book and/or in the computer database.
6. Check and organize the main stock regularly.
7. Advise the administrator when new medicines and materials are required.
8. Collect supplies of medication, stationery, and sundries from the main stock twice a week (at BMC, this occurs on Mondays and Thursdays). A request should be approved by the director and/or administrator.
9. Keep the main stock record in the store and keep the content up to date by noting changes in the stock.
10. Check shelves monthly for expired medications and remove them from the pharmacy area. Notify the clinical director or administrator.
11. Ensure that the pharmacy room is kept clean and tidy: thoroughly clean the work surfaces as required for a hygienic environment.
12. Refill the night and weekend boxes regularly. Control their content. Notify the administration regarding any anomalies.
13. Assist in preparing the annual medicine and supply order.
14. Demonstrate flexibility to meet the human resource needs of the hospital (reception, pharmacy, errands, etc.).

25.6.3 Administrative Staff

25.6.3.1 Accounting and Resource Manager

1. Prepare daily records of income and itemized expenses. Monitor prices on prescriptions.
2. File daily records (prescriptions and payment vouchers) for future reference. Safeguard these records in the administrative office.
3. Update bills for contract payments.
4. Prepare salary payments (bank transfers, checks, or cash payments).
5. Regularize fiscal and social issues (income tax payments, social security payments, registration).
6. Deliver bills monthly to insurance companies and other institutions contracted to the hospital.
7. Bill collection: monitor and collect payments from insurance companies and other institutions.
8. Procurement: make sure that stationery, sundries, medicine, and medical supplies are always available.
9. Timekeeping: provide time sheets to the security guard. Monitor the attendance of hospital personnel and regularly inform administration about excessive absenteeism.
10. Coordinate technical maintenance and communicate with external contractors in areas such as the generator, electricity, plumbing, and carpentry.
11. Chair weekly Wednesday meetings. Provide written minutes of each meeting electronically.
12. Human resources: attend to the basic needs of personnel (annual leave applications, absenteeism). Provide forms to applicants, review job applications and meet with applicants.

25.6.3.2 Human Resource Manager

1. Provide the first line of contact regarding staff recruitment and motivation.
2. Search for and screen potential candidates.
3. Conduct preliminary interviews.
4. Judge the suitability of candidates for positions.
5. Explain rules, regulations, and contracts.
6. Coordinate disciplinary measures.
7. Convey verbal warnings. (Reason, date, time, and witnesses should be verified and recorded.)
8. Convey written warnings. (Reason, date, time, and witnesses should be verified and recorded.)
9. Timekeeping: provide time sheets to the security guard. Monitor the presence of personnel in the hospital, and regularly inform administration about absenteeism.
10. Attend to basic needs of personnel (annual leave applications, absenteeism, emergency employee loans).
11. Chair weekly Wednesday meetings. Provide written minutes of each meeting electronically.
12. Prepare job descriptions for recruitment efforts and personnel reviews.
13. Prepare and pay staff salaries at the end of each month.
14. Record medical bills and staff absences.
15. Prepare the monthly roster.
16. Supervise housekeepers.
17. Plan and conduct team-building activities.

25.6.3.3 Facility Manager

1. Coordinate technical maintenance and communicate with external contractors, including generator, electricity, plumbing, carpentry, and ambulance services.
2. Write notices for public and employees regarding the state of the facility.
3. Write special medical bills for international insurances, certificates, death certificates, etc.
4. Attend to issues around volunteers: communicating with potential volunteers, selection of volunteers, briefing about accommodations, feeding, security and immigration issues in The Gambia, working hours, certification, etc.
5. Arrange purchase of cash power and diesel for generator.

6. Cross-match cashier, pharmacy, and gate records.
7. Record the facility's daily income and expenses.
8. Prepare monthly insurance and company bills.
9. Pay monthly bills from Africell CUG, Q-Cell, and Metro Trash, or the equivalent agencies.
10. Supervise the cleaning staff.
11. Procurement: make sure that stationery, sundries, cleaning materials, medicine, and medical supplies are always available.
12. Receive visitors.
13. Call FEDEX for collection of DNA samples.
14. Control payments of debts.

25.6.3.4 Cashier

1. Calculate the total sum for treatment and medicines prescribed each day.
2. Receive payments from in- and outpatients, and issue receipts for each payment.
3. Verify the validity of patients' insurance status.
4. Fill out the Daily Balance sheet.
5. Monitor and organize the payment of debts.
6. Receive records and cash from weekend and night nurses.
7. Prepare monthly bills of insurance, other companies, and individuals.
8. Hand over payment received, patient prescriptions, and the Daily Account sheet to administration at the end of each day.

25.6.3.5 Receptionist

1. Ensure that the reception desk area is kept clean and tidy at all times.
2. Assist and direct patients on their arrival.
3. Retrieve patients' medical cards and update with relevant information:
    (a) Personal information (including phone number).
    (b) Date and time of arrival.
    (c) Patient's weight.
4. Monitor closely the time between arrival and handing over to medical staff.

5. Inform the appropriate nurse of patients' arrivals and ensure that patients are comfortable and kept informed at all times.
6. Ensure that patients are seen by the doctors in the correct order.
7. Keep all files up to date and in order.

25.6.3.6 Housekeeper

1. Ensure that all floor areas are swept and washed daily.
2. Clean and wipe all surfaces regularly, except those in the nursery and laboratory.
3. Remove waste from all areas and put it into the correct containers.
4. Change curtains on doors and windows when necessary.
5. Clean sinks and toilets daily. Wash toilet floors every morning and as necessary during the course of the day.
6. Ensure toilet rolls are in the dispenser, and soap and clean towels are available at the hand-washing basin.
7. Clean windows and wash all paintwork once a week.
8. Collect all dirty linen from the wards and launder as required.
9. Make sure that clean uniforms are always available for all the staff members.
10. Iron all items and store them in relevant cupboards.

25.6.3.7 Security Guard

1. Secure all properties of the hospital, day and night.
2. Note incoming and outgoing times of all on hospital premises.
3. Ensure that water tanks are full and the hospital has running water at all times.
4. Open and close the hospital gates for incoming and outgoing vehicles.
5. Guard the key to the dressing room. Write down the time and name every time the key is used.
6. Ensure that lights and fans are off after 18.00.

25.6.3.8 Groundskeeper

1. Maintain the outside area. Maintain the gardens, water the plants, and trim along the

fence, both inside and out, on the first Friday of the month.
2. Control cleaning outside.
3. Take care of the generator: make sure it is in working order and fuel is always available.
4. Make sure that the ambulance is in working order and there is a schedule for drivers.
5. Maintain the machinery in the laundry area.
6. Take care of small maintenance issues (e.g., changing lightbulbs).
7. Supervise the security guard and make sure there are always enough forms available.
8. Assist in loading and unloading goods brought to the hospital and those to be taken away from the hospital.
9. Assist in the disposal of waste from hospital premises.

25.7 Hospital Maintenance Unit in a Standard Minimal-Resource Facility

Conserving and maintaining material resources are important aspects of BMC's aspiration to continually expand, develop, and improve its facilities (Fig. 25.3). All staff members are urged to take responsibility and report any damaged material immediately. The hospital has a liaison agreement with maintenance personnel, who will come and repair such materials upon the request of the administration. Hospital equipment should be well taken care of by all staff to ensure durability. The facility manager is responsible for handling reports about damaged materials and taking appropriate measures to maintain equipment and other material resources.

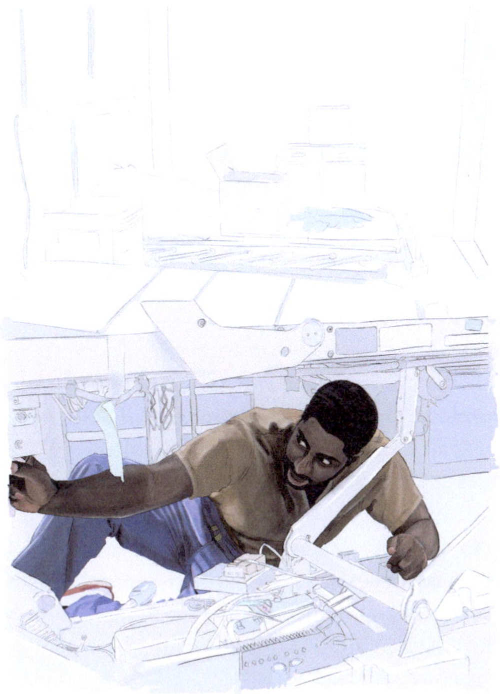

Fig. 25.3 An organized maintenance unit is essential to assure an uninterrupted provision of healthcare in a standard minimal-resource facility

The administration is responsible for recharging the electric cash power on a monthly basis. In case of electrical outage, the generator should be switched on by the groundman or another staff member who is trained in the operation of the generator. Untrained personnel should not attempt to turn it on or off. To ensure quietness for the patients and the neighborhood, the generator must not be switched on after 24:00.

25.7.2 Plumbing

The availability of safe running water is of paramount importance in healthcare delivery. It ensures hygiene and plays a crucial role in preventing iatrogenic/nosocomial infections. Any damaged taps should be reported to the facility manager. Any change in the color of the water

25.7.1 Electricity

Conservation of electricity is of paramount importance, especially as the cost is increasing. For this reason, electrical appliances should only be used when needed.

should be reported to ensure the cleaning of the tank. The hospital should cooperate with plumbing personnel, who will come and repair damaged taps and clean the tank upon the request of the management. Water is an important resource of the hospital and must be used in a rational manner.

25.7.3 Construction

There is a constant need to maintain and upgrade the hospital structures. All staff members are encouraged to make suggestions if they feel that a change in any particular structure will be good for the hospital and, in particular, patient care. When a change of structure is deemed necessary, a qualified mason will be contracted and the architectural plan will be provided to him to give an idea of what the structure will look like.

25.7.4 Carpentry

Woodwork provides an easy and reasonably convenient infrastructure. All needed changes will be thoroughly evaluated, and, if woodwork is preferred for a particular change, a qualified carpenter will be contracted to carry out the work. Staff members are encouraged to keep wooden areas tidy. This will ensure longevity and prevent repeated staining of the wooden areas.

25.7.5 Gardening

Being surrounded by a beautiful environment of greenery is one of our greatest aspirations. The grounds man is responsible for taking care of the garden. He ensures that the garden is watered and that the plants are in good health. He should notify the administration when fruit ripens, and he should be directly involved in harvesting and delivering the fruits to the hospital administration to be equitably provided to patients and employees. He is responsible for cleaning the hospital terrace on a daily basis, excepting Sundays.

25.7.6 Housekeeping and Laundry

The role of the housekeepers in maintaining quality standards cannot be overemphasized. They are responsible for making sure that the hospital is clean at all times. The housekeeping staff is composed of a dynamic team that works tirelessly in keeping the wards and various units clean at all times. They are also responsible for laundering the dirty linen. All dirty linen is conveyed to the laundry department, where the laundry team launders it and packs all items neatly for the next user.

The house keeping unit provides the clean linen or bed sheets to the nurses on a regular basis, according to demand. The work of this team is both arduous and tedious, so all staff members are encouraged to assist them by not using the bed sheets unnecessarily and by soaking stained or soiled bed sheets in a container when the laundry team is off. Taking this small step ensures that laundering the sheets the following day will be much easier.

25.8 Appendix: Checklists of Hospital Chores and Duties by Classified Department and Position

An effective delivery of healthcare services is characterized by execution of specific chores at a timely order. The timing of execution of the chores may be hourly, daily, weekly, or yearly. The execution of each chore is assigned to a particular individual, which facilitates supervision, accountability, and traceability. To maintain good standards rigor and discipline must be exercised at its fullest.

Below is a list of chores that are executed.

25.8.1 Routine Hospital Chores

Admin issues	Admin manager	Med officer	Chief nurse	Admin assistant	HR manager
Salary payment end of month					
Advance salary payments					
Emergency employee loans					
GRA tax monthly payments					
Social security monthly payments					
Retainership contracts					
Payment monthly Africell CUG					
Payment monthly phone bills					
Payment monthly trash removal					
Payment monthly security services					
Preparing job descriptions					
Yearly vehicle documents					
Receiving daily income					
Cross-matching cashier, pharmacy, and gate records					
Record daily income and expenses					
Preparing bills, insurances monthly					
Vanbreda					
Clearing imported goods					
Hospital TIN certificates					
Employee TIN certificates					
Social security employee registration					
Social security employee contribution					
Routine hospital forms					
Notices for the public					
Notices for employees					
Deciding on uniforms					
Public relations					
Volunteering issues					
Marketing					
Writing medical certificate					
Writing special med bills					
Writing death certificates					
Buying cleaning material					
Buying stationery					
Buying drugs locally					
Annual medicine order					
Receiving visitors					
Buying cash power					
Cashing cheques hospital account					
Order cheque book from GTB					

Admin issues	Admin manager	Med officer	Chief nurse	Admin assistant	HR manager
Recording staff med bills					
Payment of consultants					
Pricing surgical operations					
DNA bill payments USA					
Receiving DNA payment					
Calling FedEx for DNA sample					
Central stores: HIV, diazepam, vaccines					
Mailbox collection weekly at Serekunda Post Office					
Collection of med sup 3× week					
Printer: paper cartridge					
Permission for owing					
Controlling payment owing					

25.8.2 Human Resource Management Checklist

Human resource issues	Admin	Physician	Chief nurse	Admin assistant	HR manager
Monthly roster					
Recruitments: form filling					
Interviews					
Supervision of supervisors					
Hierarchy establishments					
Timekeeping					
Wednesday meetings					
Training arrangements					
Leave approval—leave letters					
Disciplinary actions					
Dismissals—terminations					
Team-building activities					

25.8.3 Facility Management Checklist

Facility management	Admin	Med officer	Chief nurse	Admin assistant	HR manager
Maintenance and repairs					
Construction					
Stores and their management					
Equipment repair					
Furniture repair					

25.8.4 Nursing Team Management Checklist

Nursing team	Admin	Med officer	Chief nurse	Admin assistant	HR manager
Individual duty assignment					
Dressing room					
Nursing room					
Presenting patient files in the morning meeting					
Wards					
Delivery room					
Consultation room					
Echo lap					
Laboratory					
Floor hallway					
Mosquito nets					
Drip stands					
Dustbins					
Controlling surgery area					
Arranging surgical consultation					
Arranging gynecology consultation					
Arranging radiography					
Morning "BMC-clinical flash" seminar					
ECG writing					
Preparing contract for uniform delivery					
Handing out uniforms and getting contracts signed					
Providing thermometers and BP machine					

25.8.5 Groundsman Management Checklist

Groundman	Admin	Med officer	Chief nurse	Admin assistant	HR manager
Garden: cleaning watering, pruning					
Trash corner					
Coordinating trash collection					
Outside toilet					
Prayer area					
Mortuary					
Carport					
Generator					
Generator room					
Shop area					
Hospital front yard					
Hospital backyard					
Mosquito control					
Pest (cockroach, etc.) control					
Ambulance					
Technical store					
Tap in prayer area					
Supervision of cleaners					

25.8.6 Housekeeping Management Checklist

Housekeeping	Admin	Med officer	Chief nurse	Admin assistant	HR manager
Dirty bedsheets					
Clean bedsheets					
Cleaning buckets					
Cleaning rags					
Soap for skin					
Brooms					
Laundry outsourcing (bedsheets)					

Contents

26.1   **Patient Card** 341

26.2   **Medical Report** 342

26.3   **Certificate of Good Health** 343

26.4   **Attestation of Fit to Fly** 344

26.5   **Attestation of Birth** 345

26.6   **Referral Form for Outside Treatment** 347

26.7   **Surgical and Medical Procedure Informed Consent Form** 348

26.8   **Retroviral (HIV) Test Consent Form** 349

26.9   **Surgical Operation Report** 350

26.10 **Request for Maternity Leave** 351

26.11 **Excused Duty Certificate** 352

26.12 **Antenatal Card** 353

26.13 **Obstetrical Delivery Chart** 355

26.14 **Child Health Card** 357

26.15 **Essential Medication List** 361

26.16 **Available Vaccines/Infant Immunization Schedule** 362

26.17 **Laboratory Request Form** 363

26.18 **X-ray Request Form** 364

26.19 **Medical Prescription Form** 365

26.20 **Self-Discharge Form** 366

26.21 **Certificate of Death** 367

26.22 **Job Application Form** 368

26.23 **Cash Transaction Receipts** 370

26.24 **Institutional Affiliations** 373

Bibliography 374

M. Touray, A. Touray, *Clinical Work and General Management of a Standard Minimal-Resource Facility*, Sustainable Development Goals Series, https://doi.org/10.1007/978-3-030-71032-3_26

"Communication" stems from Latin *communicare,* meaning "to share." Communication is the act of conveying meanings from one entity or group to another through the use of mutually understood signs, symbols, and words. Communication is central to all human activities and especially so to activities pertaining to healthcare provision. In the medical professional setting, communication represents a way of exchanging information. Communication signifies our capability to express our knowledge and thought process and to transmit these to others for a mutual benefit.

During clinical work in a team, to assure proper communication and transmission of information, words must be used accurately. Accurate use of words minimizes ambiguity, allows precise transmission of patient condition, assures patient safety, and improves clinical outcome. Hence the significance of learning the accurate meaning of words and using the learnt words correctly cannot be overemphasized.

It is estimated that during the four to six years of preclinical and clinical formal medical education, a student encounters over thirty thousand words. Of these, the student may be required to know about three thousand to successfully go through the various academic assessment schemes. Once in routine active healthcare service, using three hundred medical words accurately may be sufficient to describe, discuss, and transmit most clinical scenarios.

In this chapter we present a glossary, consisting of three hundred medical words we deem necessary for all healthcare workers to be familiar with. Because of the complexity of the medical profession, this list is in no way comprehensive. It represents what the authors judge most useful.

Specific examples of documents written by clinicians are presented in subsequent sections. The quality of the documents generated by the clinicians directly impacts on clinical outcome of the patient (Fig. 26.1).

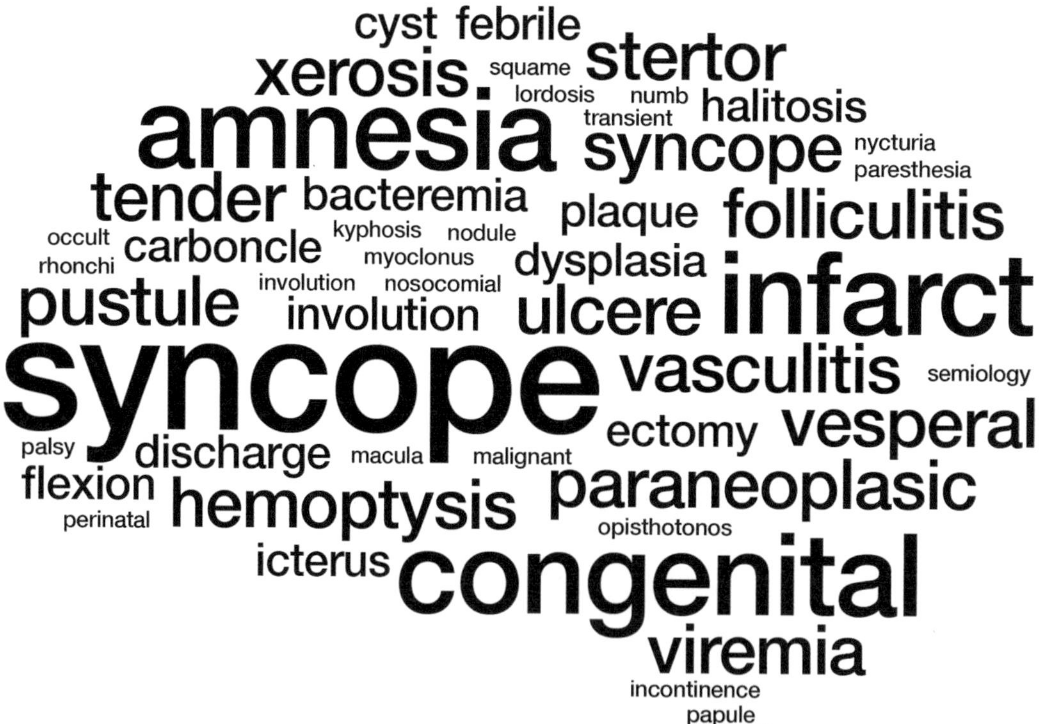

Fig. 26.1 Clinical communication: illustration depicting the large number of words that need to be mastered for a good interprofessional communication. These are common words that health professionals should know. The meaning of words should be clear and known to healthcare providers in order to facilitate professional communication

26.1   Patient Card

The patient card is a very important and confidential document where the consulting physician notes his historical, physical, and laboratory findings. The formulated diagnostic and differential diagnosis as well as the management plan are noted in the patient file. Although legally the file belongs to the patient, for convenience they are safely filed in the hospital under key.

Patient's Card

Bijilo Medical Center
Care
Compassion
Commitment

Bijilo, Near CSE, Tel: 4464868, Fax: 4464867

Name: .... Surname: .... Date of Birth: ....

Address: .... Occupation: ....

Date

26.2 Medical Report

A medical report is a document that entails patient identity, medical history, diagnosis, treatment plan, and clinical outcome. It may also contain various propositions. It serves to assist subsequent healthcare givers to have a comprehensive medical knowledge of the patient concerned. A medical report denotes the quality of the institution that issues it as well as the expressive knowledge or capacity of the physician that authored it.

✚ BMC
Bijilo Medical Center
PO Box 3349
Serekunda
The Gambia
Telephone: +220 xyz   Date...............

Medical Report

Re: Mr/Ms XY   **DOB: ....**
Diagnosis:
1. xxx
2. xxx
3. xxx
History
Mr/Ms XY was hospitalised at BMC from ... to ...
Mr/Ms XY presented with xxxxxxxx ....
Physical
(Evaluation of the physical state)
Laboratory
(Laboratory test values)
Chest X-Ray:xxxx
Echocardiography *Date....... see reports*
Conclusion and Proposition
xxxx
Medication:
xxxxx

Dr XX
BMC

26.3   Certificate of Good Health

Health is *a state of physical, mental, and social well-being, not just the absence of disease or infirmity (WHO).* Good health enables people to live a full life and perform professional duties: Good health is also required to be engaged in physically and mentally exertional hobbies.

Before embarking on a new employment, a curriculum in an institution, and participating in a sporting event, some institutions request for certificate of good health. Based on medical history, physical findings, and laboratory results, the physician attests to the physical and mental capability of the candidate by issuing the certificate of good health.

✚ BMC
Bijilo Medical Center
PO Box 3349
Serekunda
The Gambia

Telephone: +220 xyz

Date

Certificate of Good health

This is to certify that Mr./Ms. XY, DOB …..is in good health. Based on medical history, physical examination and paramedical investigations performed on this Date………….., Mr./Ms. XY is mentally and physically fit to execute his professional duties.
There is no evidence of contagious disease.

Sincerely

Dr XX
Bijilo Medical Centre

26.4 Attestation of Fit to Fly

A Fit to Fly certificate is a medical document that is completed by a clinician to attest that a traveler can sustain the physiological and psychological stress associated with flying without adverse repercussions.

The attesting physician should familiarize him/herself with the physiology during flight. To enable attestation, a thorough systematic clinical review of the patient should be performed considering cardiovascular or respiratory diseases. Risk factors for deep venous thrombosis, gestational age, anemia, ear-nose-throat pathologies, post-surgical conditions, trauma and orthopedics, psychiatric or neurological illness, and contagious infectious diseases should be evaluated. Diabetic patients should be provided special advice.

✚ BMC
Bijilo Medical Center
PO Box 3349
Serekunda
The Gambia
Telephone: +220 xyz   Date

Fit to Fly

Re: Mr./Ms. XY
D.O.B. ……..

Based on medical reasons, we advise that Mr./Ms. XY is fit to fly on……………
We remain at your disposal for any further clarification.

Yours sincerely,

Dr. XX
BMC

26.5 Attestation of Birth

(a) Every birth at a standard minimal-resource facility is attested by the gynecologist or midwife. This document is presented to the appropriate health authority for the issuance of the official national birth certificate. The birth attestation report should contain the bio-data of the child: notable birthweight, length, sex as well as date, time, and place of birth.

✚ BMC
Bijilo Medical Center
PO Box 3349
Serekunda
The Gambia
Telephone: +220 xyz

Date....

Attestation of Birth

This is to certify that the child, XY, was born at Bijilo Medical Centre, Bijilo Village

Date and time of birth: ....

Weight at birth: ....

Length at birth: ....

Place of birth ....

Gender: ....

Mother's name: ....

Dr XX
Bijilo Medical Centre

(b) Births that occurred at home are generally certified by the midwife with the acknowledgment of an appointed communal author-ity. The form below is used for registration of births at home.

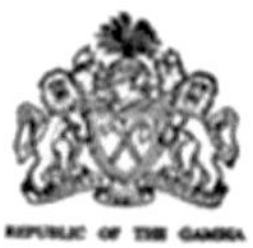

BIRTH'S ATTESTATION

TO WHOM IT MAY CONCERN

Annex F

NAME OF VILLAGE /TOWN..DISTRICT..

DATE..Region...

I.. the Alkali of.. do hereby attest to

the birth of ....in ....

He/She was born on the day.............................month............. ....year.....................................

His / her father's name... who was born in.................

...............................Village/town in the Republic of.. Whose Nationality

is..NIN/PC/BC#...

His/Her mother's name... who was born in................

.... village/town, whose nationality is ....and her

NIN/PC/BC #..Both parents were married/ Unmarried at the time of

his/her birth.

Father's occupation is / was............................The parents of the said applicant are personally   known to

me and presently resident in .... I am aware/ not aware the birth of the said applicant.

Informant: **Alikalo**

Signature/ thumb print..   signature /thumb print..................................

NIN/ PC/BC#..   NIN/PC/BC...

Address...   mobile /telephone#..................................

Mobile/Telephone#..   Stamp

District Chief's Stamp

26.6   Referral Form for Outside Treatment

Referring patients from one health faculty to another is a regular occurrence. The reasons for referrals are multiple. To assure good clinical patient outcome, a standard minimal facility should establish a list of referral centers. The healthcare workers on the wards should be familiar with the different referral options. A good working relation should be nurtured between the referring center and the receiving center. Below is an example of the center we frequently refer patients to for various reasons.

The referring physician needs to complete this form which entails patient identity, relevant clinical date, and the reason for referral.

Bijilo Medical Center
PO Box 3349
Serekunda
The Gambia
Email: drmusa@bijilomedical.org
Telephone: +220 6665555 / +220 9980371

BMC REFERRAL FORM

Patient name   ....

Date of birth   ....

Diagnosis   ....

History:

Physical examination:

Additional investigation:

Medication:

Proposition:

Please take care of this patient. We would highly appreciate your feedback.

Signature   Date

....

26.7   Surgical and Medical Procedure Informed Consent Form

Consent implies that a lucid person voluntarily agrees to the diagnostic or therapeutic proposal of a healthcare provider.

Medical and surgical procedures must be preceded by a consultation where the medical officer, surgeon, or other qualified medical personnel formally explains the planned diagnostic or surgical procedure, its outcome, and its possible side effects or negative outcome.

Signing this document attests that the patient has been informed and accepts the procedure. The signee should be medically and psychologically fit during the process of explaining and signing.

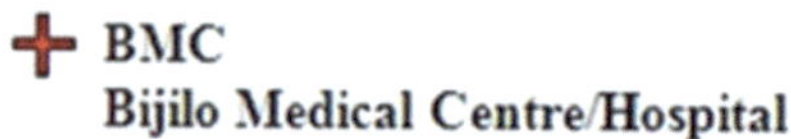

BMC
Bijilo Medical Centre/Hospital

CONSENT BY PATEINT / NEAREST RELATIVE

I ....

Of ....

Hereby consent to the operation of ....

On myself / my husband / my wife / my child ....

The effect and nature of which has been explained to me by

Dr / Mr ....

I also consent to such further or alternative operative measures as may be found to be necessary during the course of such operations and to the administration of local or other anaesthetic for any of these purposes.

No assurance has been given to me that the operation will be performed by a particular Surgeon

Signed ....

Date: ....

I confirm that I have explained to the patient / nearest relative the nature and effect of this operation

Signed ....

Date ....

26.8   Retroviral (HIV) Test Consent Form

Before conducting an HIV serology, a patient must be counseled and sign this consent form acknowledging full acceptance of performing the test.

BMC
Bijilo Medical Centre/Hospital   **VCT SERVICES**

<u>Consent of client</u>   I have / have not consented to HIV testing

Date:......./......./200.... VCT No:...................   Signature:....................................

Name of Counsellor:...............................   Signature:....................................

26.9   Surgical Operation Report

✚BMC
Bijilo Medical Center
PO Box 3349
Serekunda
The Gambia
Telephone: +220 xyz

Date....

Surgical Operation Report

Preoperative diagnoses:
xxxx
xxxx
Postoperative diagnoses:
xxxx
xxx

Operation:	xxx
Date:	xxx
Estimated blood loss:	xxx
Transfusions :	xxx
Drains :	xxx
Spécimen :	xx

Description of procedure: xxxx

Using his knowledge of anatomy, the instruments available the surgeon precisely describes the procedure as carefully as possible.

Dr. XX
Bijilo Medical Centre

26.10 Request for Maternity Leave

Maternity leave is the time a mother takes off from work for the birth of a child. Different legislatures accord different duration for this leave. Very often, employers will request a letter from a medical institution to define the leave.

+ BMC
Bijilo Medical Center
PO Box 3349
Serekunda
The Gambia
Telephone: +220 xyz

Date..........

Request for Maternity Leave

Reference: Ms. XY   **DOB: ....**

I hereby present to you the application of Ms XY for her maternity leave as specified below.
Expected Delivery Date: ....
Start Date of Maternity Leave: ....
Last Date of Maternity Leave: ....
Resume Date to Work: ....

I remain at your disposal for any further clarification.
Sincerely,

Dr XX
Bijilo Medical Centre

26.11 Excused Duty Certificate

An employed individual who cannot perform his duties because of a medical condition needs to present a document certifying that effect to be presented to the employer within 24 h. It is the responsibility and discretion of the attending physician to fill out this form and hand it over to the concerned patient.

✚ BMC
Bijilo Medical Center
PO Box 3349
Serekunda
The Gambia
Telephone: +220 xyz

Date........

Excused Duties

This is to certify that due to medical reasons, we advised that Mr/Ms ....
DOB........................., should be excused from his/her duties from................................... to
....

We remain at your disposal for any further information.

Yours sincerely,

Dr XX
Bijilo Medical Centre

26.12 Antenatal Card

Soon after testing positive for pregnancy, all women are encouraged to join the antenatal program. The pregnant woman presents this card during each antenatal visit (page 1 of 2).

BMC

Bijilo Medical Centre / Hospital

Ante Natal Card

Surname: ___________________ Given Name: ___________________

Address: ___________________

Parity Gravida ___________________ Para

Age: ___________________   Married ☐ Single ☐ Divorce ☐

Serological Tests	1st Trimester	2nd Trimester	3rd Trimester
Haemoglobin			
VDRL Test			
Sickle Cell Test			
HIV Test if Necessary			
Blood Sugar Test			
Urinanalysis			

Tetanus Injection			
1st Dose			
2nd Dose			
3rd Dose			
Booster Dose			
X-ray			
Scan / Ultra Sound			

Medical History & Family History

			OBS/Gynae History		
Diabetes	yes ☐	no ☐	Pre-Eclampsia	yes ☐	no ☐
Hypertension	yes ☐	no ☐	Abortions	yes ☐	no ☐
Twins	yes ☐	no ☐	Prem Delivery	yes ☐	no ☐
Sickle Cell Anaemia	yes ☐	no ☐	Still Birth	yes ☐	no ☐
HIV/AIDS	yes ☐	no ☐	Caesarian	yes ☐	no ☐
Tuberculosis	yes ☐	no ☐	Other Com Disease	yes ☐	no ☐
F/Planning Method used .	yes ☐	no ☐	Abnormal Deliveries	yes ☐	no ☐
Heart Disease .	yes ☐	no ☐			
Surgical Ops .	yes ☐	no ☐	Date Of LMP		

Ante Natal Visits and Examination

Date	Wght	B/P	HT/Wks	FH	Presentation	Position	Lie	Medication	Next Appt

Antenatal card, page 2

26.13 Obstetrical Delivery Chart

This chart comprehensively notes all relevant physical maternal and fetal/baby findings during the course of labor. Medications and methods of delivery applied are indicated.

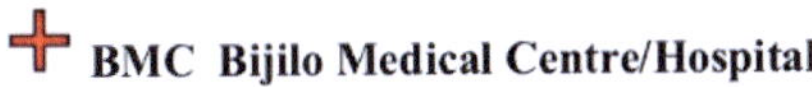

BMC Bijilo Medical Centre/Hospital

DELIVERY RECORD CHART

Name   **D.O.B.**   **Address**

First Stage Summary
Time of Onset................Induced................Accelerated...................

Time Membranes Ruptured.............Spontaneously........Assisted................

Colour of Liquor......................   Pitocin Used...........................

Second Stage Summary

Time Second Stage Confirmed........... Time of Delivery...........................

Indication for C/S or Instrumental Delivery...

Perineum...... INTACT   TEAR   EPISIOTOMY
How Sutured.............................. By Whom...................................

Lidocaine Given .... % .... Mls...............

Erogmetrine or Pitocin Given..................... I.M. or I.V.......................

Placenta..... Healthy   Complete   Abnormalities

Time of Delivery or Third Stage ....Blood Loss.................................

Delivered By   ....R M Midwife

BABY   Alive   Innd   Fresh SB   Mac SB

Sex ....Weight ....APGAR at 1 Min..............

Vit B Given.........Abnormalities Seen...................................

Blood Pressure   ....
Pulse   ....
Temp   ....
Uterus   ....
Lochia   ....
Bladder   ....

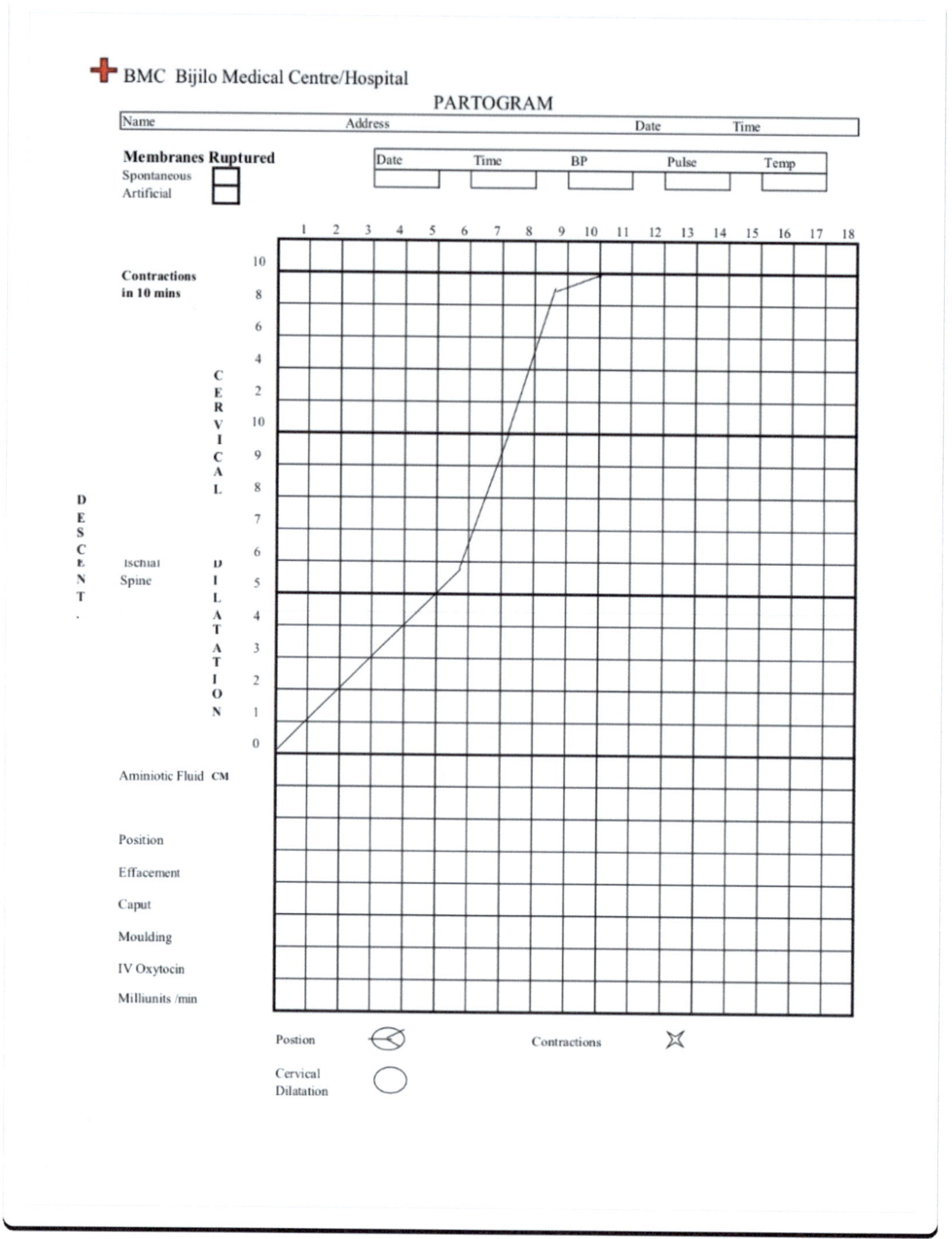

Obstetrical partogram: This is a key antenatal document. The attending gynecologist and midwife use the partogram to carefully note key data (maternal and fetal) during labor. It notes the delivery process on a single sheet of paper.

26.14 Child Health Card

Every child obtains this 4-part hardcover card that contains all relevant clinical information about the child. The mother presents this card at each health visit. The attending healthcare giver is expected to succinctly note his findings and the medication prescribed in this card.

+BMC
Bijilo Medical Centre / Hospital
P.O. Box 1049 Serrekunda, The Gambia
Tel: (220) 4464866 Fax: (220) 4464867 Mobile: (220) 9080071

A. PERSONAL HISTORY   **CHILD'S NUMBER:**

Child's Name	Date of Birth:
Mother's Name	Birth Register No:
Father's Name	Place of Delivery:
Address / Name of Village and Compound	Health Facility ☐ Home ☐
	BBA ☐ TBA ☐ Other ☐
Tel:	Sex
Welfare Clinic:	

B. IMMUNISATION RECORD: **DATE REQUIRED**   **DATE RECEIVED**

ANTI-TUBERCULOSIS AND HEPATITIS IMMUNISATION
BCG injection   (at birth or soon after)
Date of recognizing BCG scar
Hepatitis B   (at birth or soon after)

POLIOMYELITIS IMMUNISATION
Polio 0   (at birth or soon after)
Polio 1   (at the age of 2 months) or soon after)
Polio 2   (one month after second dose)
Polio 3   (one month after third dose)
polio 4   (at the age of 9 months or later)
Booster   (at the age of 18 months or later)

PENTAVALENT IMMUNISATION (DPT-HEPB-Hib)
Pentavalent 1   (at the age of 2 months or soon after)
Pentavalent 2   (one month after first injection)
Pentavalent 3   (one month after second injection)
DPT Booster   (one year after third injection)

PNEUMOCOCCCAL CONJUGATE IMMUNISATION
Pneumo 1   (at the age of 2 months or soon after)
pneumo 2   (one month after first injection)
pneumo 3   (one month after second injection)

ROTA IMMUNIZATION
rota 1 (at the age of 2 months or soon after)
rota 2 (one month after the first dose)
rota 3 (one month after the second dose)

MEALESES IMMUNZATION
Mealeses 1   (at the age of 9 months or soon after)
Mealeses 2   (at the age of 18 months or soon after)

YELLOW FEVER IMMUNIZATION
Yellow Fever   (at the age of 9 months or soon after)

Vitamin A	Date Received	Mebendazole	Date Received	Received LLIN	
1st Dose 100,000 IU at 6 months		1st Dose at 12 months		Date:	
2nd Dose 200,000 IU at 12 months		2nd Dose at 18 months			
3rd Dose 200,000 IU at 18 months		3rd Dose at 24 months		Yes: ☐ No: ☐	
4th Dose 200,000 IU at 24 months		4th Dose at 30 months		(TT - MOTHERS ONLY)	
5th Dose 200,000 IU at 30 months		5th Dose at 36 months		Dose	Date
6th Dose 200,000 IU at 36 months		6th Dose at 42 months		TT 1	
7th Dose 200,000 IU at 42 months		7th Dose at 48 months		TT 2	
8th Dose 200,000 IU at 48 months		8th Dose at 54 months		TT 3	
9th Dose 200,000 IU at 54 months		9th Dose at 60 months		TT 4	
10th Dose 200,000 IU at 60 months					

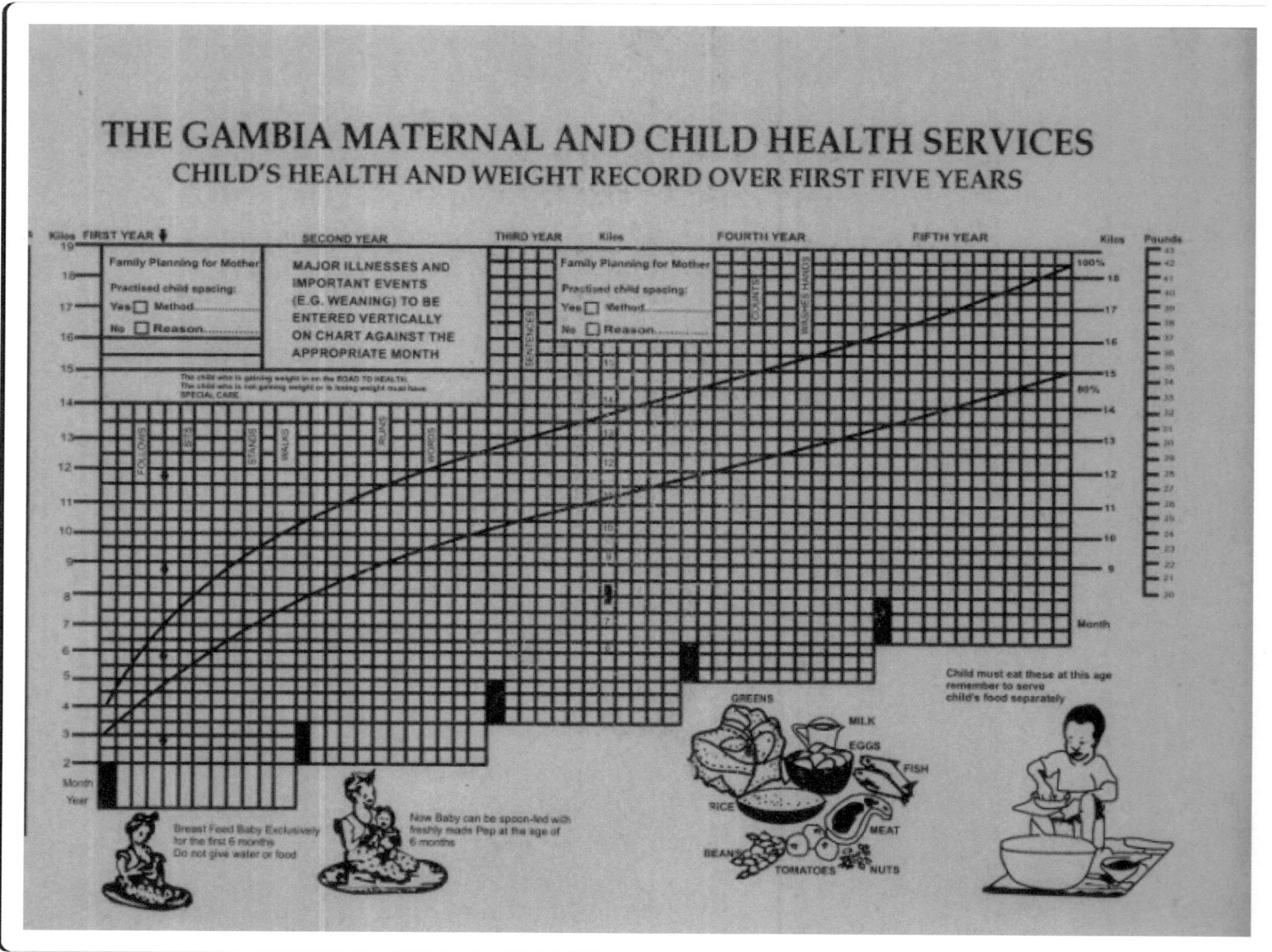

Child health card, page 2

1st Routine Post Partum Examination (1 week after delivery):

Mother   B.P:______________________   Newborn   Tempt:______________________

Wt:______________________   Eyes:______________________

Temp:______________________   Cord:______________________

2nd Routine Post Partum Examination (4 week after delivery):

Mother   B.P:______________________   Newborn   Tempt:______________________

Wt:______________________   Eyes:______________________

Temp:______________________   Cord:______________________

CHILD HEALTH VISITS

Date	Treatment Centre	Complaint, Treatment, referral	Investigation	Initials

Child health card, page 3

CHILD HEALTH VISITS

Date	Treatment Centre	Complaint, Treatment, referral	Investigation	Initials

Child health card, page 4

26.15 Essential Medication List

A regular pharmacy stock: This list is representative of the permanent sustained stock of medication that is present at all times in the pharmacy of a standard minimal-resource facility.

✚BMC Essential Medication List

Antibiotics
Amoxicillin: 250mg, 500mg
Benzybenzathin: 1.2 mio unit
Cephalexin: 500mg
Ciproxin 250mg 500mg
Co-Amoxicillin 625mg
Doxycycline 100mg
Erythromycin 250mg
Metronidazole 250mg 500mg
Penicillin-G2.4mio unit

Antifungal
Benzyl benzoate cream (Whitfield cream)
Clotrimazole
Flutinizole 150mg
Griseofulvin 250mg 500mg
Ketoconazole cream

Anti-Helminthes
Albendazole
Mebendazole 400mg

Anti-Malarial
Artesunate adult and pediatric dose
Doxycycline 100mg
Fansida
Mefloquine (Lariam)
Plasmotrim
Quinine 300mg (tabs) 600mg (iv)

Anti-Hypertensive
Atenolol 50mg 100mg
Enalapril 5mg
Furosemide 40mg 20tabs
Hydralazine 100mg
Hydrochlorothiazide 25mg
Nefidipin 20mg
Spironolactone 25mg

Anti-diabetics
Glybenclamide 5mg
Insulin act rapid
Metformin 500mg

Anti-allergies (anti-inflammatory)
Beta-methasone 500mg
Dexamethasone 4mg
Hydro-cortisone cream

Anti-emetics
Metaclopramide 10mg
Promethazine 4ml

Antacids
Magnesium tricyclique
Omeprazole 20mg

Laxatives
Five fruit a day
Bisacodyl
Movicol

Vitamins and supplements
Fefol (ferrous sulfate + folic acid)
Ferrous sulfate
Folic acid
Multivitamins
ORS (oral rehydration solution)
Vitamin B complex

Psychiatric drugs
Amitriptyline 10mg
Benz diazepam 10mg
Fluoxetine20mg
Haloperidol 20mg

Analgesic and NSAIDS
Aspirin 100mg 300mg
Buscopam 10mg
Co-codamol
Diclofenac 25mg

Ibuprofen 200mg 400mg
Morphine 30mg
Naproxen 250mg
Tramadol 100mg

Intravenous fluids
5% Dextrose
50% Dextrose
Normal saline

Vaccines
Tt
Hepatitis A
Hepatitis B
Measles vaccine
Polio
Vitamin A

Miscellaneous
Loperamide

Bronchodilator
Salbutamol

Antitussive
Bromohexadine

Mariama Touray, August 2013

26.16 Available Vaccines/Infant Immunization Schedule

A poster that sensitizes the public and also educates healthcare workers about available vaccines in the country. It is an official document issued by the local health authorities and displayed at most standard minimal-resource healthcare facilities.

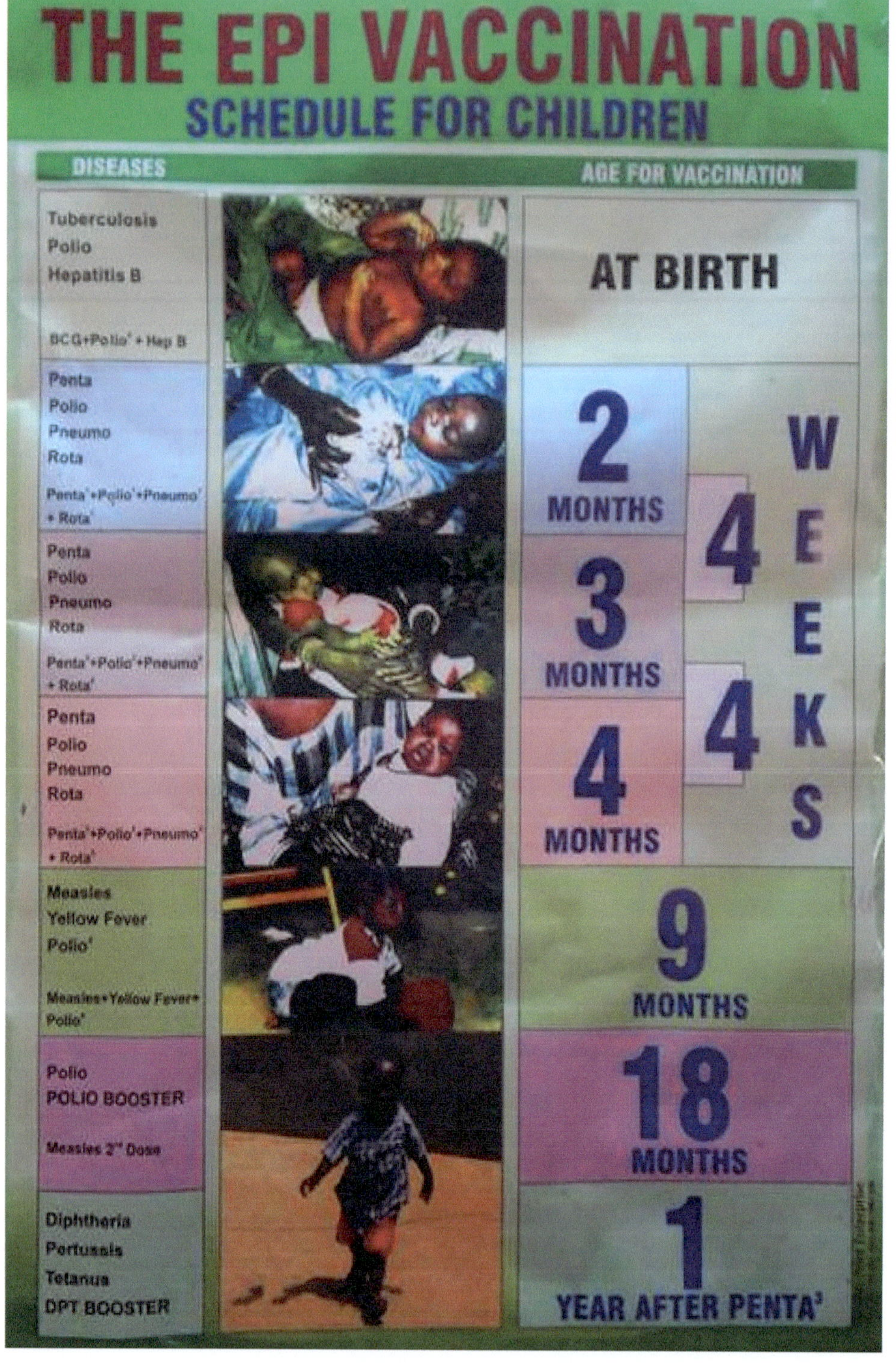

26.17 Laboratory Request Form

Based on the patient history and physical examination, a physician reflects on the diagnostic laboratory tests that need to be performed. These are marked on this laboratory request form and submitted to the laboratory for execution.

| Name: | | Surname: | Lab Number: |
| Date : | | Date of Birth | Male / Female: |

Analyse	Unit	Norm	Date and Results							
Coagulation										
TP		70–100 %								
Hematology										
Erythrocytes		3.80 – 5.20 10^{12}/l								
Haematocrit		0.35 – 0.47 l/l								
Hemoglobin		117 – 157 g/l								
Leucocytes (WBC)		3.8 – 10.0 10^9/l								
MCH		27 – 34 pg								
MCHC		3101 – 360 g/l								
MCV		81 – 99 fl								
Thrombocytes		150 – 350 10^9/l								
ABO-Blood Group		A, B, AB, O								
Urine Stix										
Leucocytes		negative								
Nitrite		negative								
Uroglobuline		negative								
Protein		negative								
PH		6.5								
Blood		negative								
Glucose		negative								
Ketone		negative								
Bilirubin		negative								
Serology / Endo										
HIV 1/2		negative								
VDRL		negative								
Hbs Antigen		negative								
TSH		0.4 – 5.0 mU/L								
Urine-Beta HCG		negative								
Malaria Search		negative								
Chemistry										
ALT (GPT)	U/L	M: < 41 F: < 32								
AST (GOT)	U/L	M: < 40 F: < 33								
Creatinine	µmol/L	M: < 90 F: < 80								
Glucose	µmol/L	2.5 – 5.5								
Potassium	mmol/L	3.60 – 5.10								
Cholesterol	µmol/L	< 6.5								
Bilirubin (total)	µmol/L	< 17								
Uric acid	µmol/L	M: < 416 F: < 339								
Amylase	U/L	< 100								
Alkaline phosphatase	U/L	M: < 270 F: < 240								
Urea	mmol/L	2.78 – 7.64								
Gamma GT	U/L	M: < 11-50 F: < 7-32								
Creatinine Kinase (T)	U/L									

26.18 X-ray Request Form

For a radiographic examination to be done, a physician should thoroughly examine a patient and fill out this form meticulously. The form is given to the radiography technician who then performs the test.

✚BMC
Bijilo Medical Center
PO Box 3349
Serekunda
The Gambia
Telephone: +220 xyz

Date...........................

Medical Imaging Request Form

Imaging modality
3. Standard radiography ☐
2. Ultrasonography ☐
3. Echocardiography ☐

Name of patient, DOB:...

Indication/History/Diagnosis...
....
....
....
....
....
....

Prescribing Doctor: ....

Performed by: ....

Interpretation/observations..
....
....
....
....
....
....

Interpreting physician: ....   Date: ....

26.19 Medical Prescription Form

A physician lists the names and mode of administration of the medicines in accordance with evidence-based medical practice. The prescription is presented to the drug dispenser for dispensing out the medicine to the patient and/or his escorts.

+BMC

Bijilo Medical Centre / Hospital   N⁰ 0043322

P.O. Box 3349 Serrekunda, The Gambia
Tel: (220) 4464868. Fax: (220) 4464867. Mobile: (220) 9980371

To ....

.... Date .... No ....

Code	Prescription	Amount

26.20 Self-Discharge Form

Patients who for one reason or the other would like to leave the hospital against the informed advice of a qualified medical personnel are made to sign a self-discharge form. This is an important legal document and is filed in the patient file.

✚ BMC
Bijilo Medical Center
PO Box 3349
Serekunda
The Gambia
Telephone: +220 xyz

Date..................

Self-Discharge Form

I, Mr/Ms .... hereby discharge myself/my child ....
from Bijilo Medical Centre on this .... day of ...., I have taken this action on my own accord against the advice of the doctor/ nurse at Bijilo Medical Centre. I understand that Bijilo Medical Centre will not be liable for any repercussion this action may cause to the medical condition of myself or my child.

Patient/ Guardian
Signed: ....
Print: ....
Date: ....

Doctor/Nurse
Signed: ....
Print: ....
Date: ....

26.21 Certificate of Death

Death is a permanent cessation of all vital functions in an individual and it marks the end of life.

Every death that occurred in the hospital is recorded in a designated registry. For various reasons, family members do request for certificate of death. A certificate of death must mention the identity of the disease, date of birth, date and time of death, and the principal cause of death. If the death is not natural, this should be indicated. The certificate of death is a legal document that families use to claim heritage and lineage.

✚ **BMC**
Bijilo Medical Center
PO Box 3349
Serekunda
The Gambia
Telephone: +220 xyz

Date..............

Certificate of Death

Reference: **Mr/Ms** Name/Surname   **DOB:**   ....

This is to certify that Mr. Name/Surname, DOB ...., died at Bijilo Medical Center, Bijilo Village, on Date................., Time.................

The cause of this natural death is xxxxx.

Dr . XX
Bijilo Medical Centre

26.22 Job Application Form

Applicants fill out this form. It serves as a first checkpoint determining the suitability of the applicant for the applied position. The administrators hand out the form to the applicant, who has 15 min to complete it. That is followed by a fifteen-minute spelling test in which the administrator dictates 15 words to the applicant.

+BMC

Bijilo Medical Centre   Date: ___________

JOB APPLICATION FORM

Position applied for: _______________________________

From which date are you available? _______________

Personal information

Surname : _______________________   First Name : _______________________

Date of Birth : __________   Civil State : __________   Tel. : __________

Address : ____

Education

Name of institution	Date of graduation	Certificate obtained

Tell us something about yourself that you feel would make you an asset to the Bijilo Medical Center :

Present employer

Name :____   Salary :______________

Start date:____________   Reason for leaving :________________________________

Duties / responsibilities :____

____

____

____

Past work experience

Name	Dates	Duties / responsibilities	Reason for leaving

Please provide the contact information for at least two referees, including your current employer :

1.

2.

Spell Check

____________   ____________   ____________   ____________

____________   ____________   ____________   ____________

____________   ____________   ____________   ____________

____________   ____________   ____________   ____________

____________   ____________   ____________   ____________

Signature :______________________________   Date :__________

Job application form (page 2)

26.23 Cash Transaction Receipts

All monetary transactions are documented with receipts that are filled by the cashier and submitted appropriately to the administration.

✛ BMC

Bijilo Medical Center / Hospital
P. O. Box 3349, Serrekunda. The Gambia.
Tel: (220) 4464868 Fax: (220) 4464867 Mobile: (220) 9980371
E-mail: drmusa@bijilomedical.org

№ 005017

No:..

Payment Voucher

Date: ....

Ref:..

Payment:..

Amount: D...

In words:...

Cash / Cheque:...

Signed:...   Print:...

Authorised by:...   Print:...

Signature of Recipient:...

Print:...

Date:..

+BMC

Bijilo Medical Centre / Hospital
P.O.Box 3349 Serrekunda, The Gambia
Tel: (220) 4464868 Fax: 4464867 Mob: (220) 9980371
Email:info@gambiahealth.org

Date:................................   **Receipt**   No:.006141...........

Received from:...

The sum of:...

....

In payment of:...

....

Signature

26.24 Institutional Affiliations

All patients who regularly attend the facility are issued an affiliation card. This is a highly appreciated document which the patient carries and presents to the receptionist at each visit.

+ Bijilo Medical Centre/Hospital

Dr. Musa Touray MD – PhD
Specialist in Internal Medicine
Clinical Director
PO Box 3349
Serekunda
The Gambia

Telephone: +220-6665555
Mobile: +220-9980371

e-mail: drmusa@bijilomedical.org
www.bijilomedical.org

personal data:
registration nr.
name
surname
DOB   telephone
address
employer
insurance

Facilities at BMC:
- Comprehensive medical team
- 30 bed modern clinical ward; private and general
- Outpatient-policlinic unit without long waiting periods
- X-Ray and Ultrasound facilities
- Modern clinical diagnostic laboratory
- ECG investigation
- Echocardiography
- Physiotherapy
- Surgical theatre
- Antenatal, maternity, delivery and child healthcare unit
- Immunisation-vaccination services
- 24-hour ambulance service

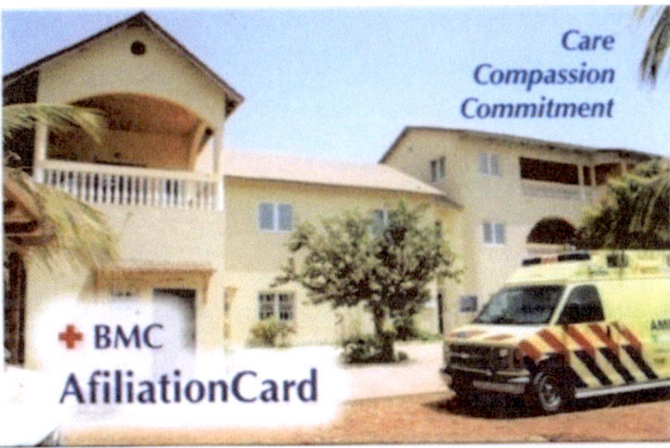

Bibliography[1]

1. Papadakis MA, McPhee SJ, Rabow MW. Current medical diagnosis & treatment 2019. New York: McGraw-Hill Education; 2019. https://accessmedicine.mhmedical.com/book.aspx?bookID=2449.
2. Buckingham TA. Effective medical writing. 1st ed.
3. Armitage M. From clinical practice to medical writing: a career transition guide (medical writing for clinicians).
4. Ultimate guide to medical manuscript writing—medical writing (themedwriters.com).
5. Preclinical and clinical lecture notes of the curriculum of medical studies, Faculty of Medicine, University of Lausanne, Course year 2015–2021.
6. Mirali S, Seneviratne A. Essential med notes, 2020: comprehensive medical references and review for the United States Medical Licensing Exam (USMLE) step II and the Medical Council of Canada Qualifying Exam (MCCQE) Part 1. 36th ed.
7. WHO model list of essential medicines, 20th list. World Health Organization. Mar 2017, Amended Aug 2017. https://apps.who.int/iris/bitstream/handle/10665/273826/EML-20-eng.pdf?ua=1.
8. Cornuz J, Pasche O, Kermode-Noppel T. Compas: Stratégies de prise en charge clinique, Médecine interne générale ambulatoire. Lausanne: Institute of Social and Preventive Medicine; 2010.

---

[1]The material presented in this book originates from the efforts of the authors to converge various sources of medical information to constitute this book. The invaluable lecture notes and handouts received through the medical curriculum of the University of Lausanne, Switzerland, where both authors trained, has been very useful. Personal notes taken during many years of clinical work in medical wards and outpatient units are incorporated. Finally, these two crucial sources of medical information are complemented by selected classical medical literature listed below.

Appendix

Glossary

Below is a list of words and their common meaning. This list is not comprehensive by any standards. However, the list constitutes a basis for effective communication among clinicians and paramedical personnel. It represents most of the common words that health professionals should know. The meaning of words should be clearly known to healthcare providers in order to facilitate professional communication.

© The Author(s), under exclusive license to Springer Nature Switzerland AG 2021

M. Touray, A. Touray, *Clinical Work and General Management of a Standard Minimal-Resource Facility*, Sustainable Development Goals Series, https://doi.org/10.1007/978-3-030-71032-3

Glossary[1]

Abatement Diminution, decrease of symptomatology.

Abduction Movement of a limb or a limb segment away from the body axis.

Abrasion Superficial skin lesion, epidermic erosion.

Abscess Dermal or hypodermal encapsulated bacterial collection, not linked to a hair follicle (unlike furuncle).

Abulia Difficulties or impossibility of exercising one's will, particularly in taking action, with a tendency to procrastinate.

Acute Of abrupt onset, short in duration, rapidly progressive.

Adduction Movement of a limb or a limb segment toward the body axis.

Agnosia Inability to recognize an object or a shape.

Akathisia Hyperkinetic movement disorder, extrapyramidal symptom characterized by restlessness, an impossibility to sit or remain in a seated position, can also result in a feeling of inner anguish slightly relieved by a change of position.

Akinesia Reduction in the initiation and movements execution, independent of paralysis and hypertonia.

Algia: omalgia, gonalgia… Suffix meaning pain, e.g., omalgia is pain in the shoulder, gonalgia is pain in the knee.

Algomenorrhea Pain associated with the onset of menstruation.

Allodynia Pain caused by a non-painful external stimulus, lowering of the pain threshold (contact of the skin with a piece of clothing or simply touching the affected area is unbearable).

Amenorrhea Primary: absence of menstruation from 15 to 16 years of age with complete or partial development of secondary sexual organs (investigation of $1°$ amenorrhea) or absence of menstruation from 14 years old associated with impuberism (conduct investigation of pubertal delay); secondary: absence of menstruation corresponding to the duration of the last three cycles, absence of menstruation for 6 months.

Amnesia Total or partial loss of episodic memory.

Amyotrophy Muscle wasting.

Analgesia Suppression/attenuation of sensitivity to pain.

Anhedonia Impairment in the ability to experience pleasure.

Anorexia Total or partial loss of appetite.

Anosmia Loss of olfaction (smell).

Antenatal Period preceding birth, period of pregnancy.

Antiseptic Chemical product or procedure applied on tissues or surfaces to eliminate, kill microorganisms or inactivate viruses.

---

[1] Basic vocabulary for clinical communication.

Anuria Absence of urine in the bladder, urine retention should be ruled out.

Aphasia Acquired language disorder secondary to a brain injury (usually located in the left hemisphere).

Apnea Involuntary or voluntary interruption of breathing.

Apoptosis Cell death process; contrary to necrosis, it is not accompanied by an inflammatory reaction; characterized by DNA fragmentation and chromatin condensation.

Apraxia Inability to perform voluntary goal-directed movements in the absence of motor, sensory, or comprehension impairments.

Aptyalism Decrease or cessation of salivary secretion with permanent mouth dryness.

Arrhythmia Abnormality in the regularity or frequency of heart contractions.

Ascites Collection of fluid located in the large peritoneal cavity, except pus (peritonitis) and blood (hemoperitoneum).

Asialia Lack of saliva by reduction or suppression of its secretion.

Asphyxia Severe reduction of oxygen supply to tissues due to the inability to breathe normally; Three mechanisms: inadequate concentration of oxygen in the environment, absent or insufficient respiratory movement, airflow obstruction in the airways.

Asterixis Also known as flapping tremor, when wrists are extended, successive movements of flexion-extension of the wrists and flexion-lateralization of the fingers, slow, irregular and of great amplitude, caused by the abrupt and brief inability to maintain postural tone.

Asthenia Widespread and long-lasting fatigue.

Asymptomatic Which presents no pathological manifestations perceived by the patient, a patient who has no visible clinical symptoms manifestation of any kind.

Ataxia Motor coordination disorders that affect the direction and amplitude of voluntary movement, postural maintenance, and balance.

Atrophy Decrease in the volume and size of part or all of an organ or tissue.

Bacteremia Presence of bacteria in the bloodstream.

Benign A disease that progresses in a noninvasive way and without severe consequences.

Bradycardia Slow heart rate, less than 60 beats/min in adults.

Bradykinesia Slowness of movement, observed especially during confusion, stuporous states (predominantly melancholic, catatonic, and emotional) or neurological conditions (Parkinson's disease, typical sequelae of encephalitis lethargica, adverse effects of neuroleptics, sometimes with paradoxical kinesis).

Bulla Intraepidermal or mucous cavity of serous, sero-purulent, or hemorrhagic content, >0.5 cm in diameter, larger than a vesicle, has thin walls.

Cachexia State of emaciation observed after severe and prolonged dietary deficiency and in the terminal phase of infectious or malignant neoplastic diseases.

Callus New bone that forms at the fragmented edges of a fractured bone and restores its integrity.

Carbuncle Conglomerate of several furuncles.

Cardiomegaly Abnormal increase in heart size.

Catarrh Acute or chronic inflammation of the nasopharyngeal mucosa associated with hypersecretion.

Caudal Which relates to the tail or the posterior part of the body.

Cellulitis Dermo-hypodermitis, acute purulent infection of the epidermis, dermis, and hypodermis, while erysipelas is located in the superficial dermis.

Chorea Abnormal movement most often generalized, brief, unpredictable, and uncoordinated, involving the proximal or distal part of the limbs, the trunk, neck and face muscles; may be associated with: hypotonia, motor impersistence, athetosis.

Chronic Slowly progressing disease with no tendency to heal.

Circadian rhythm Rhythmic processes that occur over a 24-h period.

Clinophilia Substantial amount of time spent in a reclining position without sleeping.

Clubbing Deformation of the fingers and often of the toes, associating a very marked curvature, both longitudinal and transverse, of the nails (watch-glass appearance), hypertrophy of the soft parts of the distal phalanges (drumstick appearance), and inconsistent local cyanosis.

Congenital An individual particularity present from birth, which may be morphological, psychological, physiological, or pathological.

Congestion Increase in the volume of blood in the vessels of a tissue (hyperemia) or excessive accumulation of mucus in cavities.

Constipation Difficulty or delay in evacuating hardened feces after a prolonged stay in the large intestine.

Contralateral Refers to the opposite side of the body.

Crackles Discontinuous adventitious noise reflecting the abrupt opening of the airways and a decrease in lung compliance (e.g., edema, pneumonia, fibrosis); subdivided into fine and coarse crackles/rales.

Cramp Sudden, involuntary, painful, and transient contraction of a muscle or muscle group.

Cranial/cephalic Which concerns the head, as opposed to caudal (tail/posterior part of the body).

Crust Desiccation of a serous/hemorrhagic/purulent exudate, outer layer covering a wound or skin excoriation, easily detachable in a single piece with a curette.

Cyanosis Dark blue discoloration of teguments, indicative of severe hypoxia, due to a higher concentration of deoxygenated hemoglobin; central (tongue and peripheral tissues), peripheral (extremities and lips).

Cyst Benign tumor consisting of a cavity filled with a liquid, soft or rarely solid substance and lined with an epithelial surface.

Debilitating Refers to disease turning someone physically weak.

Dementia Syndrome associating multiple acquired cognitive deficits, occurring in the absence of a confused state; by definition, intellectual disability, confusional state, and isolated cognitive deficit are excluded.

Dermatome Cutaneous territory limited and defined (the Voigt or Futcher lines) that is innervated by the sensory fibers coming from a posterior nerve root, which corresponds to the embryological or metameric somites.

Diagnosis Determination of a person's condition or disorder.

Diarrhea Emission of liquid stools of excessive frequency and abundance.

Diascopy Blanchability test used in dermatology; consists in applying pressure on the skin lesion with a glass blade or a finger and observing change in color.

Disinfectant Chemical product or process applied to an inert medium in order to eliminate, kill microorganisms or inactivate viruses.

Diurnal Occurring during the daytime.

Dullness Muffled sound heard at percussion of a compact organ or a liquid effusion.

Dysentery Intestinal condition characterized by abdominal pain and associated with diarrhea, frequently accompanied by blood and mucus.

Dysesthesia Unpleasant subjective sensation perceived in a cutaneous territory, without external stimulus.

Dysphagia Disorder of the pharyngeal-esophageal transit of food and/or liquids.

Dysplasia Abnormality in the development of a tissue, organ, or part of an organ.

Dyspnea Subjective symptom corresponding to an unpleasant sensation of difficulty in breathing.

Dystonia Alteration in the function of a smooth or striated muscle, nerve, or group of nerves, or a decrease, increase, or defect in its tone.

Dysuria Difficult urination resulting in a low stream of urine, regardless of the cause.

Ecchymosis Flat intracutaneous bleeding, interstitial hemorrhage within a tissue, skin hematoma larger than 10 mm.

Echolalia Stereotypy, which consists of the repeated involuntary, virtually automatic and pointless repetition of the last words heard.

Echomimy Stereotypy, which consists of the repeated involuntary, virtually automatic and pointless repetition of the mimicry or attitudes of others.

Echopraxia Stereotypy, which consists of the repeated involuntary, virtually automatic and pointless repetition of the acts and gestures of others.

-Ectomy Suffix used to refer to the ablation of an organ: mammectomy, splenectomy, hysterectomy, prostatectomy.

Ectopia Abnormal location of an organ or part.

Edema Excess fluid in interstitial tissues and/or serous cavities.

Emesis Vomit, hematemesis (vomiting of blood), hyperemesis (incoercible vomiting), hyperemesis gravidarum (pregnancy complication).

Empyema Purulent collection in a natural cavity: nasal sinus, gall bladder, pleura, uterus.

Endemic Persistence of a disease in a region or community, either permanently or periodically.

Enthesopathy Enthesis disease (insertions of tendons, ligaments, and joint capsules), of inflammatory (enthesitis) or mechanical nature.

Enuresis Lack of control over miction, during the day or more often at night.

Epidemic Spread to a population of an infectious disease with human-to-human transmission.

Epiphora Symptom characterized by an excess of tears leading in overflow.

Epistaxis Nasal bleeding most frequently related to an erosion of the anterior part of the mucous membrane of the nasal septum (Kiesselbach area).

Erosion Superficial cutaneous or mucous loss of substance, that does not result in scar formation.

Eructation Noisy emission of gas from the stomach through the mouth.

Erysipela Skin infection limited to the superficial dermis and involving drainage lymphatic (lymphangitis), common infection in the elderly.

Erythema Elementary cutaneous lesion characterized by congestive, localized, or diffuse redness, linked to vasodilatation and disappearing with diascopy, observed in a large number of dermatoses of which it sometimes represents the major symptom.

Etiology Study of the causes of diseases.

Excoriation Superficial skin ulceration of traumatic origin.

Expectoration Mouth serous/mucous/purulent/mucopurulent secretions from the respiratory tract.

Exudate High-density, protein-rich liquid (fibrin) containing cells (leukocytes) and cellular debris.

Extension Movement of the joint to align the components of the joint at the widest angle.

Fasciculation Short involuntary contractions or twitching, rarely isolated, most frequently grouped in muscle bundles, spontaneous or triggered by cold or percussion, may be physiological or pathological (reflecting peripheral neurologic lesions).

Febrile Related to fever.

Fecaloma Fecal mass in the large intestinal lumen with impaired possibility of peristaltic evacuation, caused by abnormal sphincter tone and results into dilatation of the rectal ampulla.

Fibroma Benign tumor consisting of entangled bundles of well-differentiated spindle cells, fibrocytes, and fibroblasts mixed with collagen fibers of varying abundance.

Fissure (rhagade) Linear loss of substance.

Fistula Pathological acquired or congenital orifice or duct.

Flexion Position or movement in which a limb segment or part of the body forms a more or less pronounced angle with the neighboring segment.

Folliculitis Hair follicle inflammation, most often of infectious etiology.

Fracture State of what is broken.

Furuncle Deep necrotizing folliculitis of the entire pilosebaceous follicle; cf carbuncle = conglomerate of several furuncles.

Galactorrhea (1) Overabundant milk flow during the lactation period; (2) abnormal flow of milk outside the lactation period.

Galenic formulation Presentation of a medicinal product resulting from the combination of one or more active ingredients and an excipient.

Gangrene Disease process involving tissue death, generally caused by partial or total interruption of the vascularization of the tissue, resulting in acute ischemia in the injured area.

Generic Generic drugs contain the same active substance as the original drugs or reference pharmaceutical products.

Haem-, haemo-, hem-, hemo- Blood: hematemesis, hematocrit, hemophilia, hemoptysis, hemorrhoid…

Halitosis Bad breath of oral or other origin.

Hallucination Sensory perception (visual, auditory, tactile, olfactory, or gustatory) in the absence of a detectable stimulus.

Hematemesis Vomiting of blood.

Hematochezia Rectal passage of bright red undigested blood, mainly observed during inflammatory disease or acute colitis.

Hematoma Localized blood effusion outside of blood vessels.

Hematuria Macroscopic: visible presence of blood in urine; microscopic: presence of excessive red blood cells in urine.

Hemianopia Decrease or suppression of vision in one half of the visual field of both eyes.

Hemoptysis Often during a coughing spell, a quantity of blood from the subglottic portion of the respiratory tract is released through the mouth.

Hemothorax Blood pleural effusion.

Hiccup Spasmodic contraction of the diaphragm, triggering an inspiratory thoracic movement promptly interrupted by contraction of the glottis with vibration of the vocal cords.

Hyperhidrosis Excessive production of sweat which is not necessarily secondary to excessive exertion or heat.

Hypersomnia Pathological tendency to excessive nocturnal or diurnal sleep.

Hypertrophy Increase in volume of a tissue, organ, or part of the body.

Hypoplasia Failure of an organ, limb, or tissue to develop fully.

Hyposmia Decrease in olfactory function, decrease in the ability to smell.

Iatrogenic Caused by a physician/healthcare professional, secondary to the treatment undertaken by a physician.

Icterus Jaundice, yellow coloration of variable intensity of the skin, mucous membranes, and conjunctiva following their impregnation by bile pigments.

Idiopathic Of unknown etiology and origin, without apparent cause.

Illusion Deformed sensory, visual, or auditory perception of a real object.

Impetigo Infection (or secondary infection of chronic dermatosis), localized in the epidermis, more often of the face than of the limbs; follows this sequence: vesicle, pustule, honey-colored crust.

Impotence Disability, physical impairment making certain movements impossible to perform; the term only applies to the motor function.

Incidentaloma Neologism referring to a tumor-like mass accidentally discovered in radiology in an asymptomatic patient.

Incontinence Involuntary emission of feces or urine; can be qualified as diurnal or nocturnal; when referring to children: primary or secondary (child has been continent for >6 months).

Induration Pathological hardening and thickening of organic tissue.

Infarct Circumscribed site of ischemic tissue necrosis, with or without blood infiltration, related to arterial, more rarely due to venous obliteration by thrombosis or embolism.

Inflammation A set of defensive reactions of the organism against an aggression (infection, trauma, etc.), which can manifest in various signs: dolor (pain), tumor (swelling), calor (heat), rubor (redness), and functio laesa (loss of function or disturbance in function).

Inflammatory syndrome Set of clinical manifestations: pain (dolor), redness (rubor), heat (calor), swelling (tumor) in reaction to various aggressions.

Ischemia Decrease or deprivation of blood supply to a tissue or organ.

Isomenorrhea Succession of regular menstrual cycles of constant duration.

Jaundice Icterus, yellow coloration of variable intensity of the skin, mucous membranes, and conjunctiva following their impregnation by bile pigments.

Lichenification Thick, shiny, and leathery aspect of skin, accentuation of skin folds, typically associated with severe pruritus/chronic scratching.

Luxation Dislocation, total or partial loss of normal anatomical relationships between the extremities of a joint; by extension, displacement of an organ out of its normal lodge or position.

Macro/micro-vascular Refers to large and small blood vessels respectively.

Macula Cutaneous flat spot without infiltration, can form a plaque when confluent.

Malignant Refers to a disease of high severity or a cancerous tumor tending to infiltrate the surrounding tissue, metastasize with a high potential of fatality.

Marasmus Deep deprivation by undernourishment during a long illness or food shortage (famine, cancer, anorexia nervosa).

Melena Black thick stool with a tar-like appearance or more or less mixed with feces.

Menorrhea Menstruation, period, periodic blood flow due to uterine mucosa discharge.

Meteorism Abnormal abdominal bloating due to gas accumulation distending the intestine.

Metrorrhagia Endo-uterine hemorrhage occurring outside the menstrual period.

Myoclonus Brief muscle twitches, manifesting as involuntary and sudden movements.

Necrosis Cell or tissue death as a result of deprivation of nutritional and vital supplies.

Neonatal Pertains to the newborn/the 4 first weeks after birth.

Nocturnal Relating to the night.

Nodule Circular, protruding, palpable skin lesion, diameter >1 cm; resulting either from edema or from an inflammatory or tumoral infiltrate; can be dermal or hypodermal.

Nosocomial Relating to infections that develop during and as a result of the hospital stay.

Nychthemeral cycle Alternation of a day and a night that corresponds to a 24-h biological cycle.

Nycturia Complaint of having to wake up at night with the urge to urinate.

Occult Hidden, not visible to the eye; example: occult blood in the stool.

Odynophagia Painful swallowing.

Oliguria Decrease in the volume of urine emission per unit of time, less than 500 mL/24 h for adults.

Opisthotonos Type of tetanus contraction prevalent in the extensor muscles, with the body and head tilted backwards and the limbs extended.

Otorrhea Serous, mucous, or purulent discharge exuded through the external auditory canal.

Palpitation More or less distressing sensation of precordial shock due to abnormal perception of the heartbeat.

Palsy Refers to various types of paralysis.

Pandemic Epidemic that affects many countries or the entire world or that affects most individuals in a single country.

Papule Small cutaneous lesion (<0.5–1 cm of diameter), well delimited, elevated, and solid (does not contain any liquid).

Paralysis Abolition of motor function (skeletal muscle), can be described as flaccid or spastic.

Paraneoplastic (syndrome) Set of symptoms associated with cancer, but not directly related to the tumor itself.

Paresis Incomplete paralysis, incomplete suppression of contraction of one or several skeletal muscles.

Paresthesia Uncomfortable or even painful sensation, of varied nature, usually compared to tingling, prickling, numbness.

Patch (plaque?) Broad elevated cutaneous area.

Pathognomonic Refers to a characteristic symptom or sign of a specific disease.

Perinatal Which relates to the circumstances surrounding the birth.

Petechia Punctiform stain which does not disappear with diascopy due to the presence of extravasated blood in the dermis.

Phlegmon Pyogenic inflammation of connective tissue or dermis; infection without collection, unlike the abscess that is collected.

Phlycten Blister, bullae containing a liquid of variable content: serous, hemorrhagic, purulent, can be indicative of a second-degree superficial burn.

Plegia Suffix describing a certain paralysis.

Pleural friction rub Dry, rough, superficial noise auscultated at inspiration and expiration, indicating an alteration in the regularity and smoothness of the pleural surface.

Pneumothorax Spread of air between the two layers of the pleura, which may be spontaneous or caused by a disease process, trauma, or by therapeutic insufflation of a gas (iatrogenic).

Pollakiuria Excessive frequency of urination, not to be mistaken for polyuria.

Potomania Psychogenic eating disorder characterized by the constant need to ingest large quantities of fluids, usually water, and accompanied by polyuria.

Prenatal Period preceding delivery.

Prognosis Prediction, after diagnosis, of the degree of severity and subsequent course of a disease, including its outcome, taking in consideration the course usually observed for similar disorders in other patients.

Pronation Rotation movement of the forearm from outside to inside.

Pruritus Itch.

Pseudarthrosis Non-union, failure to consolidate a fracture within the normal time frame.

Ptyalism Pathological increase in salivary excretion.

Puerperal Pertaining to the period following childbirth or miscarriage.

Purpura Hemorrhagic stain which does not disappear with diascopy due to the presence of extravasated blood in the dermis, confluence of petechiae.

Pustule Small cavity filled with pus, may be follicular or non-follicular.

Pyuria Presence of pus in urine.

Reflux Passage of a liquid in a direction opposite to that of the physiological flow.

Remission Temporary alleviation or disappearance of the symptoms of an acute or chronic disease.

Reservoir (1) Living or inert medium (animal, plant, or external environment), ensuring the prolonged survival of a microorganism and making it transmissible to different hosts; (2) geographic area where a disease is observed with a higher prevalence and incidence than other areas, to which it could potentially spread.

Retraction Permanent shortening of a soft tissue that prevents it from returning passively to its normal length.

Rhonchi Continuous low-pitched sound due to the vibration of the walls of the airways of intermediate size, can often be altered or even disappear after coughing.

Rigidity Form of muscular hypertonicity characterized by resistance to passive motion.

Scale Whitish thin flake indicating a thickening of the corneous layer of the epidermis.

Scurvy Disease caused by vitamin C deficiency with the following symptoms: follicular hyperkeratosis with perifollicular hemorrhages, ecchymotic purpura, erythema and hemorrhages of the interdental papillae, hemorrhagic hypertrophic gingivitis and loose tooth.

Semiology Study of signs and symptoms and their diagnostic and prognostic significance.

Sepsis Inflammatory state accompanying a clinically plausible or microbiologically proven infection.

Sign Objective manifestation of a disease, observed by the physician through the clinical examination.

Spasticity Contraction of a muscle presenting all the characteristics of a spasm: involuntary, usually of short duration, painful or painless.

Splenomegaly Increase in the volume of the spleen, appreciable by palpation at clinical examination.

Sporadic A disease occurring in isolated cases, as opposed to endemic, epidemic, or pandemic cases.

Squame Flake of dead skin tissue, thickening of the stratum corneum, can be detached by light tangential scraping.

Stertor Inspiratory noise that signals narrowing at the oro-pharyngeal level; the pharynx being a flexible tube that can easily collapse, a minor obstruction is enough for it to occur.

Stimulus Any physical, chemical, or biological element capable of triggering nervous, muscular, or endocrine phenomena.

Stridor Pathognomonic acute inspiratory/ expiratory/bi-phasic noise signaling a narrowing of the laryngotracheal region; given the relative rigidity of these structures, a narrowing of $\geq 50\%$ is required for it to occur.

Subcutaneous Beneath skin layer.

Subfebrile Slightly higher than normal body temperature.

Supination Movement of rotation of the forearm from inside to outside.

Symptom Pathological manifestation perceived by the patient, as opposed to signs observed during the examination.

Syncope Transient loss of consciousness and postural tone resulting from acute and diffuse cerebral hypoperfusion, complete and spontaneous recovery.

Syndrome A set of clinical symptoms and signs and pathological changes, always associated and that represent a disease.

Systemic Which refers to a system; affecting the whole body, as opposed to localized diseases.

Tachycardia Heart rate above 100 beats per minute in adults.

Tender Sensitive to touch or feel.

Tenesmus Severe abdominal pain with false urges to expel feces, indicating an inflammatory or infectious pathology of the colon or rectum.

Teratogen Capable of inducing embryonic malformation by disrupting organogenesis.

Tinnitus Misperception of a sound inaudible to others.

Tonus: hypo, hyper State of tension.

Transudate Low-density liquid, poor in protein and containing little to no cellular debris.

Tumefaction Cf edema.

Tympany Increase in thorax or abdomen resonance detected by percussion, and due to an excess of air or gas.

Ulcer Localized cutaneous or mucous loss of substance arising from trauma or necrosis; when cutaneous reaches at least the superficial and deep dermis, cannot heal without leaving a scar.

Umbilication Presence of an umbilicus-shaped depression in the middle of a skin lesion or a tumor.

Urticaria Sudden cutaneous eruption of itchy, edematous, and circumscribed papule; their localization, size, and shape are very variable, fugace (lasts <24 h).

Vaccination A method of prevention of human or animal diseases of a bacterial, viral, or parasitic nature, aiming to develop active immunity by introducing a vaccine into the body by oral or parenteral routes.

Vasculitis Generic term for an inflammatory disease of the blood vessels of various etiologies and sizes.

Vector Host that actively transmits the parasite to the next host.

Vesicle Intraepidermal or mucous cavity of serous, sero-purulent, or hemorrhagic content, <0.5 cm in diameter, has thin walls.

Vesperal In the evening, at sunset.

Viremia Temporary or permanent presence of virus in blood.

Wasting Process by which a disease leads to progressive physical weakening and a decrease in muscle and fat mass.

Wheezing Audible sound at prolonged expirium reflecting vibrations in narrowed airways, may be heard in case of bronchial obstruction or asthma.

Xerophthalmia Extreme dryness of the eyes.

Xerosis Dryness of the skin or mucous membranes of the mouth or eyes.

Xerostomia Sensation of dryness in the mouth (psychiatry).

Zoonosis Infectious or parasitic disease transmissible from wild or domestic animals (usually a vertebrate) to humans.

Bibliography[2]

1. Papadakis MA, McPhee SJ, Rabow MW. Current medical diagnosis & treatment 2019. New York: McGraw-Hill Education; 2019. https://accessmedicine.mhmedical.com/book.aspx?bookID=2449.
2. Preclinical and clinical lecture notes of the curriculum of medical studies, Faculty of Medicine, University of Lausanne, course year 2015–2021.
3. Scientific-Units-Recommendations-Formulas (SURF), guidelines 2020. Médecine Interne General. Philippe Furger en collaboration avec Thierry Fumeaux et le SURF-team.
4. Pocket Book of Hospital Care for Children. Guidelines for the management of, common, childhood illnesses. 2nd ed. Geneva: World Health Organization; 2013.
5. Mirali S, Seneviratne A. Essential med notes, 2020 Comprehensive medical references and review for the United States Medical Licensing Exam (USMLE) step II and the Medical Council of Canada Qualifying Exam (MCCQE) Part 1. 36th ed.
6. WHO model list of essential medicines, 20th list. World Health Organization. Mar 2017, Amended Aug 2017. https://apps.who.int/iris/bitstream/handle/10665/273826/EML-20-eng.pdf?ua=1.
7. The Gambia standard drug treatment guidelines. 2nd ed. Department of State for Health & Social Welfare, The Republic of the Gambia; 2001. http://apps.who.int/medicinedocs/documents/s22418en/s22418en.pdf.
8. Cornuz J, Pasche O, Kermode-Noppel T. Compas: Stratégies de prise en charge clinique, Médecine interne générale ambulatoire. Lausanne: Institute of Social and Preventive Medicine; 2010.
9. Diseases and conditions: comprehensive guides on hundreds of conditions. Mayo Clinic. https://www.mayoclinic.org/diseases-conditions.
10. https://www.uptodate.com.
11. https://www.cdc.gov/ncbddd/actearly/milestones.
12. https://www.who.int/biologicals.

---

[2]The material presented in this book originates from the efforts of the authors to converge various sources of medical information to constitute this book. The invaluable lecture notes and handouts received through the medical curriculum of the University of Lausanne, Switzerland, where both authors trained, has been very useful. Personal notes taken during many years of clinical work in medical wards and outpatient units are incorporated. Finally, these two crucial sources of medical information are complemented by selected classical medical literature listed below.

Index

A

Abdominal pain, 11, 19, 64, 86, 88–91, 95–98, 101–105, 124, 126, 129, 131, 140, 146, 174, 178, 181, 224, 228, 307, 308, 379, 383
    in pregnancy, 126
Acne, 128, 137, 141, 158, 159, 168, 181, 184, 275
Acute coronary syndrome (ACS), 56, 57, 60, 63
Addiction, 204, 205, 273
Adenopathy, 11, 19, 44, 51, 82, 87, 119, 145, 172, 175
Adjustment disorders, 204, 205
Adrenal insufficiency, 88, 89, 180, 181, 314
Adult congenital heart disease, 56, 58
Allergic conjunctivitis, 47, 190, 194
Alopecia, 158, 159, 165, 179, 184, 275
Amenorrhea
    primary, 127, 377
    secondary, 128, 281
Anal fissure, 86, 90, 91, 93
Anemia, 12, 28, 61, 76, 87, 95, 99, 101, 102, 104, 105, 124, 125, 127, 130, 137, 138, 168, 171–174, 177, 186, 226, 262, 263, 285, 308, 312, 313, 344
Anesthesia, 167, 183, 253, 254, 257–259, 261, 274
Angioedema, 158, 160, 174
Anisocoria, 190, 192
Ankylosing spondylitis, 150–152, 156
Anorectal infections, 86, 91
    proctitis, 86, 91
Antenatal card, 353, 354
Antibiotic-associated colitis, 86, 91
Anxiety disorder, 70, 203–206, 296
Aortic aneurysm, 56, 58, 59, 119, 121, 145
Ascites, 86, 89, 90, 92, 93, 105, 176, 378
Asthma, 11, 18, 47, 48, 73, 74, 76, 78, 125, 174, 185, 226, 227, 277, 384
Astigmatism, 190, 200, 202
Atrial fibrillation, 28, 56, 60, 70
Attention deficit hyperactivity disorder, 204–206
Autism spectrum disorder, 204, 206

B

Bacterial skin infections, 158, 160
Balanitis, 108–110
Bartholin duct cysts and abscess, 124, 128
Behcet syndrome, 152
Benign prostatic hypertrophy (BPH), 108, 110, 120
Bilharziasis, 86, 104
Birth attestation, 15, 345
Bleeding in pregnancy, 124, 128
Blepharitis, 163, 189, 190, 193, 194
Blood transfusion, 259, 263, 266, 285, 286
Brain tumors, 25–27, 31, 39, 127
Bronchiectasis, 74, 77, 78
Bronchopneumonia, 77, 237
Burns, 5, 53, 108, 158, 160, 168, 194, 222

C

Candidiasis, 108, 110, 124, 129, 146, 163, 175
Carcinoma of the cervix, 124, 129
Cardiac arrythmias, 56, 61
Cardiac failure, 55, 56, 61, 75, 180
Cardiac insufficiency, 218, 226, 248
Cardiomyopathy, 56, 61–63, 135, 226
Cardiovascular arrest, 56, 62
Care of mother and baby immediately after delivery, 124, 130
Cataract, 183, 189, 190, 193
Cellulitis, 46, 47, 66, 158, 159, 161, 166, 378
Cerebrovascular accident, 26, 28, 55, 168, 174, 237, 248
Certificate of good health, 15, 343
Checklist of hospital chores, 334–338
Chest pain, 11, 18, 55–57, 62, 63, 65–67, 70, 73, 75, 78, 80–82, 97, 101, 102, 174, 175, 228, 275
Chief complaint, 10, 11, 13, 157
Child abuse, 204, 207, 232, 244
Child health card, 357–360
Choking child, 218, 227
Cholecystitis, 63, 86, 89–91, 103, 121, 176
Cholelithiasis, 86, 92
Chronic hepatic disease, 86, 92, 165
Chronic obstructive pulmonary disease (COPD), 60, 74, 79, 277, 286, 287, 289
Chronic pain disorder, 204, 207
Chronic pain syndrome, 26, 28
Clubfoot, 218, 231
Compartment syndrome, 150, 152, 169

Confusional state, 379
    acute, 26
Congenital neurological defects, 26, 29
Conjunctivitis
    allergic, 47, 190, 194
        bacterial, 190, 192
        viral, 189, 194
Constipation, 85, 86, 88–91, 93, 99, 102, 120, 126, 132,
        140, 186, 224, 236, 262, 273, 278, 297, 379
COPD, *see* Chronic obstructive pulmonary disease
Corneal abrasion, 190, 195
Corneal ulcer, 190, 195, 196, 199
Coronary heart disease, 56, 64, 293
Cough
    acute, 78
    chronic, 74, 78, 79, 262
Coxo-cruralgia, 150, 153
Cranio facial pain, 26
Cryptorchidism, 111
Cushing syndrome, 60, 179–181
Cutaneous hookworm, 86

D
Dacrytis, 189, 197
Death certificate, 15, 331, 335
Deep venous thrombosis (DVT), 64, 68, 75, 344
Delirium, 207, 209, 236, 297
Dementia, 29, 65, 103, 119, 145, 203, 209, 212, 379
Dental abscess, 45
Dental caries, 45, 49, 51, 98
Developmental dysplasia of the hip, 231
Diabetes
    gestational, 134–136, 141, 183, 211, 220
    insipidus, 179, 182
    mellitus, 28, 64, 97, 109, 115, 116, 127, 134, 182,
        186, 198, 293
    type 2, 182, 318
Diabetic foot, 166, 183, 261
Diabetic gastroparesis, 94
Diarrhea, 11, 19, 85, 88, 91, 94, 96–98, 100, 102, 104,
        105, 109, 127, 156, 174, 175, 222–224, 233,
        234, 273, 278, 288–290, 297, 307, 318, 379
Diplopia, 36, 191, 195, 200, 275
Diverticular disease of the colon, 95
DVT, *see* Deep venous thrombosis
Dysautonomia, 29, 63
Dysphonia, 11, 44, 49, 160

E
Eclampsia, 30, 65, 124, 130, 142, 274
Ectopic pregnancy, 88, 121, 128, 131, 141
Eczema, 47, 109, 158, 161, 174
Emergency contraception, 131
Empyema, 74, 77, 79, 261, 380
Endocarditis, 64, 65, 70, 112, 117, 133, 244
Endometriosis, 131, 141, 282
Endophthalmitis, 196
Eosinophilia, 174, 181

Epididymitis, 108, 115–117, 197
Epilepsy, 26, 30, 185, 199, 212, 229, 307, 326
Epistaxis, 49, 380
Erectile dysfunction, 20, 112
Erythema
    multiforme, 158 , 162, 163
    nodosum, 100, 105, 152, 162
Essential drugs, 4, 15, 267
Essential medication list, 361
Essential tremor, 28
Excused duty certificate, 352
Exophthalmia, 196
External otitis, 49

F
Facial paralysis, 31, 50
Falls in older persons, 26
Female genital mutilation, 19, 104, 107, 132, 248
Female genital prolapses, 132
Fever of unknown origin (FUO), 112, 133
Fibromyalgia, 32, 101, 149, 153
Fit to fly certificate, 15, 344
Foreign body in eye, 196
Fractures, 40, 46, 151, 153, 155, 167, 181, 191, 196, 232,
        250, 380
Fungal skin infection, 163

G
Gait disorders, 26, 33
Gastric tumors, 86, 95
Gastritis and Gastropathies, 86, 96
Gastroenteritis, 85, 86, 89, 96, 126, 223, 224, 278, 305
Gastroesophageal reflux diseases (GERD), 73, 86,
        97–99, 224
Gastrointestinal complaints, 63, 81, 85, 88, 95, 162, 173,
        175, 212, 237, 272, 278–280
Gastrointestinal gas, 97
GBS, *see* Guillain Barré syndrome
Genital ulcers, 113, 118, 119, 133, 144, 176
Genital warts, 108, 113, 124, 134, 232
GERD, *see* Gastroesophageal reflux diseases
Gestational trophoblastic neoplasia (GTN), 124,
        135, 298
Gingivitis, 44, 50, 98, 383
Glaucoma
    closed-angle, 195, 333
    open-angle, 190, 195, 197, 333
Guillain Barré syndrome (GBS), 26, 33, 39, 94, 164,
        176, 195
Gynecomastia, 179, 180, 184

H
Halitosis, 46, 98, 230, 380
Headache, 11, 14, 18, 26, 27, 32, 34, 35, 41, 45–48, 55,
        64, 65, 78, 99, 102, 119, 128, 142, 145, 153,
        171, 175, 178, 179, 181, 185, 195, 197, 199,
        200, 230, 273, 306–308, 313

Health
- definition, 5
- determinants, 4, 222
- facts, 6

Healthcare systems
- primary healthcare, 5, 55
- quaternary healthcare, 5–6
- secondary healthcare, 5
- tertiary healthcare, 5

Hearing loss, 19, 44, 45, 50
Heart murmur, 226
Helminthic infections, 99
Hematopoietic cancer, 174
Hematuria, 11, 88, 105, 107–109, 114, 121, 127, 173, 381
Hemophilia, 174, 198, 380
Hemorrhagic conjunctiva, 197–198
Hemorrhoids, 99, 103, 138, 262, 380
Hemostasis workup, 138, 143
Hepatocellular carcinoma (HCC), 92, 99, 319
Herpes
- herpes zoster, 63, 121, 164, 199, 309
- simplex, 31, 91, 119, 145, 158, 162, 232

Herpes zoster ophtalmicus, 164
Hiatus hernia, 63, 86, 99
Hiccup, 35, 99, 381
Hirschsprung disease, 224
Hirsutism, 128, 137, 141, 164, 179, 181, 182, 184, 275
HIV, *see* Human immunodeficiency virus
HIV (infection, test consent form), 349
- Chalazion, 189, 198

Hordeolum, 201
Horner syndrome, 192, 198, 200
Hospital maintenance, 333–334
Hot flush, 139, 185
Human immunodeficiency virus (HIV), 20, 25, 31, 33, 39, 47, 81, 94, 103, 112, 119, 129, 133, 145, 162–155, 168, 174, 175, 204, 207, 218, 234, 263, 282, 302, 303, 309, 316, 349
Hydatidform mole pregnancy, 135
Hyperbilirubinemia, 135, 176, 225, 315
Hyperkeratosis, 165, 383
Hyperopia, 196, 200, 202
Hypertension
- arterial, 59, 69
- in pregnancy, 125, 136

Hypertensive crisis, emergency, 65
Hyperthyroidism, 60, 103, 127, 168, 179, 184–187, 189, 196, 293, 316, 317
Hyperventilation syndrome, 80
Hyphemia, 191, 196, 198
Hypotension, 32, 54, 63, 67–69, 81, 88, 97, 101, 160, 169, 181, 185, 191, 233, 297, 307
Hypothyroidism, 18, 39, 60, 93, 103, 127, 168, 173, 186, 293

I

IBS, *see* Irritable bowel syndrome
Icterus, 88, 381

Immunization status, 20–21
Infant immunization schedule, 362
Infertility
- female, 107, 137
- male, 115
- primary, 132, 140, 144
- secondary, 145

Inflammatory bowel disease, 89, 100, 126, 152, 156, 162, 201, 318, 319
Insect bite, 165
Institutional affiliation card, 373
Intestinal obstructions, 90, 98, 100, 121, 224
Intracranial abscess, 35, 46
Intracranial aneurysm, 35, 192
Irritable bowel syndrome (IBS), 89, 93, 98, 101, 102

J

Jaundice, 87, 135, 172, 175–177, 225, 233, 381
Job
- application form, 326, 327, 368–369
- descriptions, 4, 327–333

K

Keratoconjunctivitis, 156, 194, 201
Ketoacidosis, 89
- diabetic, 76, 98, 180, 183, 244

L

Laboratory
- request form, 326, 363, 364
- work-up, 131

Larva migrans, 86
Leiomyoma uteri, 124, 137
Leucopenia, 174, 308
Lichen planus, 109, 146, 158, 165
Lower limb ulcer, 158, 165
Lumbago, 150, 154
Lupus erythematosus, 37
Lymphedema, 56, 66, 248

M

Malaria
- in children, 176, 177
- complicated, 177
- in pregnancy, 138, 177, 178
- severe, 34, 177, 178, 244, 290, 291
- uncomplicated, 176, 177

Malnutrition, 4, 86, 89, 102, 116, 154, 159, 160, 202, 218, 222, 248, 286, 287, 289, 307
Malocclusion, 44, 49, 50
Mania, 204, 208, 296
Maternity leave (request), 15, 351
Medical check-up, 3, 17–21
Medical documentation, 15
Medical documents, 15
Medical history taking, 9–11

Medical prescription, 15
Medical report, 15, 58, 342
Meningitis, 14, 26, 34–36, 46, 50, 163, 164, 175, 176,
        192, 199, 230, 286–288, 304, 306
Menometrorrhagia, 124, 138
Menopause, 124, 132, 139, 185
Mesenteric ischemia, 86, 88–90, 103, 121
Molluscum contagiosum, 103, 108, 116, 124,
        139, 193
Mononucleosis syndrome, 47, 84, 172
Mood disorder, 40, 119, 203, 204, 208, 248
Multiple sclerosis, 26, 28, 31, 35, 36, 54, 152,
        168, 185
Musculoskeletal chest pain, 56, 63, 66
Myocardial infarction, 18, 56, 57, 60, 63, 65, 67, 68, 88,
        89, 183, 248, 326
Myocarditis, 56, 57, 63, 66, 71, 176, 273
Myopia, 190, 197, 200, 202, 295
Myxedema, 67, 89, 180, 186

N
Nephritic syndrome, 116
Nephrotic syndrome, 89, 109, 116, 318
Neuro-cognitive disorders, 209
Neurocutaneous diseases, 37
Neurological congenital defects, 37
Non-progression of fetus, 139

O
Obesity, 28, 59, 64, 66, 68, 95, 96, 102, 103, 109, 121,
        132, 180, 181, 186, 211
Obstetrical delivery chart, 355–356
Obstetrical partogram, 356
Obstructive sleep apnea syndrome, 74, 80, 83, 213
Onchocerciases, 190, 199
Ophthalmia neonatorum, 190, 197, 199
Ophthalmic shingles, 189, 190, 199
Ophthalmic zoster, 190, 199
Oral hygiene, 44, 45, 49–51, 98
Orbital cellulitis, 46, 157, 167, 196
Orchitis, 108, 115, 116, 304
Organization of routine healthcare, 4, 340
Orthostatism, 56, 57
Osteoarthritis, 149, 150, 153, 154, 284
Osteomyelitis, 46, 65, 150, 151, 154
Osteoporosis, 139, 150, 155, 182, 285
Otitis media, 44, 50, 218, 230, 286, 287
        acute, 50, 218, 230
        chronic, 50

P
Palliative care, 5, 235–238, 295, 297
Pancreatitis, 75, 86, 89, 90, 93, 176, 316, 319
        acute, 89, 90, 93, 316
        chronic, 86, 89, 90, 92, 93, 316
Paraphimosis, 108, 117
Parkinsonism, 26, 33, 37, 209, 275

Patient admission, 244–246
Patient's card, 341
PCOS, see Polycystic ovary syndrome
Pediculosis pubis, 108, 118, 143
Pediculosis pus, 124
Pelvic inflammatory disease (PID), 107, 124, 126, 138,
        140, 145
Pelvic pain syndrome, 124, 140
Perianal pruritus, 85, 86, 103
Pericardial effusion, 56, 67
Pericarditis, 56, 57, 63, 67, 71, 76, 89, 237
Perineal fistulas, 86, 104
Periodontal abscess, 51
Peripheral arterial disease, 56, 68
Peripheral neurologic deficit, 26
Peripheral vascular disease, 56
Personality disorder, 203, 204, 209, 210
Pharyngitis, 44, 47, 51, 71, 84, 175, 218, 230, 286, 287,
        289, 309
Phimosis, 107, 108, 117, 262
Physical examination, 3, 9, 11–15, 17, 19–20, 25–28, 32,
        34, 43, 44, 55, 56, 60, 69, 74, 85, 87, 88, 108,
        110, 112, 115, 128, 133, 137, 138, 151–153,
        158–169, 171, 174, 185, 204, 219, 224, 312,
        363
Physiotherapy services, 247–250
PID, see Pelvic inflammatory disease
Pile, 86
Pleural effusion, 74, 79, 81, 93, 176, 261
Pneumonia
        community acquired, 77, 286–289
        hospital acquired, 78, 287, 288
        severe, 218, 248, 287–289
Pneumothorax, 62, 63, 74, 81, 260
Polycystic ovary syndrome (PCOS), 124, 127, 134, 141,
        184, 281
Polyneuropathy, 26, 38, 39, 195
Postnatal depression, 204, 211
Postpartum hemorrhage, 124, 141
Preeclampsia, 124–126, 130, 134–136, 141, 142, 274
Prelabor rupture of membrane, 124, 142
Premenopausal abnormal uterine bleeding, 124, 143
Presbyopia, 190, 202
Prescription form, 324, 326, 365
Preterm labor, 124, 143
Prostatitis, 108, 110, 117, 118, 144, 288, 289
Pruritus, 85, 86, 103, 109, 116, 146, 158, 168, 194, 199,
        263, 273, 308
Psoriasis, 49, 152, 156, 158, 168
Psychosis of unspecified etiology, 204, 212
Pterygium, 190, 200
Ptosis, 190, 196, 198, 200
Pubic lice, 108, 118, 119, 124, 143
Pulmonary embolism, 56, 63, 64, 68, 105
Pulmonary malignancies, 74
Pulpitis, 44, 51
Purpura, 158, 167, 363
Pyelonephritis, 89, 108, 118, 124, 126, 130, 144, 146,
        244, 288, 289
Pyodermitis, 158

R

Receipts, 324, 332, 370–372
Rectal prolapse, 93, 104
Referral form for outside treatment, 347
Refractive errors, 192, 200, 201
Refractory arterial hypertension, 69
Regulations staff, 326–327
Renal failure
    acute, 109, 127, 176
    chronic, 111, 130, 168, 237
Respiratory distress syndrome in adults, 75
    acute, 75
    Respiratory insufficiencyacute, 75, 168
    chronic, 76
Retarded mental development, 212
Retinopathy, 37, 55, 60, 183, 189, 200
Retropharyngeal abscess, 53
Rheumatoid arthritis, 18, 112, 133, 149, 150, 153, 155
Rhinitis
    acute, 46
    allergic, 47, 174

S

Sarcoidosis, 63, 82, 162, 185, 201
Scabies, 168, 169, 174
Schistosomiasis, 104, 105, 174
Schizophrenia spectrum disorder, 213
Scoliosis, 73, 231, 248
Scrotal hernia, 118
Seizure, 25, 27, 30, 39, 65, 69, 76, 130, 142, 177, 223, 224, 228, 229, 233, 306, 308
    febrile, 228, 229
Self-discharge form, 366
Seminoma, 120
Sepsis
    neonatorum, 197, 199
    perinatal, 134, 135, 149, 211, 212, 232, 382
    puerperal, 144, 383
Septic arthritis, 65, 150, 151, 153
Sexual dysfunction
    female, 133
    male, 115
Sexually acquired acute inguinal lymphadenitis, 118, 144
Sexually transmitted disease (STD), 18, 20, 108, 113, 118, 119, 131, 133, 140, 144, 145, 147, 219, 316
Shock, 31, 40, 69, 75, 76, 88, 118, 132, 144, 177, 181, 285, 297, 306
Sickle cell disease, 11, 76, 114, 125, 151, 155, 173, 178, 198, 304
Sigmoid volvulus, 86, 106
Sinusitis
    acute, 46, 48, 98, 230
    chronic, 48, 98
Sjogren syndrome, 156, 168, 201
Sleep disorder, 32, 83, 153, 208, 213
Sleep-wake disorders, 83, 213
Snakebite, 152, 169, 310
Splenomegaly, 64, 89, 172, 175, 176, 178, 225, 383

Spondyloarthritis, 149, 151–153, 156, 201
Spontaneous bacterial peritonitis, 89, 105
Squint, 200
STD, *see* Sexually transmitted disease
Stevens-Johnson syndrome, 162
Strabismus, 167, 200
Stridor, 52, 53, 74, 227, 383
Stupor and coma, 39
Sty, 201
Substance use disorders, 205, 214
Sudden infant death syndrome (SIDS), 228
Suicide and suicide risk, 214
Surgical (procedure, unit, consent form, operation report), 348, 350
Syncope, 29, 39, 63, 69, 70, 229, 383
Syphilis, 20, 31, 59, 103, 107, 113, 119, 133, 134, 144, 145, 175, 201, 225, 232, 233, 263, 287, 316
Syphilis in pregnancy, 119, 145

T

Taenia, 99, 158, 163
Talipes equinovarus, 218, 231
Tamponade, 56, 62, 63, 67
Temporomandibular joint disorders (TMD), 34, 48
Testicular mass, 120
Testicular torsion, 111, 120, 180
Thrombocytopenia, 87, 142, 167, 198, 258, 275, 313
Thyroid nodule, 180, 187
Thyroid storm, 180, 187
Tonsillitis, 44, 47, 51
Toxic epidermal necrolysis, 158, 162
Trachoma, 190, 201
Transient ischemic attack, 26, 39, 174
Traumatic spinal cord injury, 40, 44
Tremor, 26, 30, 37, 76, 87, 187, 205, 209, 378
Tuberculosis, 19, 21, 74, 75, 81, 84, 89, 112, 131, 133, 162, 303

U

Ulcerative colitis, 86, 89, 100, 105, 152, 162
Upper respiratory tract infection, 50, 74, 84, 183, 194
Urinary incontinence in the adult male, 108
Urinary infection
    lower, 146, 286, 287, 290
    upper, 121, 146
Urinary stone disease, 121, 146
Urinary tract infection, 14, 19, 107, 109, 110, 114, 121, 124, 126, 146, 218, 225, 261
Urticaria, 154, 155, 158, 160, 162, 164, 168, 169, 174, 176, 339, 384
Uveitis, 100, 105, 152, 190, 199, 201

V

Vaccines, 21, 36, 223, 266, 301–310, 336, 362
Vaginal discharge, 124, 129, 140, 146
Vaginitis, 146

Vaginosis, 124, 145–147
Valvular heart diseases, 56, 70
Varicella (chicken pox), 21, 158, 164, 168, 169, 232,
        303, 309
Venereal, 108, 113, 119, 124, 125, 134
Vertigo, 11, 41, 43, 44, 54
Vestibular dysfunction, 41, 54
Virilization, 137, 184

Visual field
    amaurosis fugax, 191
    amputation of, 191
Vulvovaginitis, 110, 124, 129, 146

X
X-ray request form, 326, 364

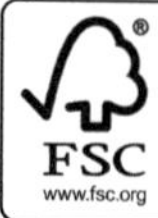